*USMLE™ STEP 2 CS: COMPLEX CASES

35 CASES YOU ARE LIKELY TO SEE ON THE EXAM

Phillip Brottman, M.D., with Sonia Reichert, M.D.

Special Flashcard Section by Eric Deppert, M.D., and Henry Ostman, M.D.

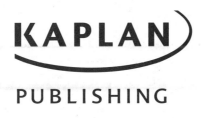

PUBLISHING

New York

*USMLE™ is a joint program of the Federation of State Medical Boards of the United States, Inc. and the National Board of Medical Examiners

Vice President and Publisher: Maureen McMahon
Editorial Director: Jennifer Farthing
Development Editors: Ruth Baygell, Sheryl Gordon
Contributing Editor: Sonia Reichert, M.D., Director of Curriculum, Kaplan Medical
Production Editor: Dominique Polfliet
Production Designer: the dotted i
Cover Designer: Carly Schnur

Published by Kaplan Publishing, a division of Kaplan, Inc.
1 Liberty Plaza, 24th Floor
New York, NY 10006

September 2007
10 9 8 7 6 5 4 3 2 1

ISBN 13: 978-1-4195-9550-9

AVAILABLE ONLINE

FREE ADDITIONAL PRACTICE

kaptest.com/booksonline

As owner of this guide, you are entitled to get more practice online. Log on to kaptest.com/booksonline to access a selection of USMLE™ clinical case walk-throughs.

Access to this selection of online USMLE™ practice material is free of charge to purchasers of this book. When you log on, you'll be asked to input the book's ISBN number (see the bar code on the back cover). And you'll be asked for a specific password derived from the text in this book, so have your book handy when you log on.

FOR ANY TEST CHANGES OR LATE BREAKING DEVELOPMENTS

kaptest.com/publishing

The material in this book is up to date at the time of publication. However, the USMLE™ may have instituted changes in the test after this book was published. Be sure to carefully read the material you receive when you register for the test. If there are any important late-breaking developments—or any changes or corrections to the Kaplan test preparation materials in this book—we will post that information online at kaptest.com/publishing.

FEEDBACK AND COMMENTS

kaplansurveys.com/books

We'd love to hear your comments and suggestions about this book. We invite you to fill out our online survey form at kaplansurveys.com/books. Your feedback is extremely valuable as we continue to develop high-quality resources to meet your needs.

If you have any further questions or comments please email medfeedback@kaplan.com.

RELATED KAPLAN MEDICAL TITLES

Contents

About the Authors

Phillip Brottman, M.D., is a board-certified emergency medicine physician. He currently serves as faculty for Kaplan Medical and teaches Step 2 CS in Chicago, where his nickname is "Dr. Phil." Prior to that, Dr. Brottman served as a medical director and as an academic physician teaching in the lecture hall and bedside. He has personally seen and supervised his students and residents in approximately 40,000 patient visits over his lifetime. Having seen so many patients—most of them in about 15 minutes—uniquely qualifies Dr. Brottman on the best practices for gaining the patient's trust and collecting the needed history/physical in a brief amount of time.

Sonia E. Reichert, M.D., served as Director of Curriculum for Kaplan Medical until summer of 2007 and is currently an Internal Medicine Resident at SUNY Downstate, Brooklyn. After completing the new Step 2 Clinical Skills (CS), she was involved in establishing Kaplan Medical's Step 2 CS facilities, training standardized patients, and helping to develop Kaplan's CS cases and grading system for Kaplan Medical's live classes. Dr. Reichert regularly attended National Board conferences to best understand all facets of the Clinical Skills exam—its structure, testing, and scoring. Because Dr. Reichert completed her medical degree overseas, she brings an international perspective that is invaluable to International Medical Graduates taking the Step 2 CS and other U.S. Medical licensure exams.

Eric J. Deppert, M.D., FACP, is associate residency program director at Graduate Hospital in Philadelphia, and president and CEO of Global Health Educators.

Henry E. Ostman, M.D., is a fellow in pulmonary medicine and former chief medical resident at Graduate Hospital in Philadelphia.

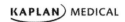

A Note from the Author

Most prefaces contain humble thanks to the many individuals who made the work possible. This volume is no exception. This is really a collaborative effort on the part of many individuals. Without the many Kaplan contributors who came before me and shaped the Kaplan method, it could not have been written. Special thanks to Sonia Reichert, M.D., and the Kaplan Publishing team who took my disjointed concepts and made them understandable.

This study guide is an outgrowth of my teaching the live lectures for Step 2 CS. Based on the questions of my students over the past year, I have begun to see what aspects of the exam cause the most confusion. I have tried to summarize what you need to do to pass this exam. At the same time, I wanted to answer common questions about various aspects of the exam.

When I attended medical school there was no Step 2 CS to focus my attention on effective communication skills or clear, relevant histories and physicals. As a result, I learned these techniques later by trial and error over 20 years and 40,000 patient encounters. How fortunate your first real patients will be as they benefit from your polished interpersonal skills!

I realize if you are reading this book you may be somewhat stressed by the formal, expensive, and high-stakes process of taking your Boards. Try to look past the exam as much as possible. The majority of people do pass on their first attempt. Try to imagine while you are studying what it will be like to be a first-year resident. The skills emphasized for Step 2 CS will make you a successful resident and attending physician if you begin to develop them now.

When you are with real patients, that will be the test that really counts! Do not think that passing Step 2 CS is an end unto itself, or that you can stop improving your skills once you pass. Because in the real world, every day is a Board exam.

Best of luck,

Phillip Brottman, M.D.

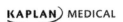

| Section One |

The Basics

THE PURPOSE OF THE EXAM

The USMLE states that the "Step 2 assesses whether medical school students or graduates can apply medical knowledge, skills and understanding of clinical science essential for provision of patient care under supervision." (usmle.org)

To accomplish this, the two USMLE Step 2 exams make sure that you have the basic skills needed to function as a first-year resident. Step 2 Clinical Knowledge (CK) exam is a computer-based theoretical exam that measures your medical knowledge base. Step 2 Clinical Skills (CS) is a clinically based exam with standardized patients to test your ability to perform as a first-year resident.

- You need to look professional, act and speak like a doctor, and have a professional bedside manner.

- You must able to collect the pertinent history and physical quickly while supporting the patient's emotional and physical needs.

- You must be able to convey your findings in written form to your attending physician.

- You are expected to have a general idea of what basic workups to order and to list some possibilities as to the diagnosis.

There are no treatments or medicines given in Step 2 CS. There is no ordering of consultants or hospitalizations. You are not being asked for the single best test. You are not being asked to narrow your diagnosis. You will not be making any life-or-death decisions.

HOW THE EXAM IS SCORED

Step 2 CS is a pass/fail exam made up of three separate subcomponents, each of which is also pass/fail. If you fail one subcomponent, you fail the entire exam and you will then need to retake the entire exam another day. The three subcomponents are:

1. Spoken English Proficiency (SEP)
2. Communications and Interpersonal Skills (CIS)
3. Integrated Clinical Encounter (ICE)

You are not graded on the basis of your passing or failing on each patient; instead, your pass/fail determination is based on your overall performance in the ICE, CIS, and SEP across all 12 cases. What this means in terms of test-taking strategy is: Never Give Up! Even if you get off to a bad start on a case, do your best and get as many points for each of the three subcomponents as possible!

Spoken English Proficiency (SEP)

This section is graded by the Standardized Patient (SP) on a rating scale that is most likely the same for all 12 cases. This score is graded while you are writing your Patient Note. The big question is: Can you understand the SP, and can the SP understand you? Clarity of verbal English communication is the key. Word pronunciation, word choice,

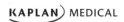

and minimizing the need to repeat questions are important. However, no human communication is perfect, and USMLE does not expect you to be perfect either.

Communications and Interpersonal Skills (CIS)

This section is also graded by the SP. Again, the checklist has been developed based on national consensus documents as to essential communication skills. It tests your bedside manner and skill in questioning the patient. Specifically, the SP is looking at your questioning skills and information-sharing skills, as well as your professional manner and rapport.

Integrated Clinical Encounter (ICE)

This subcomponent encompasses two critical skills: (1) Data Gathering, and (2) Documentation of this data (patient note). Data Gathering involves asking a relevant history and performing a focused, relevant physical exam on each patient. Data gathering is graded by the SP. Each checklist will be different for each case because each case requires different relevant history and physical to be performed. The Document portion of the ICE subcomponent refers to the Patient Note. The Patient Note will be graded by a physician—one of your peers! Legibility and quality of content are what is important to physicians. Capitalization, punctuation, and proper sentence structure are not important.

THE DAY OF THE EXAM

The following information is detailed in the USMLE Step 2 CS Content Description and General Information Booklet. Information is current as of publication; however, please visit the USMLE website for any notifications or announcements (usmle.org).

Identification

Bring with you your scheduling permit and a current government-issued photo ID that also has your signature. If the names printed on the two documents are different (except for middle name), contact USMLE well ahead of Test Day. If you have no valid ID you will not be allowed to take the exam.

What to Bring

Do bring the following:

- Your white lab coat and professional attire. Keep your wallet, car keys, and breath mints in your pants pocket.
- Your stethoscope
- A watch that is not digital
- A bottle of juice or water and nonperishable items to eat on break or at lunch. Food will be provided, but if you are a picky eater it's nice to have something you know will be nourishing.

If you have any personal medical needs, it is best to contact USMLE well ahead of Test Day to arrange for any additional items.

What Not to Bring

Do not bring:

- Digital items
- Cell phone, computer, PDA, or digital watch
- A pen (you will be provided with this)

There will be a nonlocked open space to store your overcoat. If you bring an expensive laptop you will have to leave it unlocked, so don't bring it!

Timing

You can expect to spend a full 8 hours at the test center. You will have graded 12 cases. If you have 13 cases, the extra case is for the purpose of pilot testing and will not be scored. You will not be told which of your cases is not scored, so you will have to complete them all with the same effort. However, don't worry too much about this because the case that you feel you did the worst on may in fact be the unscored case. It is more difficult to finish on time and do a good job if the case is still under development and not normed.

You will have one 30-minute lunch break and one 15-minute break to have your snack and visit the bathroom.

Each patient encounter lasts 25 minutes. 15 minutes to enter the room, introduce yourself, take the relevant history, wash your hands, do the focused physical exam, and tell the patient what will happen next (closing or summary). Then 10 minutes for you to complete the Patient Note outside of the exam room. If you finish in the patient's room early, you may leave early and have additional time to complete the Note. While you are in the patient's room, you will hear one announcement when 5 minutes are remaining (10 minutes after the beginning of the case). Good test-taking strategy indicates that if you are still taking the history at the 5-minute warning, you should wash your hands and get the most relevant physical exam completed.

Standardized/Simulated Patients (SPs)

This exam is unlike any you have taken before. It involves interpersonal skills and complex psychomotor skills. The "patients" you see are trained to portray certain disease states and are following prepared scripts. They know what to say and do depending on the actions and speech of the doctor. SPs are trained by the National Board of Medical Examiners. They do not have professional degrees in health care; in fact, many of them are actors. However, SPs certainly do know how they want to be treated by their physicians. Because the SPs grade the majority of the exam, it is impossible to pass if you don't treat them as real patients all the time. For this reason it is important that you do not speak to the SPs outside of the role of a patient.

Irregular Behavior

You do not want to be labeled as having irregular behavior, as this may be recorded in your USMLE records. The following are all considered dangerous or disruptive behavior:

- Carrying unauthorized materials, such as a pager

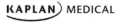

- Conversing in a language other than English at *any* time
- Talking about the content of the exam (even after the exam is over)
- Preparing any notes to take away from the test center
- Speaking to the SPs outside of their role as patients
- Continuing to write your note after the 10 minutes is finished. When you are told to stop writing, you must stop writing at that precise moment—not three or four words later.

SPOKEN ENGLISH PROFICIENCY (SEP)

SEP consists of two basic parts: Can the patient understand the doctor, and can the doctor understand the patient. The grading scale that the SP uses reflects this basic concept of understandability. No human communication is perfect. Nobody expects you to understand every word and be understood on every utterance during the 8-hour Test Day. The important point is to use the communication strategies outlined here so that you communicate most effectively with your patient. Remember, your intent and sincerity to communicate with your patient must be genuine.

Speak in English as much as possible before Exam Day. If English is not your first language, make every effort to speak as much as possible with native English speakers in the weeks and months leading up to Test Day. Just being comfortable speaking, even about nonmedical topics, will spill over as greater self-confidence on Test Day. Even if you are unsure about your spoken English, continue to speak openly and freely. Doctors who are unsure of their English skills frequently limit their use of spoken words on the exam. This is a mistake—it is sure to come across as detached and uncaring, and may affect your communications skills (CIS) score. You may also find that you are not able to collect all of the historical information needed to pass the Integrated Clinical Encounter (ICE).

Do not be concerned about any accent you may have. SPs are used to hearing a variety of accents and do not expect you to speak with the same accent as they do. They are looking for understandability. If you enunciate your words clearly, your accent will not matter. If you mumble, however, it will be difficult for the SP to understand you—accent or no accent.

Word choice is important. Three words that repeatedly get doctors into trouble are "feel," "good" and "okay." If you say "good or okay" after performing a physical exam maneuver, the patient might take it to mean that the exam was normal. During the history, if you say "good or okay" after a patient answers your question, it may come across as judgmental that you agree with her behavior. Use "Thank you" or "thanks" instead of "Okay" or "good."

The word "feel" is appropriate to use in the History. "How does that make you feel?" is perfectly acceptable. Try not to use the word "feel" during the physical exam, as it often has sexual connotations that are inappropriate. Prior to palpation of the chest wall, say, "Now I am going to push on your chest." It would be wrong to say, "Now I'm going to feel your chest."

Tips for Being Understood by Your SP

Tip 1. Speak slowly.
If you speak really quickly, patients will not understand.

Tip 2. Speak loudly.
Some hearing loss is common in the general population. If your patients cannot hear you, you will not be understood. Also, a very low volume of voice comes across as meek, uncertain, and not confident. If you come from a part of the world that considers loud speaking to be rude, consciously practice raising the decibels of your voice.

Tip 3. Use short sentences.
Patients are nervous and have limited short-term memory. For example, "Do you have chest pain?" is much better than "Now I'm going to ask you, if that is okay with you, have you ever had, now or in the past, any chest pain, discomfort, or sense of impending doom now or any time in the past?" Besides being better understood, short questions have the additional advantage of not taking up so much time.

Tip 4. Use simple vocabulary.
Not including your medical training, you are likely to be much better educated than many of your patients. Minimize the excessive syllables—that is, use shorter words.

Tip 5. Use body language.
Use hand gestures to explain ideas whenever possible. If you say to a patient, "Please show me where it hurts," you will more likely be understood if you hold out your index finger at the same time. The patient will get the idea he should point to where it hurts.

This technique works especially well when having the patient go through the range of motion of any joint. Saying, "Do this," and demonstrating the movement you want the patient to do, is a lot more efficient and understandable than saying, "Please extend your wrists."

Tip 6. Memorize suggested Kaplan phrases for the History and Physical.
Memorizing a range of possible questions for the History and commands to give during the physical exam can greatly improve your speed, communication, and confidence. Be careful not to become too robot-like in your delivery. Speak to the SP as if he has never been asked these questions before.

Tips for Understanding Your SP

Tip 1. Pay attention.
Listen! This is the most common problem in communication. Doctors do not listen to their patients. While the patient is speaking, look at him or her as much as possible and concentrate on what he or she is saying. Do not think about what your next question will be. If you have to write yourself a note on the clipboard, look down at it only briefly. Many doctors score low on SEP because they were not listening, not because of any deficiencies in their English language skills.

Tip 2. Look at your SP's body language and acting.

If the patient is crying, grimacing, or doing any other acting, it is part of the case! Comment on it and the SP will think you an excellent communicator.

Tip 3. Nod occasionally when the patient is speaking.

Head bobbing up and down means YES. Shaking head from side to side signals disapproval or NO.

What if the patient says, "I do not understand"? The key here is to not ignore the patient. Telling a patient who doesn't understand you that it "doesn't matter" is not the correct response. It is best to respond by asking the same or a very similar question in another way. For example:

> **Doctor:** "Do you have any ischemic symptoms?"
>
> **Patient:** "I do not understand?"
>
> **Doctor:** "Do you have any chest pain?"
>
> **Patient:** "I still do not understand."
>
> **Doctor:** *(Pointing to the patient's sternum)* "Does it hurt here?"
>
> **Patient:** "Ohh … no, Doctor …"

Throughout this exchange with the patient, be sure not to get flustered, angry, or defensive. Keep a caring, professional demeanor the entire time.

What if you do not understand the patient? If you have no idea at all what the patient has said, you could ask the question in another way. Without getting a history, it is impossible to select the correct physical exam elements to perform, and impossible to write an accurate note. In other words, you cannot pass the ICE component without understanding the majority of the history.

The most important thing here is to paraphrase and find out what the patient has to say. Paraphrasing means repeating back to the patient what you think he may have said. It is a technique to check your understanding, and is not a sign of weakness or failure. Paraphrasing will improve your CIS score, SEP score, and ICE score!

If you are unsure of what the patient said, just guess and repeat it back to the patient! The whole idea is to make the patient say it again for you to hear. For example:

> **Patient:** "I have had a cough and fever for 3 days."
>
> **Doctor:** "You have chest pain and cough for 3 days. Is that right?"
>
> **Patient:** "No chest pain, just 3 days of cough and fever."
>
> **Doctor:** "Oh, 3 days of cough and fever, no chest pain?"
>
> **Patient:** "Yes."
>
> **Doctor:** "Thank you. Have you had any sputum?"

COMMUNICATION AND INTERPERSONAL SKILLS (CIS)

The CIS component relates to treating the patient with respect and showing empathy for the patient's condition. This section of the exam is just as important as SEP or ICE. Having an excellent bedside manner is necessary for success in the real world as well as on Board exams.

The guiding principle is to treat patients the same way you would want your mother treated by a physician. You would demand that your mother's physician do everything in his ability to make your mother comfortable physically as well as emotionally and, at the same time, gather all the personal information and perform the physical exam required to make an accurate diagnosis.

Emphasis is placed on the introduction at the beginning of the patient encounter and the closing or summary at the end of the encounter. The introduction allows the doctor to make an excellent first impression on the SP. A good closing allows the doctor to make an excellent last impression on the SP. This is always nice, as the next thing the SP is going to do is grade the doctor!

Fortunately, we have a concrete list of objectives and communication techniques to share that will help you pass the CIS component. While you will memorize and practice these techniques, the most important idea is that each patient should be able to sense your desire to help. If the patient realizes you are there to help and you will not cause any unnecessary pain or embarrassment, you are well on your way to passing Step 2 CS and having a satisfying career.

The Introduction

The introduction can be subdivided and thought of as five tasks:

1. Entering the room
2. Greeting the patient
3. Offering a handshake
4. Draping the patient
5. Asking the first question

Task 1: Entering the Room

At the beginning of the case, you will be standing outside the door with your clipboard. You will hear the overhead announcement, "Your patient encounter will now begin." Do not write on your clipboard until you hear the starting announcement. Slide open the little cabinet that contains the Doorway Information.

Read the Doorway Information carefully and take up to 45 seconds to collect your thoughts about the case. When you are ready to enter the patient's room, knock twice loudly on the door. Take a deep breath, let it out, smile, and enter. There is no need to wait for the patient to respond verbally before you enter. The time it takes for one breath and a smile will be enough for the patient to make any quick adjustments with her gown to protect her modesty.

When you enter the room, walk toward the patient before beginning to speak. If you begin speaking while your hand is still on the doorknob, it gives the patient the impression that

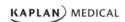

you are terribly rushed (this might be true, but don't let on). Observe the patient as you walk in. If she is smiling and in no obvious distress, keep smiling. If she is any physical or emotional distress, drop the big smile. If you are responding to a patient as you would to a real patient in distress, your face will reflect this. For a patient not in distress, 3 to 5 feet is good conversational distance. For a patient in severe physical distress, standing even closer is comforting. Position yourself so you can make good eye contact.

Task 2: Greeting the Patient

Saying hello and telling the patient your name is always a good start and may begin the process of putting the patient at ease. Below are two correct ways to do a greeting.

Greeting A
   Doctor: "Hello, my name is Dr. First-Name Last-Name."

Don't worry if you're still a fourth-year medical student and not officially a doctor yet.

Next you'll need to establish a doctor-patient relationship.

   Doctor: "I will be your physician today."

This is certainly a direct, short, and simple statement that will be understood by all patients.

This is not the only way to begin an interview. Some physicians prefer to check the patient's name right at the beginning of the interview. For example:

Greeting B
   Doctor: "Hello, Mrs. Smith?"

   Patient: "Yes, Doctor."

   Doctor: "My name is Dr. William Osler."

   Patient: "Please call me Mary."

   Doctor: "All right, Mary, I will be your physician today."

One advantage of taking a Board exam is that you are always in the correct patient's room. With this in mind, Greeting A is slightly shorter and still gets the job done. Greeting B allows the patient a chance to introduce herself. Always use the appropriate title (Mr., Mrs., Ms.) unless the patient specifically gives you permission to use the first name.

Task 3: Offering a Handshake

The handshake is a traditional greeting. Handshaking is the normal accepted convention regardless of the gender or age of the patient or of the doctor. Deciding on whether to shake hands or not can be simplified into three general rules.

Rule 1. Always shake hands if the patient offers. It would be considered rude to refuse.

Rule 2. Do not initiate a handshake if the patient has any emotional or physical distress. You would not want to extend your hand to someone with a possible myocardial infarct as he would feel obligated to shake back even though it might make his chest pain worse. If the vital signs are abnormal you can consider the patient to be in distress. It is always embarrassing to make someone shake hands when he has a fractured clavicle. Similarly, a patient in emotional distress will typically not appreciate the contact. Looking at the patient's face will help you decide if a handshake is helpful or not.

Rule 3. When in doubt, leave it out. You may occasionally meet a patient from a cultural background where you may not be sure about the handshake. If you aren't sure, it's better to err on the safe side and leave it out.

If you decide to shake hands, offer your hand when you say "Hello."

Task 4: Draping the Patient

There will be a white sheet clearly visible in your test room, most typically folded on the chair or patient table. It is your responsibility to give it to the patient and to all SPs dressed in patient gowns at this point of the introduction so that you do not forget. There is no need to offer—nor should you offer—a drape to the guardian(s) of the patient who are wearing regular street clothes (such as a grandmother of a pediatric patient).

For a patient in no distress, simply pick up the drape, unfold it one or two folds, and say, "Here is a drape for you." Simply drop the sheet on his lap. There is no need to tuck the drape in or even touch the patient at all. As soon as you let go of the drape, the patient will adjust it the way he wants.

For a patient in distress, perhaps someone lying in pain with a broken hip, adjust the drape for him to be sure he is comfortable. Having him adjust his own drape might make him move his broken femur and induce more pain.

> **Doctor:** "I have a drape for you. May I cover your legs?"
>
> **Patient:** "Yes, please."
>
> **Doctor:** "Here you go. *(Adjusting the drape)* How is that?"
>
> **Patient:** "Fine."

During the physical exam, the drape might get displaced when the patient rolls over or when you do physical exam maneuvers. You are responsible for seeing that the drape stays in place if it falls to the side.

What should you do if you realize halfway through the encounter that you forgot to offer the drape? Offer the drape with great poise when you think of it, and present it to the patient with a smile.

Note: Make sure you provide the drape to the patient before you begin the physical examination.

Task 5: Asking the First Question

The first question must always be an open-ended question; in other words, a question that cannot be answered with a simple "Yes" or "No" response.

> **Doctor:** "How can I help you today?"

This is an excellent way to begin the interview. It shows that you are caring and want to help. Here are three of many alternative ways to begin:

Doctor: "What brings you in today?"

or

Doctor: "What can I do for you today?"

or

Doctor: "I see you have *(state the symptom listed on the doorway)*. Please tell me all about it."

The key here is to be sure it is an open-ended question. Do not begin the interview by making small talk, commenting about the weather, or complimenting the patient on her nice clothes.

After you ask your opening question, be quiet, listen, and let the patient tell you her story.

The Closing or Summary

The summary is completed after you finish your physical exam. This is your last chance to make a good impression on the patient. Before beginning the summary, ask the patient to sit up if it isn't uncomfortable to do so. Stand or sit so you have good eye contact. A complete closing consists of seven tasks:

1. Making the transition
2. Paraphrasing
3. Giving knowledge
4. Telling what you are going to do
5. Counseling as needed
6. Asking for questions
7. Saying goodbye

Task 1. Making the Transition

This is to let the patient know that you have finished your physical exam and now want to tell him what you think.

Doctor: "Let me tell you what I am thinking."

Task 2. Paraphrasing

The purpose of this is to highlight the key historical points and the key physical findings. It is your last chance to make sure you have the information correct. There is no need and no time to repeat everything the patient told you.

Doctor: "You told me you have had 3 days of cough and 1 day of shortness of breath. Is that correct?"

Patient: "Yes, Doctor."

Doctor: "On physical exam I found that you have a fever and you are breathing fast."

Task 3. Giving Knowledge

This is where you explain in lay language one or two possible diagnoses. It is perfectly acceptable to be unsure of the exact diagnosis. After all, you have not even done any tests yet or written your note!

> **Doctor:** "I think you may have *(name one possibility)*, or it could be *(name another)*."

Task 4. Explain What You Are Going to Do

In this section, be definite. While you're yet unsure of the final diagnosis, you can be certain about what tests you are going to order. It is also very important to tell the patient that you will meet again to go over the test results.

> **Doctor:** "I am going to take a picture of your chest to find out why you are coughing. I am also going to take a blood test to look for infection. When the test results are back I will call you so we can discuss them and make a treatment plan."

Enjoy the role-playing aspect of Boards. If the case involves someone who is very ill, you could pretend the tests will be back very soon. For example:

> **Doctor:** "I am going to take a sample of your blood to find out why you are so short of breath. I will have the results in a few minutes. Could you wait here? I'll be back as soon as possible."

Task 5. Counseling

If you have found any behaviors that affect a patient's health, this is the time to advise the patient on the importance of treatment. Smoking, alcohol abuse, drug abuse, addiction of any kind, safe sex practices, depression, domestic violence, weight loss, and management of chronic diseases such as hypertension and diabetes would all be appropriate here.

How should you counsel? It is appropriate to counsel the patient on behaviors that are detrimental to his health. The key here is to have the patient see the "counselor."

For Smoking
> **Doctor:** "Your health will improve if you stop smoking. I'd like you to attend nonsmoking classes run by our counselor."

For Alcohol
> **Doctor:** "For your health, it is important that you stop drinking. I would like you to speak with our alcohol counselor. I will bring you her number."

For Recreational Drugs
> **Doctor:** "Please stop using drugs. They are hurting your health. I know it can be difficult, so I would like you to speak to our drug counselor."

For Sexually Transmitted Diseases
> **Doctor:** "Do not have sex until all your treatment is finished and your partner(s) are treated as well. Then I want you to use a condom every time to prevent infection in the future."

Task 6. Asking for Questions

> **Doctor:** "Do you have any questions?"

Task 7. Saying Goodbye

This is the last step in the closing. Too often, the closing seems to be the time when you find out precisely what concerns the patient most. Answer whatever questions the patient asks. If he has none, gather up your stethoscope and clipboard and make a parting comment.

> **Doctor:** "Call me if you have any problems or any other questions before our next meeting."
>
> **Patient:** "Okay, 'bye."
>
> **Doctor:** "Goodbye, *(patient's name)*."

or

> **Doctor:** "Call me anytime with any concerns, otherwise I'll call you when the tests are back."
>
> **Patient:** "Yes, Doctor."
>
> **Doctor:** "Goodbye, *(patient's name)*."

Turn around and leave, and close the door behind you.

What Should You Do If You Run Out of Time? At the end of the 15 minutes with the patient, you will hear the announcement, "This encounter is now over." As soon as this announcement is made, you stop earning points. You will not get credit for any additional history you obtain, physical you do, or counseling you give.

Even worse, the clock is now running on the 10 minutes that remain for you to write your Note. So you need to get out of the room—fast. The SP also wants you to make a rapid exit. The SP has to grade you, set up the exam room, and get ready for the next doctor. If your exit takes too long, a proctor will come into the patient room to ask you to leave.

Picture the following scenario. A doctor has finally gained the trust of a patient who is just beginning to reveal a very personal and sensitive problem:

> **Patient:** "Well, Doctor, I think it's safe to tell you. My problem is ..."
>
> **Overhead Announcement:** "This encounter is now over."
>
> **Doctor:** *(Says nothing, since the case is over, and walks out of the room)*

This type of interaction will make the SP feel depersonalized and cheated. All the empathy that you have shown for 15 minutes is now gone. A better approach would be the following:

> **Patient:** "Well, Doctor, I think it's safe to tell you. My problem is ..."
>
> **Overhead Announcement:** "This encounter is now over."
>
> **Doctor:** "I'm sorry; I have to answer this emergency page. I'll be back as soon as I can."

Patients expect busy physicians to get emergency pages that must be answered immediately. They generally don't take offense and do accept this explanation. As you turn to leave, the SP is thinking, "What a nice doctor."

The Communications and Interpersonal Skill (CIS) checklist as well as the Spoken English Proficiency (SEP) checklist will be the same for each of the 12 patients you see on Test Day.

Bedside Manner

In addition to the items mentioned in the introduction and closing, the following will give you an excellent bedside manner.

1. Wear Professional Attire

In addition to your clean white lab coat, your clothing should be clean, relatively wrinkle-free, and neat. Expensive new clothes are not necessary or advantageous. Shoes should be polished and in good repair. Do not wear high heels or sandals. Instead, wear traditional leather shoes.

Hygiene: Take a shower and use deodorant on the morning of Test Day. Patients want their doctors to smell clean or have no odor at all. Cologne or perfume may offend some patients or, even worse, may trigger an attack in an asthmatic patient. Consider bringing some quick-dissolving breath mints and putting a couple in your pocket for after lunch.

Jewelry: Wear whatever you normally wear. Piercings are fine except for tongue-piercing, which interferes with pronunciation and could hurt your SEP score.

Religious/Ethnic Dress: If you normally wear a head covering, religious symbols on your jewelry, or ethnic clothing, then you may do so on Test Day as well. Be yourself!

Men: Wear long pants that are not denim or blue jeans. No shorts. All men need to wear collared shirts with ties.

Women: Wear long pants that are not denim or blue jeans. No shorts. A knee-length dress or skirt is perfectly acceptable as well. No t-shirts, tube tops, or spaghetti straps. Any other type of blouse or shirt is fine.

Clothing for men and women should be free of any commercial logo or printing.

2. Make Eye Contact

It is important to make eye contact the majority of the time with your SP. This is especially important during the introduction and closing, as well as when doing any counseling or discussing personal topics. During the physical exam, you should observe the patient's face when palpating and percussing to see if there are any simulated physical findings of abdominal pain.

You are not expected to have eye contact 100% of the time, though it's best any time you are speaking with the patient. It is normal to look down occasionally at your clipboard when you write notes. If you nod up and down slightly when writing on your clipboard, it gives the impression you are still listening.

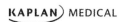

3. Pay Attention to the Patient

If you make eye contact most of the time, paying attention and concentrating on the patient is automatic. If you look at your clipboard most of the time, the patient will think you are not interested in him; he will think you care only about the medical record.

You will lose this point if you appear distracted, looking about the room randomly. Do not look at your watch repeatedly. This gives the message that you would rather be somewhere else. And if you ask the exact same question twice in row, it suggests to the SP that you are not listening.

> **Doctor:** "Do you have vomiting?"
>
> **Patient:** "Yes."
>
> **Doctor:** "Do you have vomiting?"
>
> **Patient:** "I said YES!"

Asking the same question twice in a row can annoy your SP. What the doctor above meant to ask the second time was to get a description of the emesis. Better communication would be the following:

> **Doctor:** "Do you have vomiting?"
>
> **Patient:** "Yes."
>
> **Doctor:** "How many times have you vomited?"
>
> **Patient:** "Three times."

The process of making eye contact and looking concerned goes a long way in building empathy and passing your CIS component.

4. Do Not Interrupt the Patient

If you ask a question, let the patient answer. Do not speak again until the patient is finished speaking! Yes, this can be hard to do.

The cases are designed and scripted to be doable in the 15 minutes allotted. Interrupting, besides being seen by the patient as rude, often slows you down and makes finishing on time difficult. For example:

> **Doctor:** "How can I help you today?"
>
> **Patient:** "I have pain in my chest ..."
>
> **Doctor:** *(Interrupting)* "Is it a sharp pain?"
>
> **Patient:** "No."
>
> **Doctor:** "How long have you had the pain?"
>
> **Patient:** "Three weeks."
>
> **Doctor:** "How long does it last?"
>
> **Patient:** "A few minutes."

Doctor: "How often does it happen?"

Patient: "A few times each week."

If you hadn't interrupted, the same case might have gone like this:

Doctor: "How can I help you today?"

Patient: "I've had pain in my chest for the last three weeks about the size of an orange. It's right under my breastbone. It only happens when I run in the cold weather. It lasts for a few minutes each time and stops a minute after I stop exercising."

In the first example the patient stopped talking spontaneously as soon as the doctor interrupted. It will take minutes now to collect the information needed—if you can obtain it at all. In the second example the doctor did not interrupt and was rewarded immediately with most of the information needed for the History of Present Illness (HPI).

Patients are often intimidated by their physicians; patients are sitting practically naked in your exam room, and as they undress, they know they must confess the most personal details of their lives in order to receive help. They are afraid of what you might tell them about their mortality. Painful, expensive, disfiguring treatments might be needed. You are the authority figure. They are vulnerable. If you realize this is what patients are experiencing, it's easier to let them finish their thoughts. If you allow them to speak, they will feel you are interested in them as individuals and not just organisms from which to collect and tabulate data.

However, there is one exception when it comes to not interrupting your patient: the situation where your patient is rambling and talking about unimportant, perhaps tangential, issues. It is a challenge to you—and part of the case—to see if you can gently redirect the interview. You need to collect a complete history and there's little time. Let the patient talk long enough that you realize the SP is not portraying a psychotic or manic patient. Then apologize, acknowledge, and redirect.

Doctor: "How can I help you today?"

Patient: "Oh, Doctor, thank you so much for seeing me today. I called the office and your nurse was so nice."

Doctor: "Thank you. I see my nurse wrote that you have a sore foot. Can you tell me about it, please?"

Patient: "I had a dog once with a sore leg. Spot was her name. I'll get a picture and show you."

Doctor: *(Interrupting)* "I'm sorry, I need to interrupt. I know you want to show me the picture but I would like to focus on you today. Please point and show me exactly where it hurts."

This is a case that may be easier on the Board exam than in real life. If you say you are sorry and acknowledge that you are interrupting, the SP will give you credit for passing this communication challenge. The rest of the case may be scripted such that the SP will answer questions more directly, allowing you to collect the history you need in a timely manner.

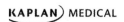

5. Keep a Professional Demeanor

SPs are looking to see if you are calm, confident, concerned, and caring. Verbal and non-verbal communication are important.

You will appear nervous if you constantly tap your pen, touch your hair, or twist your ring. Be conscious of how you stand or sit. Tapping your foot like a musician is a dead giveaway that you are nervous. Nervous physicians make for nervous patients. Patients start to wonder if the doctor really knows what he is doing when he acts nervous.

Don't worry if your hands are a little sweaty or if you have a little twitch on Test Day because of nerves. The SP will not grade you down for this. You can begin to relax because you are prepared for the exam and know generally what to expect.

How you stand or sit also projects calmness or nervousness. Stand with your feet flat on the floor and don't move a lot, shifting your weight back and forth. Keep your hands at your sides and not in your pockets. Be especially careful not to cross your arms, as this projects disapproval to the patient. Finally, do not hide behind the clipboard. Hold it so it does not cover your face or mouth.

Facial expression is part of nonverbal communication. Generally, if the patient is in no distress or is smiling, you should be smiling as well. You can tell if the patient is in distress certainly by the chief complaint and vital signs, but it's easier just to look at her and react to her facial expression and behavior as you walk in the door. If she is smiling, you should be smiling.

If the patient is in distress, is in pain, has respiratory distress, or is crying, you should drop the smile and look calm, caring, and confident. You do this by pretending this is a real-life patient whom you want to help. Your facial muscles will then take care of themselves.

Your tone of voice is also important. Never be angry, be condescending, or appear uncomfortable when you ask delicate questions. Practice the parts of the History several times until you can ask the Sexual History with the same ease as the History of Present Illness (HPI).

Finally, what you say in response to the patient is important. Here is an example of what not to do:

> **Doctor:** "Are your partners men, women, or both?"
>
> **Patient:** "Both."
>
> **Doctor:** "REALLY!"

You should not appear shocked by anything the patient says. Keep the same even tone of voice when asking personal questions. If you are genuinely surprised at a response, you can always thank the patient for sharing personal information while you regain your composure.

Here is a better interaction:

> **Doctor:** "Are your partners men, women, or both?"

Patient: "Both."

Doctor: "Thank you. Have you ever been tested for sexually transmitted disease?"

You also do not want to appear alarming. Here is another example of what not to do:

Doctor: "Has there been any change in your weight?"

Patient: "Yes, I've lost 20 pounds in the last 4 months."

Doctor: "Wow! That could be cancer! Oh, my!"

Your CIS score will be better if you keep your anxiety about the patient's diagnosis to yourself.

Doctor: "Has there been any change in your weight?"

Patient: "Yes, I've lost 20 pounds in the last 4 months."

Doctor: "Have you been on a diet?"

Patient: "No, I just can't keep the weight on."

Doctor: "Has there been any change in how much you sleep? *(Besides cancer maybe this patient is dealing with hyperthyroidism, diabetes, depression, drug abuse, or homelessness)*

6. Express Empathy

As part of your role as doctor to the SP, you will need to be empathetic. Being empathetic means being sensitive and understanding of the patient's emotional and physical state. By your actions and words, you show the patient that you understand how she feels and that you respect her concerns. You demonstrate by your actions and speech that you want to work together and help improve her comfort and health. No patient wants to be dismissed as someone whose problems are not worthy of your attention.

Empathy is built up during the 15 minutes with the patient. The concept of treating a patient the same way you would want your parent treated usually works. Some of the actions you can take to show empathy are:

- Make the patient as comfortable as possible.
- Check that the drape is always protecting the patient's modesty.
- Pull out the leg rest before a patient lies back.
- Assist the patient when he/she needs to change position during the physical exam.
- When the patient is ready to stand up, pull out the footrest and offer to help him down.
- Offer water when a patient is thirsty or when you do a thyroid exam.
- Offer to dim the room lights if the patient is photophobic.
- Offer a tissue to a patient who is crying.
- Be attentive to making a painful exam as brief as possible while explaining the need for the maneuver.
- If the patient is hard of hearing, always stand in front of him so he can read your lips.
- Stand behind the patient if he seems dizzy and about to fall.
- Sit in silence for a couple of seconds when a patient is emotional.

Verbal Empathy

Sample expressions of verbal empathy are the following:

"Tell me more."

"The more you tell me, the better I'll be able to help."

"Remember, I'm here to help."

"I want to be sure I understand. You told me *(paraphrase here)*. Is that correct?"

"I imagine that must be *(hard/sad/frustrating/painful)*."

Example #1:

Patient: "I don't like to talk about my problem. It's personal."

Doctor: "I can see that it's hard for you to talk about." *(Patient shrugs shoulders and is silent)*

Doctor: "Tell me about it, and together we can figure out what to do."

The patient here communicates in a nonverbal manner, which the doctor needs to recognize. It might also help with a reticent patient to state that everything you are about to discuss is confidential.

Example #2:

(Patient is pacing back and forth in the exam room as you enter. Before you can even say hello, the patient speaks angrily.)

Patient: "What took you so long?"

Doctor: *(Showing great empathy)* "I can see that you're upset. I'm sorry I took so long to see you."

Patient: *(Who was expecting an excuse and is pleasantly surprised by the simple apology)* "Oh, that's okay."

Doctor: "Let me introduce myself. My name is Dr. ..."

This scenario illustrates three points: (1) Always answer the patients' questions immediately. Most questions are verbal. However, if the patient makes a face to indicate pain, confusion, or any other emotion, it is best to comment also that you noticed. (2) Apologizing to the patient is not a sign of weakness. It shows the patient that you respect his time. It makes the doctor more approachable. Apologizing defuses a confrontational situation. (3) After you answer the patient's question, get back to your agenda. In this case, the doctor started his introduction.

Empathy through Appropriate Touch

It is sometimes appropriate to use touch to get the patient's attention. This is especially useful when a patient is crying. With your fingertips, touch the patient for no more than 3 seconds and make an empathic statement.

Touch only the shoulder or forearm—never the leg. Do not grab, pat, squeeze, or rub the patient. Never sit on the patient's bed.

(Patient is crying uncontrollably after being told she has cancer.)

Doctor: *(Begins appropriate touch)* "I know you are upset by the bad news. *(Releases touch now that doctor has patient's attention)* I was upset also when I read the report. The good news is that we have treatment available for your condition."

Ask Only One Question at a Time

This is a key skill that will also improve your SEP score. It helps by keeping the questions short. Quite simply, patients cannot remember multiple questions. You will find that you can ask questions fairly quickly and wait for a patient response. If you ask several questions at once to save time, you end up wasting time trying to get the patient's true meaning.

The following are sample patient responses to multiple questions:

Doctor: "Do you have now or have you in the past experienced any chest pain, shortness of breath, nausea, or vomiting?"

Patient: "What?"

* * *

Doctor: "Do you have now or have you in the past experienced any chest pain, shortness of breath, nausea, or vomiting?"

Patient: "Yes."

The doctor here would be entirely unclear on what the patient means by "Yes." To which symptom is he responding? Instead, the most efficient way to ask multiple questions is one at a time:

Doctor: "Have you ever had chest pain?"

Patient: "No."

Doctor: "Any shortness of breath?"

Patient: "No."

Doctor: "Nausea or vomiting?"

Patient: "No."

By the end of this encounter you won't require complete sentences, as the patient will have realized that you just want to check for several different symptoms.

7. Use Open- and Closed-Ended Questions

You will need to use a combination of open- and closed-ended questions. Closed-ended questions are those that can be answered with a simple "Yes" or "No." One example: "Do you have chest pain?" This type of question is useful when you need to go through a list of possible symptoms quickly.

Open-ended questions are questions that cannot be answered "Yes" or "No." Rather, an explanation is required. For example, begin your interaction with an open-ended question, i.e., "How can I help you today?" Open-ended questions allow the patient to tell his story in his own words. This is often the quickest way to obtain the history.

In general, ask open-ended questions to start and closed-ended questions to fill in the gaps of information you need to collect.

8. Use Lay Language When Speaking with Patients

Lay language means nonmedical terminology. Speak to patients as much as possible with lay terminology. Patients are often shy or intimidated by a doctor's technical and highly educated speech. In addition, it is inadvisable to give long technical explanations. Just use the lay terms to describe medical tests and procedures. It is usually not necessary to translate the lay term into medical terminology for the patient, unless, of course, he asks.

> *Incorrect: "I'm going to take a picture of your brain. It is called computed tomography, or computerized axial tomography. You lie still on the x-ray table and the camera moves about. The pictures are fed into a computer and ..."*

> *Correct: "I'm going to take a picture of your head to find out why you have headaches."*

The SP will pretend not to understand when you use medical jargon. You can use a technical term only if the patient uses it first. Even if the SP is portraying a physician who is a patient, do not use medical jargon.

Almost every physician makes an occasional mistake with medical terminology. If you get caught by your SP, simply explain yourself and move on.

> **Doctor:** "I'm going to get an echo on you."
>
> **Patient:** "A what?!"
>
> **Doctor:** "A sound wave picture of your heart."
>
> **Patient:** "Oh, okay, like when they take pictures of unborn babies?"
>
> **Doctor:** "Yes."

If you realize you have made a mistake, you can correct yourself.

> **Doctor:** "I'm going to ask for a CBC—that is, a blood test to look for infection and anemia."

More likely, the SP will catch your mistake before you can correct yourself. Remember not to interrupt the patient.

> **Doctor:** "I'm going to ask for a CBC."
>
> **Patient:** "What's that?"
>
> **Doctor:** "It's a blood test to look for infection and anemia."

The best way to tell the patient is without using medical terms at all.

> **Doctor:** "I'm going to take a blood test to look for infection and anemia."
>
> **Patient:** "Okay."

The average patient does know the names of a few organs. Heart, brain, kidney, liver, appendix, lungs, stomach, and bowel are acceptable lay terms. Try to use lay terms to describe different body parts. Head, neck, chest, belly or tummy, arm, leg, hand, foot, finger, and toes are acceptable lay terms.

Finally, it is best to use lay terms when speaking with your patients and medical terms when writing your note.

9. Be Nonjudgmental

One of the ethical tenets of being a physician is to be nonjudgmental. Even if we personally disapprove and find patients' habits undesirable, we are not to reveal our personal feelings. We treat and care for everyone with the same respect. Speech is the easiest thing to control, but it's important to keep your facial expression, body language, and tone of voice from showing any disapproval as well.

If the patient feels he is not being judged, he'll be more receptive to counseling.

> **Doctor:** "How many sexual partners have you had in the last 6 months?"
>
> **Patient:** "Ummm … eight or nine."
>
> **Doctor:** "Do you use a condom every time?"
>
> **Patient:** "Sometimes I forget."
>
> **Doctor:** "I want you to practice safe sex and use a condom every time."

If you give this advice with same professional demeanor that you've shown during the rest of the interview, it will be well received.

In the context of counseling, there is no conflict between counseling and being nonjudgmental. We are expected to help patients change behaviors that can be damaging to their health. The key is that we are basing our recommendations on medical science and, hopefully, are offering realistic advice with which our patients can comply.

10. Try Not to Ask Leading Questions

A leading question is one in which the patient guesses what answer will please you. A patient will often say what he thinks the doctor wants to hear, even if it isn't the truth. Leading questions are often judgmental as well. Doctors often slip into leading questions by mistake when they ask about habits and social conditions at home.

> *Leading question: "You work, don't you?"*
> *Nonleading question: "Do you work?"*
>
> *Leading question: "You don't use recreational drugs, right?"*
> *Nonleading question: "Do you use recreational drugs?"*
>
> *Leading question: "Your spouse has never hit you. Is that correct?"*
> *Nonleading question: "Have you ever been hit by your spouse?"*

If you do not assume or presuppose the answer to a question, you can avoid this pitfall.

11. Use Transitional Statements

Transitional statements inform the patient of what is coming next in the encounter. You are not asking permission from the patient; you are merely telling her what to expect next. Here are examples of the most common times transitional statements.

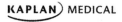

Before the Past Medical History (PMH)

Correct: "Now I'm going to ask you about your health in general."
Correct: "Now I'm going to ask you about your health in the past."

Incorrect: "Now I'm going to take your Past Medical History."

Before the Family History (FH)

Inform the patient that you are no longer talking about her but now want to know about her family.

Doctor: "Now I'll ask you about your family's health."

Before Starting the Ob/Gyn, Sexual, and Social Histories

Inform the patient about confidentiality. If you do not do this, the patient may not provide all of the information you need. Typically, confidentiality needs to be stated just once. Occasionally you will meet patients who will not give you the HPI until you assure them your conversation is confidential.

Doctor: "I'm going to ask you some personal questions. Everything we talk about is confidential."

Before the Physical Exam

While you are washing your hands, you can tell the patient what is going to happen next.

Doctor: "Now I will do your physical exam."

You may have noticed that the first part of the closing or summary is also a transitional statement.

Doctor: "Let me tell you what I am thinking."

At a minimum, use the family history, confidentiality, and closing transitions. If you use more than that, however, you'll find that it will help the patient to understand you, resulting in a higher SEP score. Keep the statements short. All you need to say is *what* is going to happen next; you are not explaining the reason *why*.

Incorrect: "I am going to ask about your family's health because I want to know about any possible genetic disease to predict what you might have."

Correct: "I am going to ask about your family's health."

Finally, do not use transitions in the form of a question.

Incorrect: "May I ask you about your family's health?"

Asking a question requires you to pause and wait for the patient's response. You can assume that the patient has already given permission for the general history, physical, and tests.

12. Pitfalls of Being Reassuring

All patients like physicians who are reassuring. The problem is, it is tempting to promise that you can cure the patient.

> **Patient who has some ominous symptoms:** "Am I going to be okay?"

> **Doctor:** "Sure, don't worry about it. We will make you all better. I promise."

This is incorrect for Step 2 CS—and for real life as well. You really don't know what the future will bring. In Step 2 CS, you are the junior member of the health care team. The case has not been presented yet to your senior physician via the Note. No workup or test results are available. The diagnosis is not yet fixed, so no definite prognosis can be made at this time.

Also, many patients are sophisticated enough to realize they have just been made a promise that cannot be kept.

You're better off reassuring the patient that you:

1. Understand his concerns
2. Will do everything you can to make him feel better
3. Will do everything you can to find out what is wrong
4. Will get him the best treatment available
5. Will remain his doctor and will always be available to help

HISTORY TAKING

General Approach

The history you need to take on your Step 2 CS exam is different from what you did in medical school. In medical school, you were taught to do a complete history. For Step 2 CS, you will take only the relevant history. In other words, you are going to skip sections of the history that are not important in making a diagnosis, ordering tests, and counseling the patient.

Furthermore, no two histories will be the same. Sometimes the family and social histories are not important. There are even situations where there is very little history of present illness to obtain. The doctor is responsible for deciding what to ask. Always consider what parts of the history are most likely on the SP's history checklist. That is what you should be asking next! Asking nonrelevant history is not penalized, though you could have been spending your time asking relevant questions. As you practice, you see that you need an organized approach and a general idea about what is relevant in different situations.

Without further introduction, here is the main history mnemonic that needs to be memorized.

SIQORAAA and PAMHRFOSS

HPI Mnemonic	Stands For	PMH Mnemonic	Stands For
S	Site/symptom	P	Previous episodes of chief complaint
I	Intensity/quantity and quality	A	Allergies
Q	Quality of the symptom	M	Medications (birth control, OTC, herbal, vitamins)
O	Onset of symptoms	H*ITS*	Hospitalizations, illness, trauma, surgery
R	Radiation	R*UGS*	Review of symptoms (urinary, GI, sleep)
A	Aggravating factors	F	Family history
A	Alleviating factors	O	Ob/Gyn
A	Associated symptoms	S	Sexual history
		S	Social history

After the introduction, and after the patient tells her story to you, the doctor, you should complete the parts of SIQORAAA PAMHRFOSS history that are relevant. This can be accomplished with a combination of open- and closed-ended questions. If the chief complaint is "pain" somewhere in the body, you'll usually need some information about each point of SIQORAAA PAM and only parts of HRFOSS. There is no absolute correct order in which to ask the questions. The SPs will not lower your grade if you ask about the Onset of a pain before you ask about the Intensity. The memory tool is just a way for you to stay organized and collect the information rapidly.

On every SP checklist you will be graded on whether you have questioned the patient about allergies and medications. Be sure to ask this of every patient every time. Another required question is for post-menarche female patients: be sure you ask each one about her last menstrual period (LMP).

You do not have to ask every question directly to get credit. If the patient volunteers that the pain is located exactly on the fifth toe of the right foot, you will get credit for knowing the site even if all you did was say hello.

Specific Phrasing for Each Part of the History: SIQORAAA

<u>S</u>IQORAAA: Site/Symptom

You may ask the site of symptoms by simply asking where it hurts. However, you need to know the precise location in order to help narrow your diagnosis.

Doctor: "Where does it hurt?"

Patient: "My head."

Use body language to help show the patient what you need. Using body language even helps with SEP.

Doctor: "Could you point and show me where?"

Having the patient point is especially useful for headache, since sinusitis pain, temporal arteritis, and temporomandibular joint pain are only centimeters apart. Having the patient point is also important for abdominal pain.

Try to identify the location of the pain as specifically as possible, and use paraphrasing to make sure you have it correct. Sometimes patients say "right" to mean the opposite of left, and sometimes "right" means correct or, as in this example, "centered."

Doctor: "Where does it hurt?"

Patient: "My back."

Doctor: "In the lower back?"

Patient: "Yes."

Doctor: "On one side?"

Patient: "No, right in the middle."

Doctor: "Thanks, so that's lower back pain in the middle."

Patient: "Yes."

If the case does not have a site of pain (such as chest pain or sore throat) but has a symptom, e.g., fatigue, fever, or shortness of breath, have the patient begin talking about the problem.

Doctor: "Please tell me about your symptoms."

Patient: "Well, I've had vomiting and diarrhea for the last 12 hours."

S*IQ*ORAAA: Intensity/Quantity and Quality

Intensity of Pain

If the patient's chief complaint is pain, have the patient rate it on the pain scale.

Doctor: "On a scale from 1 to 10, with 10 being the worst pain, how would you rate your pain?"

Patient: "8/10."

Pain is a subjective finding, and you should put in your note whatever the patient tells you. If the patient says it's a 10/10 pain but you think he looks comfortable, you can say so in the General Appearance (GA) section of your note. For example:

HPI: 10/10 pain
GA: Pt appears in no distress

The most important thing to remember when asking about the pain scale is don't rush the patient. You have to pretend this is a real patient who hasn't been asked this question hundreds of times before.

Ask the patient to point on his own body, not on your body or that of another person in the room.

Have a list of differential diagnoses of common causes of pain for every part of the body. That way you'll spend a minimum amount of time outside the doorway and be more confident inside the patient's room.

Have a list of common differentials for commonly presenting symptoms, such as shortness of breath, diarrhea, fatigue, fever, weight loss, vaginal bleeding, and dysuria.

If the patient says it's the worst headache of his life, think subarachnoid hemorrhage. If he says it's the worst sore throat of his life, think adult epiglottis, peritonsillar abscess.

Intensity of a Symptom

The pain scale is only for pain and is not used for symptoms. There are several ways to determine the intensity of a symptom: You could ask how bad the symptom is, or you could ask how the symptom is affecting the patient's life, if that is more appropriate.

Doctor: "How is this weakness affecting your life?"

Patient: "Well, I lost my job because I missed so much work."

Another way to measure the intensity of a symptom is to ask questions about functional impairment. This is especially useful with chronic problems such as dementia, depression, and Parkinson's. It is also useful in any disease that might cause one to lose the ability to live independently. These questions are known as the DEATH questions: Dressing, Eating, Ambulating, Toilet, Hygiene.

Doctor: "Are you having any problems getting dressed?"

Patient: "No."

Doctor: "Are you able to prepare your own food and eat it?"

Patient: "Yes."

Doctor: "Are you having any falls?"

Patient: "No."

Doctor: "Any problems getting off and on the toilet?"

Patient: "Yes."

Doctor: "Are you able to bathe or shower by yourself?"

Quantity of a Symptom

If the symptom has a volume, what we really want to know for Intensity is the quantity, or "How much has this been happening?"

Vaginal Bleeding:

Doctor: "How many pads or tampons do you use a day?"

Patient: "Three or four on a heavy day."

Sputum:

1 teaspoon ~ 5 cc;
1 tablespoon ~ 15 cc.

Doctor: "How much sputum do you have?"

Patient: "About 3 teaspoons a day."

Doctor: "What color is it?"

Patient: "Yellowish."

Doctor: "Any blood?"

Patient: "No."

Emesis and Diarrhea:

Find out the number of times, how much each time, the color, the consistency, and if there is any blood:

> **Patient:** "I have diarrhea."
>
> **Doctor:** "Are your bowel movements watery?"
>
> **Patient:** "Yes."
>
> **Doctor:** "How many times a day?"
>
> **Patient:** "Six times today."
>
> **Doctor:** "How much?"
>
> **Patient:** "Don't really know."
>
> **Doctor:** "What color is it?"
>
> **Patient:** "Kind of greenish."
>
> **Doctor:** "Any black or red?"
>
> **Patient:** "No, there is no blood; I know black or red vomit or bowel movement means bleeding!"

Quality of a Pain or Symptom

Ask every patient with pain in the body what the pain or symptom feels like. "What does it feel like?" is on almost all SP checklists.

SIQORAAA: Onset

Knowing the onset of any pain or symptom is very important in determining possible causes of the symptom. Sudden chest pain would suggest pneumothorax, pulmonary embolism, or perhaps a rib fracture. Slowly developing, sharp pain would be more characteristic of infection such as pneumonia or pleurisy. Even with just the Doorway Information and site/symptom, you have a differential diagnosis that you start to rank order in your mind as you continue with the rest of the history.

Onset questions that are sometimes very revealing are the following:

> "When did it begin?"
> "What were you doing when it started?"
> "Did it come on slowly? Suddenly?"

For patients who are not sure when a chronic symptom began, try the following:

> "When were you last completely well?"

Onset also includes the duration, course, and frequency. These questions are often essential in figuring out the diagnosis.

1 cup = 8 oz = 240 cc.

Ripping or tearing chest pain tends to be aortic dissection. Heavy, tight, or squeezing pain is acute coronary syndrome, and sharp pain can be everything else from pneumo-thorax, pulmonary embolism, or pneumonia to costochondritis or pleurisy

Duration

"How long does the pain last?"

"Does the pain ever go away?"

"When was the last time you didn't have pain?"

Frequency

"How often does it happen?"

Course

"Is it getting better or worse?"

"Does the pain come and go?"

For example, if the patient is getting RLQ pain every month, it is unlikely to be appendicitis.

SIQO_R_AAA: Radiation of Pain

Another question that is appropriate only when the patient has pain that radiates is the following:

"Does the pain move anywhere?"

A common pitfall with this question is using the word *radiation*.

Doctor: "Does the pain radiate anywhere?"

Patient: "What? I need radiation?!"

Doctor: "Oh no, I just want to know if the pain moves anywhere."

Patients are often under stress when they see the doctor, and misunderstandings are frequent. It is helpful to remember where a few pains radiate to.

Type of Pain	Typically Radiates To
Ischemic chest pain	Arms, neck, back, jaw
Kidney stone	Groin and testicle
Gallbladder	The tip of the right scapula
Spleen injury	Top of the shoulders (diaphragm irritation)
Testicular torsion	Lower abdomen
Abdominal aortic aneurysm	Back
Pancreatitis	Back
Posterior penetrating gastric ulcer	Back
Sciatica	Down leg
Pharyngitis pain	Can radiate to ear

Sometimes, depending on the case, the SP may ask you for more specific information. For example:

Doctor: "Does the pain move anywhere?"

Patient: "Like where?"

Doctor: "How about your arms?"

Patient: "No."

Doctor: "Neck?"

Patient: "No."

Doctor: "Back?"

SIQOR*A*AA: Aggravating Factors

"Does anything make it worse?"

Aggravating and alleviating factors are present on most SP History checklists. You will need to ask these two questions of almost all patients in the exam. It is helpful to know common alleviating and aggravating factors.

Common aggravating factors are the following:

- Ischemic heart disease: exertion, walking up stairs, sexual intercourse
- Asthma: physical exertion, exposure to cold air, dust, smoking, animals
- Ulcer: eating food, taking aspirin or ibuprofen (NSAIDs)
- Meningitis: movement, jumping up and down
- Migraine: exposure to sound or light
- Muscle contraction headache: stress
- Gallbladder: eating fatty foods
- Pancreatitis/gastritis: alcohol ingestion
- Polymyalgia rheumatica: gel phenomenon (stiff, sore joints after resting for a few hours)
- Musculoskeletal pain: moving about

SIQORA*A*A: Alleviating Factors

"Does anything make it better?"

Common alleviating factors are the following:

- Angina pectoris: rest
- Pericarditis: sitting forward
- Renal colic: moving about
- Muscle contraction headache: massage
- Migraine: dark, quiet room; caffeine ingestion
- Ulcer–GERD: antacids or eating food
- Gastric outlet obstruction: vomiting
- Musculoskeletal pain: keeping still and not moving

You may also ask the patient directly about activities that you suspect should make her symptoms better or worse.

Doctor: "Does anything make it better when you have the pain?"

Patient: "Yes, when I sit and rest for a few minutes."

Doctor: "What happens when you walk fast or climb stairs?"

Patient: "Oh, I know not to do that to keep the pain from returning."

SIQORAA<u>A</u>: Associated Manifestations

Associated manifestations are symptoms that commonly occur in the diagnoses you are considering. Negative findings are just as important as positive findings. These are symptoms that a patient might have based on the diagnosis you have made. If you do not have a diagnosis in mind yet, you can ask good associated-symptom questions based on the chief complaint and the preceding history alone.

For example, if you suspect that a patient with chest pain has acute myocardial infarction, you would also ask about palpitations, syncope, shortness of breath, diaphoresis, nausea, and vomiting.

However, if you have no idea what was causing the chest pain, your list of associated symptoms would be similar but a bit longer. To those listed above, you might add cough, sputum, and fever.

Associated manifestations for cough: Fever, sputum, shortness of breath, chest pain, hemoptysis.

Associated manifestations for joint pain: Redness, swelling, heat, and loss of function are the signs of inflammation.

Don't forget to ask about rash and fever in joint-pain cases. This may be a tipoff that you're dealing with a rheumatology case, specifically systemic lupus erythematosus.

For an abdominal pain case, try asking about fever, anorexia, emesis, diarrhea, dysuria, and jaundice. Add the question, "Are you passing gas?" if you suspect bowel obstruction.

Associated-manifestation questions can help you confirm diagnoses already in mind, or help you think of the diagnosis for the first time.

Be very careful here not to ask multiple questions at once. It is fine to ask a series of brief closed-ended questions.

Doctor: "Do you have any loss of appetite?"

Patient: "No."

Doctor: "How about any vomiting?"

Patient: "No."

Doctor: "Diarrhea?"

Patient: "No."

Doctor: "Have you noticed any yellowing of the skin?"

Patient: "No."

Doctor: "Are you having any problems urinating?"

Patient: "Yes."

Doctor: "Tell me about it."

Patient: "I have to go urinate every 2 hours, but there are only a few drops. Once I saw blood."

Doctor: "Any burning?"

Patient: "Oh, yes!!!"

You'll notice that the doctor above used closed-ended questions until she got a positive response. Then she used the open-ended "Tell me about it" question to elicit more information about the symptoms. When the patient was finished, the doctor went back to closed-ended questions to get the remaining urinary questions answered.

Specific Phrasing for Each Part of the History: PAMHRFOSS

PAMHRFOSS: Previous Episodes of the Chief Complaint

"Have you ever had this before?"

You may already know the answer to this important question from asking about the symptom's frequency during the Onset questions. If you find yourself asking this question earlier in the interview, that is completely fine. This is just a memory device to make sure that you know this information before you leave the patient's room.

If a patient has multiple episodes of identical recurrent headache, for instance, the diagnosis is more likely to be migraine or muscle contraction headache. If it's a new-onset headache in an older adult who doesn't typically have headaches, then consider other diagnoses such as temporal arteritis, tumor, hydrocephalus, or any hemorrhage.

PAMHRFOSS: Allergies

"Do you have any allergies?"

This is the basic question that must be asked of the patient in *every* case. All patients need to be asked about drug allergies. Even though there is no treatment with drugs on the exam, it is essential to ask—and later document—this information. When this question is asked, patients frequently think about prescription medication allergies first, and they may or may not tell you about allergies in other categories. The four categories are:

- Medications
- Foods
- Plants or animals
- Environmental sources

If the case might be that of an allergic reaction—a rash, shortness of breath, runny nose, watery eyes, anaphylaxis, bee sting—a more detailed allergy history is indicated.

"Do you have any allergies to prescription medication?"
"How about any bad reaction to over-the-counter pills?"
"Any bad reactions to food?"
"Do you have any allergies to animals or plants?"

If you aren't sure you covered all the categories, you may also ask:

"Anything else you can tell me about allergies?"

PA<u>M</u>HRFOSS: Medications

"Are you taking any medications?"

Medication history is essential to all histories. By knowing the medications that a patient takes every day the physician has good idea of what the chronic illnesses are going to be. The physician needs to know all drugs the patients are taking in addition to the prescription medication(s). The three categories are:

- Prescription
- Over-the-counter (OTC)
- Vitamins and herbs

A more complete line of questioning for medications is the following:

"Do you take prescription medicines?"
"How about over-the-counter pills?"
"Do you take any vitamins or herbs?"

For most cases you don't need the dose, frequency, or route. You need only the name of the drug. Use whatever name the patient gives you; the trade name or generic name is acceptable.

If you are not familiar with a particular medication, ask the patient why he is taking it. Also, many medications are prescribed for multiple indications. This question is also a natural lead-in to the past medical history that comes next.

"What do you take that for?"

If you still do not recognize what the patient is saying, ask:

"Could you spell that for me, please?"

If the patient seems to be having a hard time remembering the names of his medicine(s), ask if he has the bottles with him. If he does, you can simply read the labels.

It is not a sign of weakness to keep asking questions until you are sure of the medications. It shows the patient you are concerned enough to understand his situation completely.

Checking compliance is important in some cases. Some patients on the exam will be sicker because they are not taking their medications regularly. The classic example here is the chronic congestive heart failure patient who stops taking his medicine and now is short of breath.

Doctor: "Are you taking the Lasix regularly?"

Patient: "Well, no—I stopped it 2 weeks ago."

Doctor: "When did the shortness of breath start?"

Patient: "Just in the last 3 or 4 days."

With this history, you would be justified to include "noncompliance with medications causing CHF exacerbation" in your differential. Compliance is also checked because medicine *can* make you sick! Some patients take their medicine exactly as prescribed

Common Medications and Their Side Effects

Nonsteroidal Anti-inflammatory Drugs (NSAIDs)

Common names	Motrin, ibuprofen, naproxen
Adverse reactions	Gastrointestinal (GI) bleeding, ulcer, allergic reaction, renal insufficiency

Diuretics

Common names	Lasix, Furosemide, HCTZ, hydrochlorothiazide, spironolactone, Bumex
Adverse reactions	Renal failure, hypotension, electrolyte disorder, syncope. Gout is caused by thiazide diuretics.

Digoxin

Common names	Digoxin/Lanoxin
Adverse reactions	Arrhythmias, headache, dizziness, fatigue, nausea/vomiting

Beta Blockers

Common names	Atenolol, metoprolol, Toprol XL (anything that ends in "-ol")
Adverse reactions	Bradycardia, depression, erectile dysfunction, hypotension, wheezing

ACE Inhibitors/Angiotensin Receptor Blockers (ARBs)

Common names	Lisinopril, captopril, Avapro (irbesartan), enalapril
Adverse reactions	Renal failure, hyperkalemia, cough, angioedema

SSRIs

Common names	Fluoxetine, Prozac, Paxil
Adverse reactions	Confusion, fever, anxiety, hyperreflexia, tremors, insomnia, tachycardia, hypertension (serotonin syndrome)

Statins

Common names	Atorvastatin (Lipitor), simvastatin (Zocor)
Adverse reactions	Rhabdomyolysis—muscle pain, renal failure. Liver failure-jaundice

and as a result have side effects. There certainly could be a case of side effects from medication presented to you.

As with the noncompliance case, find out the timeline of when the medicine was started or dosage was increased, and when the side effects began.

Patients also commonly take herbal medications to self-treat conditions. It may be useful to know a few common preparations and why patients might take them. Of course, to be sure, you should ask the patient why he is taking it.

- Saw palmetto: benign prostatic hypertrophy
- Cranberry: urinary tract infection
- Echinacea: upper respiratory infection
- Ginseng: stress and memory
- St. John's Wort: depression

PAM<u>H</u>RFOSS: Past Medical History (PMH)

The PMH can be divided into four components:

1. Hospitalizations (H)
2. Major illness (I)
3. Significant trauma (T)
4. Surgical history (S)

Hospitalizations

"Have you ever been hospitalized?" or "Have you ever stayed overnight in the hospital?"

You need just a one- or two-word description of why the patient was hospitalized. There is no need for the name of hospital, attending physician, or date. If a hospitalization, surgery, or procedure was recent (i.e., within the last month), it's possible that the current case may more likely be a complication or progression of disease.

Major Illness

"Have you ever had any major illness?"

In questioning adult patients about risk factors, ask about specific diseases individually:

"Have you ever had high blood sugar?"
"Have you ever had high blood pressure?"
"How about high cholesterol?"

Make sure you wait for the patient to answer "Yes" or "No" before asking the next question.

Trauma

"Have you ever had any major injuries?"

Usually, if there have been major injuries, you will find out about them when asking about hospitalizations or surgery. If it is a mental-status-change case, you could phrase the question as follows:

"Have you had any head injuries?"

Surgery

"Have you ever had any operations?"

Record on your Note all of the operations the patient has had. Not all operations are performed in hospitals these days, so ask this even if you already know all the hospitalizations.

Occasionally, during the physical exam you will find a surgical scar you did not expect. Ask the patient the following:

(Pointing to or touching the scar) "What is this scar from?"

Be sure to pay attention to what the patient is telling you.

Doctor: "Have you ever been hospitalized?"

Patient: "Yes, I had my gallbladder out 5 years ago. That's it."

Doctor: "Have you ever had any major illness?"

Patient: "No."

Doctor: "Have you ever had any bad injuries?"

Patient: "No."

Doctor: "Have you ever had any operations?"

Patient: "Yeah, I told you about the gallbladder, weren't you listening?"

Doctor: "I'm sorry, I meant any other operations."

However, this miscommunication could have been avoided by asking the following:

Doctor: "Besides the gallbladder, have you had any other surgery?"

PAMH<u>R</u>FOSS: Review of Systems (ROS)

Review of systems is the time to ask screening questions. It is the time to see if there are other major problems that you have not yet uncovered. You can ask about any organ system that you feel is relevant, but focusing on three systems is sufficient for most cases. Those three main categories are the following:

1. Urinary
2. Gastrointestinal
3. Sleep

Urinary ROS Questions

"Do you have any problems urinating?"

If the patient says "No," go on to another organ system or the family history. If she says "Yes," go through your urinary complaint questions.

"How often do you urinate?"
"How many times do you get up at night to urinate?"
"Do you have any burning with urination?"
"Any blood?"
"Is the stream weak?"
"Do you ever have any accidents?"

If the chief complaint was dysuria, all of the questions above would have been asked in the HPI.

Gastrointestinal ROS Questions

Two high-yield questions to ask the SP about weight and diet are the following:

"Has there been any recent change in your weight?"
"Are you on any special diet?"

The diet question frequently uncovers vegans with B12 deficiency.

Have prepared by Test Day the short differential for weight gain and weight loss:

- *Weight gain* can commonly be from depression, eating disorders, hypothyroidism, Cushing's, and edematous states such as liver failure, heart failure, or nephrotic syndrome.

- *Weight loss* is seen with depression, eating disorders, cancer, hyperthyroidism, and amphetamine use, as well as many chronic diseases.

Sleep ROS Questions

"Has there been any change in how much you sleep?"

- *Increased sleep* may be due to depression, hypothyroidism, sleep apnea, or drugs.
- *Decreased sleep* may be due to depression, hyperthyroidism, mania, or drug use.

PAMHRFOSS: Family History

The family history is relevant only if the diagnosis you are considering has a genetic or familial component. Do not ask the family history if it isn't relevant. If you do need a family history, do the transitional statement first. Then ask as many of the following examples as are appropriate.

"Does anyone in your family have what you have?"
"Does anyone in your family have high blood sugar?"
"How about high blood pressure?"
"Does anyone in the family have any serious illness?"

In some cases it may be important to express condolences. However, it is not generally necessary to express condolences to the patient about the death of a parent many years ago. Do offer condolences if the death was less than a year ago or if the patient's facial expression suddenly becomes sullen.

Patient: "My mother died last month."

Doctor: "Oh, I'm so sorry."

Patient: "Thank you."

Doctor: "What health problems did she have?"

Patient: "Pancreatic cancer."

Doctor: "And how is your father's health?"

PAMHRFOSS: Obstetrical and Gynecology History

You should ask about Last Menstrual Period (LMP) with all women past the age of menarche; however, only women with complaints of abdominal pain, abnormal vaginal bleeding, dysuria, discharge, and perhaps syncope (ectopic pregnancy) will require a more detailed Ob/Gyn history.

Obstetrical History

How to determine a patient's GPA status:

G = Number of times pregnant; ask "How many times have you been pregnant?"
P = Number of live births; ask "How many times have you given birth?"
A = Number of miscarriages and abortions; ask "Have you had any miscarriages or abortions?"

For example, G2P1 describes a woman who is pregnant now and has had one live birth. G3P2Ab1 describes a woman who is not pregnant now and has had two live births and one miscarriage or abortion.

Gynecological History

Components of a comprehensive gynecological history are the following:

- Regularity
- Cramps/pain
- Flow
- Cycle length
- Age of menarche/age of menopause
- Spotting
- Vaginal discharge
- Last Pap smear

Suggested questions are:

"When was your last menstrual period?"
"Was it normal?"
"Any change in your period recently?"
"Do you have a period every month?"
"How long between periods?"
"Are you regular? How many days do you use pads or tampons?"
"On a heavy day, how many pads or tampons do you use?"
"When did you start having periods? When did you stop menstruating?"
"Any mood swings or irritability around your period? Anything else?"

PAMHRFO_S_S: Sexual History

The sexual history or parts of the sexual history are needed only if they are relevant to the case, especially if you think the patient could have a sexually transmitted disease. Also, ask yourself if sexual function could be compromised by the diagnoses you are considering. Examples of this are angina precipitated by sexual intercourse; or erectile dysfunction caused by depression, diabetes, or beta blockers. The key is not to suddenly become nervous when asking these questions. Practice them over and over until you can ask them without embarrassment.

Standard sexual history questions are the following:

"Are you sexually active?"
"Do you use contraception?"
"How many sexual partners have you had in the last six months?"
"Are your partners men, women, or both?"
"Have you ever been tested for HIV?"
"Have you ever had a sexually transmitted disease?"
"Do you have any concerns about sexual function?"

Do not use the terms "miscarriage" and "abortion" interchangeably when talking with patients. To the lay public, a miscarriage is a spontaneous abortion, and an abortion is an elective termination of the pregnancy.

PAMHRFOS<u>S</u>: Social History

Taking a complete social history consists of asking about the following:

- Tobacco
- Alcohol
- Recreational drugs
- Diet (if not asked about in ROS)
- Exercise
- Work life
- Home life

Depending on the case, ask about parts or all of the social history.

Tobacco

An efficient way to determine smoking history is to ask the following:

Doctor: "Have you ever used tobacco products?"

Patient: "Yes, I smoked for 30 years and stopped last week. I also stopped using cigars and chewing tobacco last week."

Incorrect: "Do you smoke?"

If you asked the same patient, "Do you smoke?" he may reply "No," because he quit last week.

Even if the patient had just recently stopped smoking, he might still answer, "No, I don't smoke." In this case, you would miss the entire tobacco history!

If the patient has a disease that is caused or exacerbated by smoking, it is helpful to know the total lifetime exposure.

Pack-Years = (Number of Packs Per Day) × (Number of Years)

So 20 pack-years could mean 20 years at 1 pack per day or 40 years at one-half pack per day.

If the chief complaint were that the patient wants to receive smoking cessation help, you would need to know all the details of when he started to smoke, what he has tried to do in the past to stop, and what methods of quitting have and have not been successful for him.

Alcohol

When will you need to counsel your patient to quit alcohol? You can certainly advise "No alcohol" when it is affecting your patient's health (a jaundiced patient with hepatitis) or when there is a medical condition that requires the patient not to drink (a woman who is trying to conceive or who is pregnant).

If the patient tells you he is a "social drinker," it is hard to know whether that means one sip of champagne on New Year's or a quart of whiskey per day. A good way to ask about alcohol use is the following:

Doctor: "Do you drink alcohol?"

Patient: "Yes."

Doctor: "How much alcohol do you drink?"

"Binge drinking" is loosely defined as more than five drinks (men) or four drinks (women) on any one occasion.

Quantify the number of alcoholic drinks your patient ingests a day. It doesn't matter if the active ingredient is delivered in beer, wine, or whisky. If a man says he has more than two drinks a day, or a woman more than one, ask the CAGE questions. Also ask the CAGE questions if the patient is a binge drinker.

A positive response to any of the CAGE questions or binge drinking suggests there may be an alcohol problem, and counseling should be advised.

Courtesy of Dr. John A. Ewing. "Detecting Alcoholism: The CAGE Questionaire, JAMA 252: 1905-1907, 1984".

Recreational Drug Use

The correct way to ask about drug use is the following:

Doctor: "Do you use recreational drugs?"

Patient: "Yes."

Doctor: "What do you use?"

Patient: "Cocaine, when I can get it."

Doctor: "How do you take it?"

Patient: "I smoke it."

Doctor: "When did you last use?"

Patient: "About 20 minutes ago."

If the patient uses recreational drugs, find out the specific names, what route is used (ingested, smoked, snorted, or IV), and when the drug was last used. Many patients also need to be asked if they are willing to quit, and you should find out what methods of quitting they have tried in the past.

SPs do make an effort to avoid using slang words in their speech. However, these phrases are in common usage and so it is worthwhile for you to understand their meaning. If you don't understand the street name of a recreational drug it is fine to ask the patient.

Patient: "I use coke sometimes."

Doctor: "Is that cocaine?"

Patient: "That's right, Doc."

Common names for recreational drugs:

Alcohol:	Booze, brews, brewskis
Amphetamines:	Speed, crank, crystal meth
Cannabis:	Hash, hashish, dope, pot, reefer, bud, ganja, weed, grass
Cocaine:	Blow, coke, toot, nose candy, crack
Downers:	Generic street name for benzodiazepines or barbiturates
Heroin:	Horse, brown sugar, smack
Phencyclidine:	PCP, angel dust
'Roids:	Anabolic steroids in general

CAGE Questionnaire
1. *Have you ever felt you should **C**ut down on your drinking?*
2. *Have people **A**nnoyed you by criticizing your drinking?*
3. *Have you ever felt bad or **G**uilty about your drinking?*
4. *Have you had a drink first thing in the morning to steady your nerves or get rid of a hangover? (**E**ye-opener)*

Stay away from using the term "illicit drug," as it is considered judgmental.

Exercise

This is good question for anyone who comes in for a general checkup, annual physical, or periodic health exam. It is not necessary for a patient who presents with acute problems.

"How much exercise do you get?"

Work Life

There are situations where the kind of work the patient does may give you clues about the diagnosis. A coal miner who is short of breath, for instance, may have pneumoconiosis. Also, the patient's level of stress is important. Note that the stress level is what the *patient reports,* not how stressful you determine the job to be.

Doctor: "Do you work?"

Patient: "Yes, I'm a coal miner."

Doctor: "Are you having any stress from work?"

Home Life

There are two things you will need to know about the patient's home life:

- Who does the patient live with?
- Is there any stress at home?

You can ask about home life in the following way:

Doctor: "Who do you live with?"

Patient: "My wife and our three teenagers."

Doctor: "Is there any stress at home?"

Patient: "No, just the usual stuff with kids."

PEDIATRIC AND ADOLESCENT HISTORIES

The pediatric cases on Step 2 CS will not have any patients for you to exam. These will be surrogate cases, meaning that the parent or caretaker will come to the office or call to speak to you about the patient who is not present.

For these cases, the advantage is that no physical exam is possible. Simply leave blank the Physical Exam portion of your note. The Board knows you cannot examine someone who is not present. The adolescent case will probably be a concerned parent acting as a surrogate. It would be possible to hire SPs in their early twenties to portray adolescents as well. You have permission to talk too, and exam and order tests on everyone you encounter in Step 2 CS.

Pediatric History

The younger the child, the more important the pediatric history. Once the child is an adolescent, the pediatric history is less relevant than the adolescent questions. A good way to organize your thoughts is to complete the usual introduction. Find out the name of the patient, the name of person you are speaking with, and the relationship between the family members. Complete the relevant parts of SIQORAAA PAMHRFOSS and then the relevant parts of the pediatric and/or adolescent histories.

Pediatric history consists of six subparts:

- Prenatal
- Birth
- Neonatal
- Feeding
- Development
- Routine care

Prenatal History

Sample questions (of the mother) could include the following:

"How was your health during pregnancy?"

"Did you get regular prenatal checkups?"

"Did you smoke or drink during pregnancy?"

"Were there any problems with swelling or high blood pressure?" (preeclampsia)

Birth History

You'll want to know if the child was full-term or pre-/post-mature, as well as how he was delivered.

"Was the baby full-term?"

"Did you have a Cesarean section?"

"Were there any problems with your labor?"

"How much did the baby weigh at birth?" (All mothers know this information.)

Neonatal History

Typically, newborns stay in the hospital a day or two. A longer hospital stay likely indicates a problem.

"How long did you and the baby stay in the hospital after delivery?"

"Did the child have any medical problems when she was born?"

"Any problems with breathing?"

"Any problems with feeding, having bowel movements, or infections?"

"Any problems with yellow skin?"

Do not ask the mother for the Apgar scores.

Feeding History

"Was the child breast-fed or bottle-fed?"

If the child is a newborn, ask about the success with breastfeeding.

"Are you having any problems breastfeeding?"

If the newborn is bottle-fed, get more details.

"What formula are you using?"
"How many ounces does the baby drink? How often? What is the feeding schedule?"

If the child is a bit older, ask about his eating habits:

"When did the child start eating solid food?"
"How is her appetite?"
"Is she taking a pediatric multiple vitamins?"
"Does she have any food allergies?"

Developmental History

We do not have a growth chart on Step 2 CS, so you will have to ask about growth.

"Has your child been gaining weight normally?"
"Has there been any sudden gain or loss of physical growth?"

Ask about developmental milestones as appropriate. This is more important for a toddler and less important for a 12-year-old with an earache.

"At what age did the baby start to say a few words? To social smile? To roll over? To walk?"
"At what age was the baby toilet-trained?"

Routine Care

This consists of two questions:
"Are the child's immunizations up to date?"
"Is the child getting routine checkups?"

If the mother happens to have the immunization record in her purse, ask to see it.

Adolescent History

The typical adolescent case will hinge on the main problems of an adolescent. The cases you will most likely see will mimic real-life problems and will center on issues such as self-esteem, eating disorders, and/or drug use.

It might be easier if you break this down into the following categories: body image, eating disorders, education, friends and activities, drugs, sex, and suicide/depression. If you ask a little about each category, you have covered a lot of potential problems.

Body Image

"How is your child's body image?"
(to the child) "Do you feel bad about yourself? Do you like your body?"

Eating Disorders

"Has your teen's weight changed?"
"How much does your child exercise?"
"Does he frequently go to the bathroom during dinner?"

Education

"Has there been any change in your child's grades?"

"Is your child interested in school?"

Friends and Activities

"Do you know your child's friends?"

"Is your child secretive about his friends?"

"Does your child have friends and activities?"

Drugs

"Does your child drink alcohol?"

"Does he use recreational drugs?"

"Does he smoke cigarettes?"

Sex

"Have you talked to your child about sex?"

"Is your child sexually active?"

"Have you asked your child if he is sexually active?"

"Have you discussed contraception?"

"Has your daughter had the new shot that prevents cervical cancer?"

Suicide/Depression

"Does your child seem sad or hopeless?"

"Does your child seem to want to harm himself?"

"Does your child seem uninterested in activities?"

PHYSICAL EXAM

An Overview

HEENT
Inspection
Palpation
Eyes
Ears
Nose
Throat
Lymph glands
Thyroid

ABDOMEN
Inspection
Auscultation
Percussion
Palpation
 –Light and deep
 –Rebound tenderness

CHEST
Inspection
Palpation/Respiratory excursion
Tactile fremitus
Percussion
Auscultation

CARDIOVASCULAR
Sitting
Carotid
Auscultation
Peripheral pulses, edema, clubbing

Lying Back, Head Elevated 30 Degrees
Jugular venous pressure (JVP)
Point of maximum impulse (PMI)
Auscultate a second time

NEURO
Mental status
Cranial nerves
Motor
Sensory
Reflexes
Cerebellar

JOINTS
Inspection
Palpation
Range of motion
Motor
Reflect
Sensory
Vascular

The physical exam for the USMLE Step 2 CS is very focused on the patient's presenting complaint. This means simply that you should not do a complete head-to-toe physical exam like we were all trained to do in medical school. For most cases, you will have 4 to 5 minutes to complete the exam. No two physical exams of your 12 patients will be the same.

For the USMLE Step 2 CS, you can divide the physical into six systems.

1. HEENT (head, eyes, ears, nose, and throat)
2. Chest
3. Cardiovascular
4. Abdominal
5. Neurological
6. Joints

Your goal is to perform physical exam maneuvers that are most likely on the SP's Physical Exam Checklist. Do the most relevant organ system first. For example, if the chief complaint is abdominal pain, you'll start with the abdominal exam. If the chief complaint is headache, start with the HEENT and neurological exams. Generally speaking, you want to perform a complete or near-complete exam on the most important organ systems.

After completing your exam of the most important organ systems, go on to the secondary organ systems. You generally don't have to do all of the physical exam maneuvers on the less important secondary organ systems for that case. So for abdominal pain, the secondary organ systems might be chest, cardiovascular (CV), and HEENT. For the headache case, chest and CV may be the secondary organ systems. Some organ systems you may skip completely on some cases.

After you finish taking the patient's history, you will wash your hands and say the following:

"Now I'll do your physical exam. Let me first wash my hands."

Handwashing

Before you touch the patient for a physical exam, it is mandatory that you wash your hands. You should not wash your hands prior to giving the drape or shaking hands during the introduction.

Simply step on the foot pedal beneath the basin and the water will start. Take a squirt of soap from the dispenser and rub your hands under the water for 3 seconds. Take your foot off the water pedal, grab some paper towels, and dry your hands completely. Drop the paper towels into the garbage can and proceed with the physical exam.

Do not touch your own face after you wash your hands. If you sneeze or rub your nose, re-wash your hands before proceeding to touch the patient again.

The Patient Gown and Appropriate Draping

The drape should be given during the introduction at the beginning of the encounter. Otherwise you will lose this easy point from your CIS score.

The SP will be wearing a patient gown that ties in the back, and will be wearing undergarments. It is your job to keep the patient covered as much as possible; uncover only the part of the torso you need to examine. Then replace the gown to protect the patient's modesty.

The abdomen and chest should not be exposed simultaneously. To examine the abdomen, you or the patient must raise the gown. Raise it up to an inch or so above the costal margin and do your exam. Replace the gown when you are finished with the abdominal exam.

To examine the chest you must lower the gown to an inch or so below the costal margin. This is for both male and female SPs. The gown must be replaced and retied when the chest exam is finished.

You or the patient can lower and raise the gown, depending on the circumstances. Let the patient know what is going to happen next.

Doctor: "May I untie and lower your gown so I can examine your chest?"

Patient: "Yes."

Offer to remove the gown when it would be difficult or painful for the patient to do so herself. Perhaps she has a broken clavicle or is in respiratory distress. If the patient is in no distress, it is fine for her to lower her own gown.

Doctor: "Could you please untie and lower your gown?"

Patient: "Okay."

Remember to retie the string ties on the back of the gown as soon as the gown is replaced.

Getting the patient undressed is the only time in the exam that we ask for permission. Please wait for the patient to answer before you start undressing her! You would also need permission to remove shoes and socks. This is a common CS exam challenge—you won't find a diabetic foot ulcer (simulated physical finding) unless you look.

If the patient refuses to cooperate, explain the importance of the physical in order to determine the cause of her condition.

Physical Exam Maneuvers You Are Never Allowed to Do

You are never permitted to do the following on the Step 2 CS exam:

- Female breast exam
- Internal pelvic exam
- Rectal exam
- Genital or genitourinary exams, including inguinal hernia exam
- Corneal reflex exam

This list of forbidden maneuvers is part of the Doorway Information on each case for you to review. You also will not need to test the gag reflex or sense of smell.

There is no need to memorize lists of normal laboratory values for Step 2 CS.

A general guideline is that parts of the body covered with underwear are off-limits. If an SP has his underwear pulled up above the umbilicus and you need to examine his RLQ, you could ask him to lower his underwear slightly to the top of the iliac crests so you can do an exam.

Moreover, *do not hurt your SP.* The SP is subject to multiple exams every day. It is helpful for you to realize what is most uncomfortable for the patient.

Some other points to remember:

- Otoscopy might be the most potentially dangerous maneuver you are asked to perform. The key here is to not scratch the ear canal and give the patient a bloody ear. When you place the speculum into the external auditory canal, make sure not to insert it so deeply that the tip of the speculum touches the skin.

- When examining the pharynx, use a clean tongue blade and place it only one-third to one-half of the way back on the visible portion of the tongue. This way you will not gag your SP but will still be able to inspect the pharynx.

- Be sure to keep your fingernails off the patient's skin.

- Be sure your hands are dry after you wash them before touching the patient.

- Use a firm but gentle touch. Even deep palpation of a normal abdomen should not cause discomfort (practice on a friend before the exam).

- When checking for costovertebral angle (CVA) tenderness, do not "punch" your patient. A simple tap will do. On the pyelonephritis case, the SP will give you a simulated physical finding of pain.

Simulated Versus Real Physical Findings

This is probably the hardest concept on the exam, as many of the patients don't actually have the disease they are portraying. The SPs are skillfully acting.

Accept All Physical Findings

Accept all actual physical findings on patients as real, with the exception of the vital signs. SPs are sometimes hired specifically to portray different diseases. The Board will hire some SPs who actually have physical findings, perhaps someone who has arthritis, old surgical scars, Bell's palsy, atrial fibrillation, or thenar muscle wasting from carpal tunnel syndrome. Certainly this is not a complete list.

The vital signs are the heart rate, temperature, blood pressure, and respiratory rate. Always use the vital signs from the Doorway Information when writing your note. Even if you take the SP's blood pressure yourself, write in your Note the blood pressure listed on the doorway. When considering the differential diagnosis and diagnostic workup, think only about the doorway vital signs.

Many patients will have simulated physical findings. It will be obvious that the SP is "acting" or pretending to have physical findings. Accept all of these simulated physical findings as real. An example of this is a SP pretending to have an acute abdomen. When you palpate the abdomen, the SP will grimace and possibly complain of pain. It will probably be obvious that the patient is faking this reaction. It is a simulated physical finding. Write on your Note, "+ Abd tenderness" and think of the diagnosis that explains this simulated physical finding.

Do not think that the patient is exaggerating or feigning illness; it is highly unlikely your cases will involve malingering.

It is easy for an SP to simulate weakness, abnormal reflex or sensory exam, and gait, among other things, but some physical findings are harder to simulate. If a patient is supposed to have a loud murmur due to *Staphylococcus* endocarditis, it would be nearly impossible to hire an SP who has severe tricuspid insufficiency. When you listen you may actually hear normal heart sounds. The patient will tell you the following:

> **Patient:** "I know I have a heart murmur."
>
> **Doctor:** "Thank you for telling me."

In this case, do the following:

- Write in the history: "Pt with hx of heart murmur"
- Write in the physical: What you actually heard ("S1 S2 – nl, no rub, gallop, and murmur")
- Write in the diagnosis: "Endocarditis"
- Write in the workup: Tests for endocarditis ("blood culture × 3; echocardiogram," etc.)

The sicker a patient the SP is portraying, the more often these very artificial scenarios occur when some physical exam findings are missing.

Notice All Aspects of the SP's Presentation

Smell your patients. They may smell of beer if they are supposed to be intoxicated, or fruity if they are portraying diabetic ketoacidosis. Pay attention to their behavior. If the patient is doing something unusual when you enter, that is part of the case. The SPs are not making up things as they go along—they are following a script.

Inspect the Skin Carefully

Inspection is important! Inspect the skin and comment on any simulated physical findings that need clarification. Patients may actually appear sweaty by spraying on water before you enter the room. You may see discolorations or marks on the skin that may relate to the patient's condition:

> White powder: Pallor, anemia
> Yellow powder: Jaundice
> Purple: Ecchymoses, bleeding disorder, trauma
> Red: Infection, inflammation

Let's consider a jaundice case. The SP will have some yellow powder or makeup dabbed on her skin. She isn't jaundiced in real life, so the sclera will be normal. Neither will the yellow color be all over the body, as it would with a real patient. So you'll have to deduce that this is the jaundice case.

Doctor: "Let me take a look at your skin. I see some yellow color here." *(Pointing to makeup)*

Patient: "Oh, yes, I've noticed my skin has been yellowing lately."

The doctor here would receive credit for performing Inspection because he told the patient what he was looking for and what he noticed. The SP will role-play and confirm suspicions of jaundice.

On the Note, write "Pt has jaundice." If you think the sclera exam is important, write down exactly what you saw: "Sclera clear." This can be confusing, though it is not the Board's intent to trick you.

Properly Examine the SPs

Even though you are going to perform a brief and focused examination, it's important to do each step as you would for a real patient. This means actually listening to the heart and lungs for a few seconds. It's possible for some SPs to have crackles or wheezes. Try to appreciate in 3 seconds whether the patient has normal or hyperactive bowel sounds.

Actually do the reflexes, motor strength testing, sensory exam, and HEENT exam. Inspect, auscultate, percuss, and palpate!

Don't Worry about Missing Subtle Physical Findings

It will be very difficult to test you on certain physical findings because they are transient, are faint, or require better equipment to appreciate. The physical findings you will be expected to see generally will not be subtle. Hearing a 1/6 diastolic murmur is not on the Patient Note Checklist, whereas completing heart auscultation in four different locations on the chest wall will be on the Physical Exam Checklist for certain cases.

Another source of anxiety is ophthalmoscopy. Relax. As long as you are using the ophthalmoscope correctly, you will be fine. You may not see much, aside from the red reflex. Without a dilated pupil and a dark room, it is unrealistic to expect a detailed exam. Simply write down whatever you do see of the retina.

Position the Patient

You may examine the patient from either side of the bed. Try to minimize the number of times a patient has to sit up, lie back, and stand, as having the patient move is time-consuming. It is better, however, to move the patient multiple times than to skip vital physical exam maneuvers that will be on the SP's Physical Exam Checklist.

Communicate with the Patient during the Physical Exam

Tell the patient briefly what you are going to do next as you go through the physical exam. Do not give the patient the results of your findings now (unless, of course, the patient asks). If you think of more historical questions, you can certainly intersperse them with your exam.

Use new tongue blades, ear speculums, and cotton balls on each patient. Throw away your garbage. Try not to put the tuning fork and reflex hammer in your pocket—it is very easy to leave the patient's room with them. Also, always keep your stethoscope on your body. This way you will always leave the patient's room with it in your possession.

Once you have left the room, you will not be allowed to return. So if you left your stethoscope behind, a proctor will need to retrieve it for you.

Remember to undress the portion of the body you are going to palpate. Do not examine through the clothes.

You have already completed your focused physical exam and have the patient's vital signs from the Doorway Information. A common question is: When should the doctor take the SP's HR and BP during the exam? Since you are not going to use the results you obtain, the answer is: Very infrequently. Certainly, if an SP asks you to check the BP you would comply. Also, do take the blood pressure (BP) on any case where the patient is coming in for a blood pressure check. Otherwise, stay away from repeating the vital signs.

By the time you formally begin the physical exam, some of the exam may have already been completed. You already know the vital signs, you have an impression of the patient's general appearance (GA), and you have noted any unusual patient behavior. You may already have noted obvious visible skin findings and any other physical findings. You may also have completed the mental status and psychiatric exams. Remember to write in your note all of these physical exam findings that you identified—you have completed some of the physical exam before you wash your hands.

Remember the Order in Which to Do Your Physical Exam

Start with the most relevant system first and do it almost completely. Then do the less important organ systems less completely.

COMPLETE PHYSICAL EXAM BY ORGAN SYSTEM

The most important and challenging part of the physical exam on USMLE Step 2 CS is to know what to include in a focused examination. You will have a limited amount of time. Each maneuver should relate to determining the likely and possible cause(s) of the patient's symptoms, or to evaluating the patient's condition.

Abdominal Exam

Do a complete abdominal exam when the chief complaint includes:

- Abdominal pain
- Vomiting
- Diarrhea
- Jaundice
- Urinary tract problem
- Pelvic pain

Aspects of an Abdominal Exam
- Inspection: Look for actual scars, hernias, or makeup
- Auscultation: Listen for 3 seconds in each of the four quadrants
- Percussion: Two taps each on four quadrants; tap out liver size if you are seeing a jaundice case, liver case, or CHF case
- Palpation: Palpate all four quadrants and the epigastric area for 3 seconds each

> A copy of the patient's Doorway Information is also included inside the examination room for your reference.

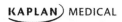

Special Tests

Perform these as needed, such as Murphy's sign for cholecystitis, CVA tenderness for kidney, and appendicitis maneuvers.

Phrasing for the Abdominal Exam

"I'm going to examine your belly. May I lift your gown?" Help the patient get comfortable, raise the patient's knees. The head of the bed may be raised 20 to 30 degrees (optional).

When you percuss and palpate, look at the patient's face. He will grimace to simulate abdominal pain.

- Inspection: "I'm looking at your belly. Have you noticed any changes?"
- Auscultation: Make sure that the SP is aware that you are warming the stethoscope before you begin auscultation. "Now I will to listen to your belly."
- Percussion: "Now I'm going to tap on your tummy."
- Palpation: Palpate the area of suspected tenderness last; otherwise, palpate from lower quadrant to upper quadrant. Say, "I need to press on your belly now."
  - For deep palpation: "I need to press a little more deeply." (No need to do deep palpation if patient has tenderness on light palpation.)
  - Do rebound tenderness palpation if you want to check for peritonitis. (No need to do rebound if the abdomen is nontender on palpation.) Positive rebound means the patient has more pain when you let go suddenly compared to when you push down slowly. Ask, "Does it hurt more when I push down or let go?"

Special Tests

Murphy's sign: Do this if you suspect cholecystitis. Place your hand gently under the right costal margin and ask the patient to take a deep breath. Positive Murphy's sign means the patient has pain with deep breathing. Say, "Take a deep breath, please."

Costovertebral angle (CVA) tenderness: Do this only if you suspect kidney stones, pyelonephritis, or other kidney pathology. You may perform this with the patient sitting, standing, lying supine, or lying on his side. Positive CVA tenderness means the patient complains of pain with a light tap. Say, "I'm going to tap on your back; please let me know if it hurts."

Tests for appendicitis: Do these only when you suspect appendicitis (RLQ pain) as part of your differential diagnosis.

Rovsing's sign: Positive Rovsing's is pain in the right lower quadrant with palpation of the left lower quadrant. Ask, "Any tenderness?" (while palpating LLQ): If it hurts ask, "Where does it hurt?"

Obturator sign: Positive obturator sign means pain in the right lower quadrant with flexion of the hip to 90 degrees and rotation of hip. Say, "I'm going to uncover your leg and bend it."

Psoas sign: Positive psoas sign means pain in the RLQ with flexion of the right hip against resistance. Say, "Please bring up your leg. Do you have any pain?"

Chest Exam

Do a complete chest exam when the chief complaint includes:

- Cough
- Shortness of breath
- Chest pain
- Respiratory tract infection
- Sputum production

Aspects of a Lung Exam

Inspection: Check the patient's hands for clubbing, cyanosis.

Respiratory excursion: To do this test, stand behind the patient. With the back of the gown open, tell the patient before you touch him, "I am going to push on your ribs." Then place both hands on either side of the lateral chest wall and say, "Now take a deep breath." Remember to say thank you after he complies.

Palpation: Check for chest wall tenderness.

Tactile fremitus: Examine both sides at once in three places on the patient's back.

Percussion: Tap two times in six places on the back.

Auscultation: Check six places on the back, four on the front. Listen for crackles, rhonchi, wheeze, or rub (listen from side to side). Listen to the back at the base of the lungs, bilaterally. Listen to the left and then the right. Next, move up and medially just below the scapula. Listen on the left and then the right. Finally, move up to about T3 dermatome level and listen between the spine and the scapula on both sides.

Phrasing for the Lung Exam

"I need to look at your back and examine your lungs. May I untie and lower your gown?"

Inspection: "I'm going to take a look at your back and chest."

Respiratory excursion: "I'm going to push on your ribs. Take a deep breath."

Palpation: "I'm going to push on your ribs." Check for chest wall tenderness. Palpate the spine, paraspinal muscles, and costovertebral angle tenderness as needed.

Tactile fremitus: "Please say, 'ninety-nine.'" When the patient speaks loudly, fremitus is increased over the major bronchi and in consolidation of pneumonia. Fremitus is decreased when the patient speaks softly, when the doctor's hands are placed farther away from the major bronchi, and in pneumothorax or pleural effusion.

Percussion: "I'm going to tap on your chest."

Auscultation: "I'm going to listen to your lungs. Breathe deeply in and out through your mouth."

Common Pitfalls in the Pulmonary Exam

Pitfall	Solution
Examining through clothing	Stethoscope should be placed directly to skin, not on underwear.
Placement of stethoscope	Don't examine over scapulae.
Comparing sides	Be sure to examine and compare right side to left side at each dermatome level.
Listening to a full breath	Listen to complete respiratory cycle on each side.
Distractions	Do not talk when you auscultate!

Cardiovascular Exam

Do a complete cardiovascular exam when the chief complaint includes:

- Symptoms to suggest a myocardial infarction
- Chest pain
- Shortness of breath
- Pedal edema
- Syncope
- Palpitations

Aspects of a Heart Exam

A complete heart exam includes two exams: one with the patient sitting up and one with the patient lying back at 30 degrees.

Phrasing for the Sitting Exam

Auscultation of neck bruit: "I need to listen to your neck sounds. Please take a deep breath and hold it." Listen for no more than 3 seconds.

Palpation of the carotid arteries: "I need to check the pulse in your neck." Note: Never palpate both carotid pulses simultaneously. You may complete this aspect of the exam in the lying-back position or sitting up.

Pulses: "I'm going to check your hands and feet." Do radial, dorsalis pedis, and post tibial, side-to-side or simultaneously. Check for atrial fibrillation (irregularly irregular pulse). This is a good time to check hands for clubbing, cap refill. There is no need to check brachial pulse if patient has strong radial pulse.

Extremities: "I'm going to check your legs for swelling."

Auscultation of the heart: "I'd like to listen to your heart. Please breathe normally." Press the stethoscope to the skin, 3 seconds for each cardiac area. Listen to as near the aortic, pulmonic, tricuspid, and mitral areas as possible.

With female patients, ask "Could you please lift your breast" if the breast is preventing auscultation of the mitral area. Do not be concerned if you are not listening in exactly the correct location. Be sure not to place the stethoscope over the clothes or underneath the clothes.

Phrasing for the Lying Back Exam

The exam table should be at a 30-degree incline.

Jugular venous distention (JVD): "I'm going to look at the vein in your neck. Please look to your left."

Hepatojugular reflux: Do this if your patient has possible congestive heart failure.

Palpation of carotid arteries: You may do the carotid exam now instead of in the sitting position.

Point of maximum impulse (PMI): "I'm going to press on your heart area."

Repeat auscultation: Listen again to all four areas.

Additional heart sounds: You can turn patient on his left side to listen for S3, S4 or to palpate PMI if it cannot be felt from the supine position (consider this in a CHF case).

Neurological Exam

Do a complete neurological exam when the chief complaint includes:

- Headache
- Dizziness
- Balance or vision problem
- Numbness or tingling
- Psychiatric problem
- Memory problem
- Muscle weakness

Aspects of a Neurological Exam

- Mental status
- Cranial nerves
- Motor
- Sensory
- Reflexes
- Cerebellar
- Specific tests

Aspects of a Mental Status Exam

There are five parts to a mental status exam:

- Orientation
- Memory
- Attention and concentration
- Language
- Obeys commands

It's best to complete all five aspects in patients with psychiatric disease, dementia, or altered mental status. You may limit the mental status exam to the Orientation only when you are not sure about the patient's mental status.

Phrasing for the Mental Status Exam
Orientation (to person, place, and time):

> "I'm going to check your memory now."
> "Could you please tell me your full name?"
> "What kind of place are we in?"
> "What is today's date?"

Memory: For immediate recall, ask the patient to repeat three simple words. For delayed recall, ask the same three words a minute later. (cat, apple, table)

Attention and concentration: Ask the patient to spell the word *w-o-r-l-d* backward.

Language: Ask the patient to name objects you point out, such as a pen or watch. Alternatively, ask her to repeat the phrase "No ifs, ands, or buts."

Obeys commands: Ask the patient to close her eyes. Be sure to have the patient open their eyes after they comply to your request.

Phrasing for the Cranial Nerve Exam
Cranial nerve 2: Use the Snellen eye chart to test vision. If the patient cannot see the eye chart, try holding up fingers to count. If that fails, see if the patient has light perception. Test peripheral vision by traditional confrontation.

Cranial nerves 2, 3: Check that pupils are round, equal, and reactive to light and accommodation (PERRLA). Check for direct and consensual reaction.

Cranial nerves 3, 4, 6 (extraocular movements): Say, "Please hold your head still and follow my finger with your eyes." For 3rd-nerve palsy, there is ptosis, a large pupil, and the eye is turned out. For 4th-nerve palsy, the patient can't look downward and inward. For 6th-nerve palsy, the eye is turned in.

Cranial nerve 5: For motor, say, "Please clench your teeth." Place your hands on the jaw and feel the muscle contract. For sensory, use the cotton balls to test light touch. Test all three branches of the 5th nerve. Say:

> "I'm going to touch your face lightly."
> "Does it feel the same on both sides?"
> "Do you feel this?"
> "Now please close your eyes. Do you feel this?"
> "How about this?"
> "Thank you. You may open your eyes."

Cranial nerve 7:

> "Show me your teeth and lift your eyebrows."
> "Please smile and show me your teeth."
> "Please raise your eyebrows." (not going to test taste)

Cranial nerves 9, 10, 12: Say, "Stick out your tongue and say, 'Ah.'" Check the palate for symmetrical movement (9th and 10th nerves). Check to see if the tongue goes out straight (12th nerve).

Cranial nerve 11: Say, "Now shrug your shoulders."

Phrasing for the Motor Exam

A general screening motor exam is good for finding gross abnormalities in a stroke patient. Say:

"Squeeze my fingers." (finger flexion is also median nerve)
"Pull me in."
"Kick out, kick out." (lower leg extension is also L4)

To begin the motor exam, say, "Now I'd like to check your muscle strength."

In some cases you may only need to check the muscle strength in the upper extremities. In other cases, just check the lower extremities.

The Motor Exam

Action	What It's Testing	Possible Phrasing
Pull arms in *Flexion of forearm*	C5, C6	"Now I'll check your arm strength. Do this *(demonstrate the action)* and don't let me push out."
Push arms out *Extension of forearm*	radial nerve	"Do this *(demonstrate the action)* and push hard."
Push wrists up *Wrist extension*	radial nerve	"Put your wrist like this *(demonstrate the action)*. Don't let me push down."
Finger flexion	median	"Squeeze my fingers."
Keep fingers together *Finger adduction*	ulnar nerve	"Put your fingers together like this *(demonstrate the action)* and don't let me pull them apart."
Keep fingers apart *Finger abduction*	ulnar nerve	"Spread your fingers apart and don't let me push them together."
Knee kick out *Knee extension*	L3-L4	"Next, I'll test your leg muscles. Please kick out."
Knee bend *Knee flexion*	S1	"Using your strength, can you pull back your legs?"
Foot bend up *Ankle dorsiflexion*	L5	"Point your foot back and hold it like that, using your strength."
Foot bend down *Foot plantarflexion*	S1	"Step on the gas, hard."
Hip flexion	L2-L3	"Pick your leg up." *(While seated, dangling feet)*
Hip extension	L4-L5	"Push your leg back down."

Aspects of a Sensory Exam

It is important to do the sensory exam if the patient is complaining of numbness or tingling, or has a history of diabetics.

- Check distal sensation for any orthopedic injury. Start distal and work proximal.
- If you have checked distal sensation and it is intact, as a rule do not also check proximal sensation.

Upper Extremity
- Tip of thumb (C6 dermatome)
- Tip of middle finger (C7 dermatome and median nerve)
- Tip of fifth finger (C8 dermatome and ulnar nerve)
- Dorsum of web space of hand (radial nerve)

Lower Extremity
- Just above patella (L4 dermatome)
- Lateral lower leg (L5 dermatome)
- Lateral foot (S1 dermatome)

Phrasing for the Sensory Exam

Light touch: When testing light touch, use cotton balls and work from side to side.

"I need to check your sense of touch."
"I'm going to touch your hands lightly."
"Do you feel this? *(pause)* Does it feel the same on the other side?"

Pain sensation (use the cotton swabs or toothpicks in the room): If using cotton swabs (sharp/dull), break a new cotton swab in half. Say, "I want to test sharp and dull feeling: This is sharp, this is dull. Please close your eyes and tell me what you feel."

With toothpicks, examine side-to-side, distal to proximal.

"Do you feel this?"
"How about here?"
"Is it the same or different?"

Do each foot, keeping each hand in one place, and work side-to-side. Move proximally if the patient can't tell the difference.

Position sense: Test position and vibration sense for diabetics or those complaining of numbness. "Tell me if I'm moving your finger/toe up or down."

For vibration sense, say: "I'm going to put this tuning fork on your toe. Please close your eyes. Do you feel a vibration?" After the patient says he has felt it, say, "Tell me when it stops." Use your other hand to stop the fork from vibrating.

Aspects of a Reflex Exam
- Compare reflexes from side to side.
- Only a couple of reflexes are needed in thyroid, suspected stroke, or suspected spinal cord lesion.

- For a suspected thyroid case, just test the biceps reflex. If the patient is hyporeflexic in the upper extremities, she will also be hyporeflexic in the lower extremities.
- For a sciatica case, just test the Achilles and patellar reflexes.
- For a stroke case, just test the biceps and patellar reflexes.

Reflexes
- Biceps: C5, C6
- Brachioradialis: C6 (only if you suspect C6 lesion)
- Triceps: C7 (only if you suspect C7 lesion)
- Patellar: L4
- Achilles tendon: S1

Aspects of a Cerebellar Exam
- Gait (most important of the cerebellar exams)
- Finger-to-nose
- Heel-to-shin
- Romberg's: Good to check in balance-problems cases. This test is considered positive if the patient loses his balance. Say, "Keep your feet together, arms out, palms up, head back, and eyes closed. I'll be behind you if you feel unsteady."

Aspects of the Specific Neurological Exams
- **Meningitis tests:** Check for stiff neck. If you have time for only one meningitis test, this is it.
- **Brudzinski:** Bring chin to chest. Test is positive if knees and hips flex spontaneously.
- **Kernig** (you'll remember because you have to touch the knee to do test): Flex the hip and knee, and try to extend the lower leg. Test is positive if there's pain and stiffness in the leg.
- **Plantar reflex (Babinski):** "I'm going to scratch the bottom of your feet." There are three possible responses: Normal response is flexion of the great toe (plantar flexion). Abnormal response is extension of the great toe and flaring of toes (extensor plantar response). This indicates an upper motor neuron lesion (in a patient older than 6 months of age). Withdrawal indicates that the reflex is too ticklish for the patient.

HEENT Exam
Do a complete HEENT exam when the chief complaint includes:

- Headache
- Eye pain
- Vision change
- Ear pain
- Dizziness
- Hearing loss
- Pharyngitis
- Throat pain
- Swelling

If you have only 30 seconds to complete your neuro exam, do the two best examinations: mental status (orientation) and gait.

Consider checking hair for brittleness, skin for texture, and hands for tremor and reflexes. You may even ask thyroid history (if not already asked), e.g., bowel, hot/ cold intolerance, weight change, or change in sleep pattern.

Aspects of an HEENT Exam

- Inspection: For scars, abnormalities, deformities, and skin changes. Say, "I'm going to look at your head."
- Palpation: For tenderness and deformities of head, face, and sinuses. Check the temporomandibular joint (TMJ) if relevant. Say, "I need to press lightly on your head and face" (palpate maxillary and frontal sinuses).
- Examine lymph glands: Submental, submandibular, anterior and posterior cervical chain, pre- and postauricular, supraclavicular as needed. Say, "I need to check your neck for swollen glands."
- Examine the thyroid: gland (note that "thyroid" is medical terminology): You can use an anterior or posterior approach when checking the thyroid. Say, "I need to check your neck now."
- Auscultate for bruit for no more than 3 seconds.
- Palpation of thyroid. Say, "I'm going to press lightly on your neck. I'll need you to swallow. Would you like some water? Take a sip and hold it in your mouth. Now please swallow."
- Test visual acuity (Snellen eye chart): Say, "I'd like to test your vision. Please stand here. Keep both eyes open but cover one eye. What's the smallest line you can read? Now the other eye, please."

Otoscope and Ophthalmoscope

The tympanic membranes can be checked only with the otoscope, and funduscopy can be done only with the ophthalmoscope. Either tool can be used as a penlight to check pupils, pharynx, and nares.

Using the Ophthalmoscope

- *Check the eyes:* Look at the pupil, direct and consensual light response; note any abnormalities. Say, "Please look at a point on the wall. I need to check your eyes." Look twice at each eye, once for direct and once for consensual.
- *Inspect the sclera:* Look for redness or jaundice.
- *Inspect the conjunctiva:* Look for pallor or discharge. Say, "I'm going to touch the skin below your eye."
- *Funduscopy:* Dim the lights (if possible). Say, "Now I need to shine a light into your eyes. Please look at this spot." Approach the patient from the side. Hold the ophthalmoscope in your right hand, hold it up to your right eye, and look in your patient's right eye. Then do the same for the left side. Hold the ophthalmoscope in your left hand up to your left eye, and look at the patient's left eye. Look for papilledema, cupping, AV nicking, and hemorrhages. In most cases you will just see the red reflex.

If the patient complains that the light is too bright, say, "Let me lower the brightness and try again. It's important I get a look." When doing funduscopy, be mindful of the electric cord so it doesn't touch the patient.

Using the Otoscope

- *Check the throat and oral cavity:* Look at the tongue. This allows for examination of the 9th, 10th, and 12th cranial nerves and pharynx at the same time. Take a clean tongue depressor, lightly place it on the anterior tongue, and say, "Please stick out your tongue and say, 'Ah.'" When you are finished, throw out the tongue depressor.

If you drop the tongue depressor or touch the end that's going to go into the patient's mouth, just get a new one. No one is counting how many you use.

- *Examine the ears:* Examine in patients with ear problems such as pain, discharge, or hearing loss. Put on a new clean ear speculum for each patient.

To inspect the pinna: "Next I'll look at your ear."

For palpation: "I'm going to touch and move your ear." Palpate the mastoid and wiggle the pinna for tenderness. Say, "Any pain? I'm going to look in your ear." Place the ear-piece just on the inside of the tragus, and do not insert it deeply. When you are finished, throw out the earpiece.

- *Examine the nose:* Say, "I'm now going to examine your nose." Push the nose up gently and look inside from a distance. Palpate the outside of the nose as needed. Say:

"Any discharge?"
"Can you breathe through both sides of your nose?"

Be careful not to touch the otoscope to the throat, nose, or eyes.

Cranial Nerve 8

Check the patient's hearing for cases of ear complaints and in pre-employment physicals.

Doctor: "I'm going to check your hearing. Tell me on which side you hear my fingers moving."

Weber and Rinne Tests for Hearing Loss

Do the Rinne and Weber tests only if there is hearing loss on history or physical examination.

- Rinne: Say, "I'm going to put this tuning fork behind your ear. Can you hear it?" Move the fork to in front of ear. Say, "Is it louder now?"
- Weber: Say, "I'm going to put this tuning fork on your head. Do you hear it? Does it sound the same or different in both ears?"

Practice using a tuning fork before test day. Do not subject the patient to overly loud sounds when doing the Rinne.

Use of a Tuning Fork to Determine the Cause of Hearing Loss: Sensorineural Hearing Versus Conductive

Diagnosis	Hearing	Rinne	Weber
Normal	Normal	AC > BC	Equal
Conductive loss	Decreased	BC > AC	Louder on the side with the hearing loss
Sensorineural loss	Decreased	AC > BC	Louder on the normal side. Softer on the side with the hearing loss.

Examining Joints

Aspects of a General Joint Exam

- Inspection
- Palpation
- Range of Motion (ROM): With active ROM, the patient moves the joint on his own. With passive ROM, the patient relaxes completely and you move the joint. Do passive ROM only if there is pain or limited mobility with active ROM. Passive ROM helps determine whether you're dealing with a problem inside the joint (intra-articular) or outside the joint from the muscle or tendon moving the joint (extra-articular). If the pain and limited mobility is the same on passive and active ROM, the problem is intra-articular. If the pain is less and range of motion better on passive ROM, the problem is extra-articular.
- Distal motor, reflex, sensation (MRS)
- Distal pulse

Aspects of a Back Exam

- Inspection: "I'll need to take a look at your back. May I untie your gown?"
- Palpation: "I'll need to push all along your back." Palpate along the bony prominences of the cervical, thoracic, lumbar, and sacral spine. Do not touch the patient's underwear.
- Range of motion: Flex, extend, lateral flexion to left and right. Rotate left and right. "Can you bend down and touch your toes? Can you lean back? Can you twist side-to-side? Any pain?"
- Muscle test of legs:
  "I need to check your leg strength."
  "Kick out."
  "Pull back."
  "Step on the gas."
  "Pull up."
- Reflex: "Now I'll tap your legs." Do patellar and Achilles reflexes.
- Plantar reflex: "I need to push on the bottom of your foot. It may tickle a little."
- Sensation: For light touch, say, "I'm going to touch your legs lightly. Do you feel that?" *(Pause)* "Now close your eyes. Do you feel that?" *(Pause)* "Is it the same or different?" Check L4, L5, S1 areas.

  For sharp/dull touch, say, "I need to check sharp and dull. This is sharp and this is dull. Now close your eyes. What's this?" Check the same areas as you did with light touch.
- Gait: "I'll need to see you walk. Let me pull out the footstool. Can I help you down? Can you walk a few steps? I'll be nearby."
- Straight leg raise: With the patient supine, lift the leg (knee extended), stretching the nerve roots. When the patient is in pain in a nerve root distribution (i.e., pain radiates below the knee and not merely in the back or the hamstrings), the test is positive. Compare left and right legs.

Consider a quick abdominal exam, and in your Patient Notes order rectal examination for tone and a prostate exam.

Nerve Root Pain Distribution in the Lower Extremities

- At L4: Pain along the front of the leg; weak extension of the leg at the knee; sensory loss about the knee; loss of knee-jerk reflex
- At L5: Pain along the side of the leg; weak dorsiflexion of the foot; sensory loss in the lateral lower leg; no reflexes lost
- At S1: Pain along the back of the leg; weak plantar flexion of the foot; sensory loss along the back of the calf and the lateral aspect of the foot; loss of Achilles reflex

Knee Exam

With any paired organ, you must compare both sides. In fact, many physicians like to examine the "normal" side first. Advise the patient that you do know which is the bad knee before you begin. Say, "I'm going to check the good knee first."

- Inspection: Look for any deformity, ecchymosis, or swelling. Compare to the other side. Say, "I'm looking at your knee. Have you noticed any redness or swelling?"

- Palpation: Say, "I'm going to push on your kneecap."
  - Check the skin for warmth.
  - Palpate the patella for fracture and ballot to check for effusion.
  - Palpate the lower femur and tibia and fibular head.
  - Palpate both menisci for tenderness.

- Range of motion: Say, "Can you bend your knee back and forth?"

Don't forget distal motor, sensation, reflexes, and pulses.

- Check pulses: Start with posterior tibial and dorsalis pedis. If these are absent or decreased, check popliteal pulse.

- Check the distal sensation: Light touch, sharp and dull, in L4, L5, and S1 distribution

- Deep tendon reflexes (DTRs): Check patellar and Achilles DTRs

- Check joint stability:
  - Anterior cruciate ligament (ACL): Check for anterior drawer sign. Bend the knee to 90 degrees, pull the tibia anterior, and see if there is any pain or laxity. Negative is normal.
  - Posterior cruciate ligament (PCL): Check for posterior drawer sign. Bend the knee to 90 degrees, push on the tibia posteriosly, and see if there is any pain or laxity. Negative is normal.
  - Medial and lateral collateral ligaments (MCL, LCL): With the patient supine, support the thigh and knee flexed 20 degrees. Check for pain or laxity.

- McMurray meniscus test: Place the patient supine, hip flexed, knee completely flexed.
  - Laterally rotate the tibia and extend the leg. This is positive if it causes pain or snapping in the medial meniscus. This indicates a medial meniscus tear.
  - Medially rotate the tibia and extend the leg. This is positive if it causes pain or snapping in the lateral meniscus. This indicates a lateral meniscus injury.

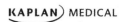

Hip Exam
Suspected Fracture

History: Patients with a fracture or a dislocated hip are typically in significant pain. Patients with previous hip replacement are more prone to dislocation.

Physical Exam: If you have a case with a fracture of the femur, the patient will not get up and walk. Be careful not to shake the leg when examining distal function; shaking the leg will make the fracture hurt. When an SP simulates a fractured hip or pelvis in the Step 2 CS, the site of fracture may be under the SP's underwear. Since all guidelines have exceptions, try asking permission and then palpating over the clothing in this case only. Do not ask permission to examine or examine over clothing on any other case.

Physical Findings: If the leg appears shortened and externally rotated, consider hip fracture or anterior dislocation. If the leg appears shortened and internally rotated, consider posterior hip dislocation.

Inspection: Say, "I'd like to take a look at your leg. May I raise your gown?"

Range of Motion: Check flexion, extension, internal rotation, external rotation, abduction, and adduction. Don't forget to check distal motor, sensation, reflex, and pulses.

Ankle/Foot Exam

Palpation: It is very important to palpate for any tenderness. Use your fingertips and palpate the small bones of the foot. With the typical inversion injury that causes a sprained ankle, also check for associated injuries. Palpate the Achilles tendon, medial malleolus, base of the 5th metatarsal, tibia, and proximal fibula.

Range of Motion of the Ankle: Check plantar flexion, dorsiflexion, inversion, and eversion. Don't forget to check distal motor, sensation, reflex, and pulses.

Hand Exam

Inspection

Palpation

Range of Motion and Strength

Distal Vascular (capillary refill)

Sensation
- Light touch, sharp, dull, and two-point discrimination
- Ulnar nerve: fifth finger pad
- Median nerve: third finger pad
- Radial nerve: dorsum of hand at web space between thumb and second finger

Motor Exam
- Ulnar nerve: finger adduction, finger abduction
- Median nerve: finger flexion, thumb opposition
- Radial nerve: wrist extension and finger extension

Carpal Tunnel Tests

Positive will give pain/tingling over medial nerve distribution

- Tinel sign: Tap on wrist over median nerve
- Phalen sign: Put dorsum of hands together

Elbow Exam

Inspection

Palpation: Pay attention to the radial head

Range of Motion: Extension, flexion, supination, pronation

Shoulder Exam

Inspection: Lower the gown and compare the shoulders; this is a good way to check for third-degree acromial-clavicular separation. Look for redness or deformity. Say, "I need to look at your shoulders."

Palpation: Say, "I need to examine your good shoulder first." Feel for heat, crepitus, and pain. Check the entire clavicle, AC joint, humeral head, humerus, scapula, and anywhere else the patient complains of pain.

Range of Motion (ROM): Check active ROM. If any pain or limited ROM, then check passive ROM.

Strength: Test external rotation with the hands behind head (as if combing the hair). Test internal rotation as if patient is touching his own scapula with his thumb. Check forward flexion; backward extension, adduction, and abduction.

Check distal function: pulse, ulna, radial and median nerve, sensation, motor and reflex (*see* Hand Exam, above).

Palpation of Bicipital Groove (test for bicipital tendonitis): Ask the patient first to sit and then to flex his arm to contract the biceps muscles. Palpate the bicipital groove to attempt to elicit pain.

Impingement Syndrome: Pain with abduction of shoulder.

Adson's Test for Thoracic Outlet Syndrome: Radial pulse is less or absent when arm is abducted more than 90 degrees.

GUIDE TO A BRIEF EXAMINATION

Now that we have studied each organ system in detail, let's review how to do quick torso and neurological exams.

Brief Torso Exam

Do a complete brief torso exam when the chief complaint includes:

- Back pain

- Rash
- Depression
- Mental status change
- Fatigue
- Extremity problem(s)

You should also do a complete brief torso exam any time a complete heart, lung, and belly exam is not indicated but you want to make sure there are no surprises.

Phrasing for the Brief Torso Exam

Transition: "I'd like to take a look at your back; may I untie and lower your gown?"

Inspection: "Now I'd like to take a look at your back."

Auscultation of the lungs: "Now I'll listen to your lungs. Please breathe in and out through your open mouth." Lungs: Listen at four places on back.

Auscultation of the heart: "Now I'll listen to your heart." Listen to four places in the heart. Don't forget to retie the gown.

Transition: "Now I'd like to look at your belly. Let me fix the bed to make it comfortable. Can you please lie back? May I raise your gown?"

Auscultation of the abdomen: "Now I'll listen to your belly." Check bowel sounds in one place for 3 seconds.

Palpation: "I need to press on your belly now." Palpate four quadrants.

For an exam with normal findings, you could write the following on the Patient Note:

"Normal-appearing chest. Lungs clear to auscultation.
Heart: regular S1, S2 without murmur, rubs, or gallop.
Abd: BS+, no bruits heard. Soft, nontender, no masses 4 quadrants."

Brief Neurological Exam (Evaluating for Gross Abnormalities)

A brief neurological exam is indicated when the chief complaint includes headache, mental status change, dementia, or head trauma. Below is a suggested exam that will cover most situations. As always, no two physical exams will be exactly alike.

Add or delete physical exam maneuvers depending on the history, the findings, and your clinical suspicions. For example, if the patient is not oriented to person, place, and time, do the rest of the mental status exam as well (that includes memory, attention and concentration, language, and commands). If you have no concerns at all that the patient's mental status is abnormal, skip the testing of mental status altogether and start with cranial nerves.

1. Mental status (person, place, and time): Say, "I need to test your memory. Can you tell me the date? *(Pause for response)* Can you tell me where we are? *(Pause for response)* Please tell me your full name. *(Pause for response)* Thank you."

2. Cranial nerves: Check cranial nerves 2, 3, 4, 6, 7, 9, 10, 12, and 5. Do the 5th nerve last. Say, "Clench your teeth," and demonstrate the action. Then check the 5th sensory with cotton balls last.

3. Sensory exam: Do a sensory exam at this point while you still have the cotton balls in your hand. Say, "I need to check the feeling in your hands"; "Now the feet." Check just the tip of the third finger on each hand and the top of the foot where the great toe and second toe meet (of the four extremities, check one place each). Check both sides at once. Ask, "Do you feel it?" (*Pause*) "Same or different?" (*Pause*)

4. Motor strength: Say, "Let me test your strength." Test both sides of the upper extremity at once. Say, "Squeeze my fingers; pull me in; kick out, kick out." Test the upper extremities at the same time but test the lower leg strength one leg at a time.

5. Deep tendon reflexes: Check brachial and patellar only. Say, "I need to tap your arm. Let me put your arm like this." Ask the patient to relax his arm if he is tense.

6. Cerebellar: Gait.

For an examination with normal findings, you could write the following on the Patient Note: "A & O × 3, cranial nerves 2–12 intact. Motor, light touch sensation intact all 4 ext. DTR nl, patella, brachial. Gait normal."

If you did not check hearing or CN 11, write, "cranial nerves 2–7, 9, 10, 12 intact."

If you find an abnormality or have more time, do a more complete neurological exam.

PATIENT NOTE WRITING

The Patient Note is a component of the ICE score and is the only component of the exam that is graded by a physician. As long as you are communicating your thoughts logically and clearly, you will score well. Physicians are not primarily concerned with grammar, punctuation, capitalization, or sentence structure. Even an occasional misspelled word—as long as it can be deciphered—is acceptable. Of course, before Test Day you should practice spelling words that are commonly misspelled, such as pneumonia, abscess, inflammation, and ischemia—or any other common medical term that gives you difficulties. However, it is better to write down something misspelled than to leave the paper blank.

Physicians grading the Patient Note are concerned with content. The key to writing a good history and physical involves putting down on paper what you asked of the patient, what exam you did, and what you observed about the patient. This includes all negative as well as positive findings you uncover. If you run through the mnemonic SIQORAAA and PAMHRFOSS in your mind while writing your Note, you will remember the interview you just completed and be able to write an excellent history. Do not write "SIQORAAA PAMHRFOSS" on your Note. Instead use the bullet-point style:

- substernal chest pain
- 8/10 intensity, heavy crushing pain

- started 1 hour ago
- radiates to L arm
- nothing makes it better, worse with walking
- positive SOB, diaphoresis, syncope. Negative vomiting, fever.

You may also write out the history in complete sentences, although that makes it more difficult to finish on time and doesn't convey additional information. The note below would be scored identically to the note above. If you were a busy attending physician, which note would you rather read?

> Patient presents with chest pain described as substernal. He rates the pain as 8/10 intensity. The pain began 1 hour ago. The pain radiates to his left arm. The patient has noticed that nothing makes the pain better. The patient complains that walking exacerbates the pain. Additionally, the patient complains of shortness of breath, diaphoresis, and syncope. The patient denies vomiting or being febrile.

Physicians are concerned with legibility. If your handwriting is not easy to read, use the keyboard provided on Test Day and type your notes on the computer. If you are writing by hand, do not touch the keyboard. If you are handwriting, you can print in block letters, use cursive, or use any combination.

The form you will write on contains four sections: History, Physical, Differential Diagnosis, and Diagnostic Workup. For most cases you will need to write something in each section. But make sure you cover all four sections—it is not in your benefit to write a detailed History for the entire 10 minutes and leave the other three sections blank. As with the scoring for the ICE and CIS components, graders use a checklist for guidance in scoring your Note.

The Note form has a black box around the perimeter. Anything you write outside the black box will not be counted. Use simple headings in the History to orient the physician grading your Note.

The suggested format for the Patient Note is as follows:

History
- HPI
- Allergies
- Meds
- PMH
- ROS
- FH
- Ob/Gyn
- SX
- SH

Physical Exam
When considering what to write on your Patient Note, follow this rule: If you observed it, asked it, and/or examined it, then write it down in your Note. Do not fabricate sec-

tions of the history and physical that you did not conduct. (In cases where the patient is not present—in a surrogate or phone case, perhaps—leave the Physical Exam section blank.)

Remember, a physician is grading your Note and is more concerned with communication of ideas than with format, punctuation, or spelling. There are many ways to write a Note, just as there are many ways to ask a question. This section will show you just one way to write an effective Note.

When considering which abbreviations to use, follow this rule: There are many abbreviations commonly accepted by the USMLE. (*See* Appendix A for a complete list.) There are other abbreviations, as well, which are frequently recognized by American attending physicians. However, when in doubt, write out the full word.

In the following paragraphs, text in **bold** is what you could write on a Note. Text in brackets is how you could describe the patient. So: **The patient is [good, bad]** means on some cases you might write **The patient is good** and on other cases **The patient is bad.** (Do not write brackets on your Note.)

When considering how to take notes, follow this rule for general headings:

VS or **Vital Signs**   **Chest** or **Lungs:** Chest
GA: General appearance   **ABD** or **Abd:** Abdomen
HEENT: Head, eyes, ears, nose, throat   **Neuro:** Neurological exam
CV: Cardiovascular   **Joints:** Joints in general

For a detailed exam of a single joint, write the name of the joint and always label it right or left. For example: **R wrist, L hand, R elbow, R shoulder, L hip, R knee, R ankle, R foot.** If the pain is in the right arm, you could use **R upper ext.** for "Right upper extremity." Be as specific as time allows.

Vital signs should be noted on every chart. Always write the vital signs that appear in the Doorway Information.

Vital Signs

"Vital Signs–WNL" or **"Vital Signs–NL."** If you are not sure if a vital sign is normal, simply write out the vital sign. You do not get a higher score for indicating a vital sign is normal or abnormal than for writing it out. You could write **"VS–NL except BP = 160/100."** Or you could just write out the vital signs that are on the doorway: **"VS 160/100, 82, 20, 37.6."**

If you think there could be confusion about the vital signs because they are abnormal, write out labels: **"VS–90/60, HR=38, RR 40,"** or **"VS: HR–100, T–102, RR–24, bp–60 systolic."**

Height and weight should be noted if relevant to the case. That would include a general physical or periodic health exam, a pre-employment physical, life insurance, or whenever you think it relevant. Since this doesn't appear on every Note, it is best to use labels such as **"WT–100 lb"** or **"Wt–100 kg."** Also, use units, as a patient can weigh 100 pounds or 100 kilograms. Height can be **"Ht–162 cm,"** **"Height–162 cm,"** or **"Ht–5ft, 2in."**

General Appearance

This is the place to describe what you see and to comment on any unusual behavior. It's fine if you have some components of psychiatric or mental status here as well. Some examples are:

- **GA: NAD** (no acute distress)
- **GA: in [mild/moderate/severe] distress from [pain/SOB]**
- **GA: no distress, A&O×3** (alert and oriented times three)
- **GA: pt is pacing about the room in [pain/anger/rage]**
- **GA: dirty, torn clothes; smells of beer and body odor**
- **GA: quiet, flat affect; will not make eye contact**
- **GA: track marks on arms, multiple bruises**

Skin

There is no reason you could not describe skin on its own instead of describing it as a part of each organ system. Describe location, color, tenderness, warmth, pattern, and flat/raised as much as possible. For example:

- **Skin: multiple blue/red rash on upper and lower ext in sun-exposed areas. Warm & tender. No streaks.**
- **Skin: jaundice; or Skin: yellow powder on face**
- **Skin: [track/needle] marks on both arms**

HEENT

Writing the note for each organ system follows the same outline you memorized for the physical exam (Inspection, Palpation, etc.). There is no need to write subheadings for eyes, ears, etc.

A normal HEENT is given below:

> **HEENT: normocephalic/atraumatic, nontender. PERRLA. Fundi–red reflex intact, EOMI. TMs, pharynx–WNL. No nasal discharge. Lymph glands, thyroid not enlarged.**

If abnormalities on the HEENT are found, be as specific as possible. For example:

- **HEENT: tender, red, swollen pre-auricular node and pinna**
- **Head: deformity, tender, and bloody nose**
- **Head: tenderness of B/L [maxillary sinus, cheek]**
- **Head: fine, thin hair. Exophthalmos [diaphoretic, sweating], large thyroid. [Tenderness, deformity, crepitus] to [nose, cheek, maxilla, jaw, zygoma, orbit, forehead].**

Further examples of HEENT note-writing:

- **PERRL:** (pupils equal, round, reactive to light)
- **PERRLA:** (the "A" stands for "and accommodation")
- **PERRLA: sclera clear, EOMI** (extraocular movement intact). **Extraocular muscles intact except [R 6th nerve palsy, R lateral gaze deficit].**
- **Visual fields intact, or R [temporal, nasal] visual field deficit**

- **Visual acuity: VA–20/20 OU** (OU = both eyes, OS = left eye, OD = right eye). **VA: 20/200 R eye, counting fingers 5 ft L eye.**
- **Visual acuity: L eye light perception only, OD–20/200. Fundi: flat** (no papill-edema), **or Fundi: Not visualized, or Fundi–NL red reflex.**

Nose

Be as specific as possible:

No nasal discharge and/or **good air entry B/L,** or **B/L thick yellow discharge or nasal septum [intact/perforated/with hole]**

Ears

- **Pinna NL. TM WNL B/L** (tympanic membrane normal bilaterally)
- **R TM red bulging, L NL.** (Right tympanic membrane is red and bulging, L tympanic membrane is normal)
- **TMs both with [perforation/holes] B/L**

Throat

- **Pharynx [clear, red, with exudates, NL]**

Teeth

- **[Dentition/Teeth], [poor/normal]**

Thyroid

- **Thyroid: [nontender/tender], [normal size/enlarged]. No nodules.**
- **Nontender, NL size, no nodules, trachea in midline; or Tender, enlarged, trachea shifted L**

Lymph Gland

You may reference specifically or generally, depending on its importance to the case.

- **Lymph glands: not swollen or tender**
- **Hard, tender supraclavicular lymph node**
- **Diffuse lymphadenopathy (seen with mononucleosis)**

You may also list the particular glands that are swollen and tender, such as the following: **[submandibular, submental, preauricular, postauricular, ant cervical, post cervical, supraclavicular, subclavicular] adenopathy.**

Chest

Remember to do the complete chest exam (inspection, palpation, respiratory excursion, tactile fremitus, percussion auscultation) and document all of your findings. Be sure to document everything that you do so you can receive a higher score.

A normal chest exam may be documented as follows:

- **Chest appears NL, nontender, NL resp, excursion, fremitus, percussion NL and equal B/L. Lungs clear to auscultation.**

- **Chest without deformity, skin WNL. Lungs clear to A&P B/L** (A&P means "auscultation and percussion").

An abnormal chest exam may be documented as follows:

- **Inspection: Increase AP diameter, or pursed-lip breathing, or chest with deformity or [ecchymoses/bruise] R flank, or thoracotomy scar**
- **Palpation: Tenderness on [R lat 8th rib, L CVA, lumbar spine, R costochondral margin]. Be as specific as possible about the area of tenderness.**
- **Respiratory excursion: Poor respiratory excursion or paradoxical chest wall excursion**
- **Fremitus: [increased/decreased] fremitus [R/L] [base/midlung field/apex]**
- **Percussion: [dull/hyperresonant] percussion [R/L] [base/midfield/apex]**
- **Auscultation: [decreased/absent] breath sounds [L/R]. Or you may have heard abnormal sounds: [wheeze, rhonchi, rub, rales] [L/R] [base/midlung/apex]**

Cardiovascular

Think about the entire cardiovascular exam and write down the parts that you conducted.

A normal cardiovascular exam may be documented as follows:

CV- S1,S2-WNL, Regular rate & rhythm. No rub/gallops/murmur sitting and supine. No JVD. PMI not displaced. No clubbing, edema. Carotid, radial, DP, PT pulse NL & equal B/L. No carotid bruits.

Note: JVD means "jugular venous distension," and JVP means "jugular venous pressure." For the normal person, you could write **"No JVD"** or **"JVP NL."** Both notations are correct.

In fact, you may also write **"CV S1,S2 WNL, RRR, no RMG."**

RRR means regular rate and rhythm. RMG means rubs, murmur, and gallop.

If abnormalities are found on the cardiovascular exam, be specific as possible.

Pulses

When documenting pulses, use the pulse grading scales as follows:

0 = no pulse
1 = decreased pulse
2 = normal pulse
3 = bounding or increased
4 = aneurysmal dilatation

You may chart an abnormal or normal pulse in the following way:

"[R/L] [radial/brachial/popliteal/DP/PT] pulse [absent/decreased/NL/bounding]"

Point of Maximal Impulse (PMI)

PMI: **PMI displaced.** If you felt the apex, you can describe its location.

For example: **PMI at anterior axillary line, 8th rib.**

Heart Rate and Rhythm

[**RRR, irregular irregularly rhythm**] (Note: An irregularly irregular heart rhythm is often atrial fibrillation.)

+ **gallop rhythm** (write this when you hear an S3 or S4 heart sound)

[**1/6, 2/6, 3/6, 4/6**] [**diastolic/systolic**] **murmur** is the basic notation for murmur. A murmur can be pansystolic, early, or late.

The grading scale for murmur is as follows:

1/6 = faintest murmur

2/6 = soft murmur

3/6 = loud murmur

4/6 = very loud murmur with palpable thrill when you check PMI

5/6 = heard with stethoscope partly off the chest

6/6 = heard with stethoscope off the chest

Abdomen

Think about the entire cardiovascular exam and write down the parts that you conducted. Remember Inspection, Auscultation, Percussion, and Palpation.

A normal abdomen exam may be documented as follows:

ABD: normal appearance, BS+ all 4 quadrants, no bruits heard, tympanic all 4 quadrants, liver size–10cm. No tenderness or masses to light or deep palpation 4 quadrants.

If you did any additional abdominal tests, be sure to list them. When all additional tests are normal, they may documented as follows:

Neg Rovsing's, psoas, obturator. No CVA pain. Neg Murphy's.

If any abnormalities are found on the abdomen exam, be as specific as possible:

- **ABD:** [**distended/obese/visible peristalsis**]. Be sure to comment on any makeup or real changes in the skin.
- **ABD: R subcostal scar, ecchymosis periumbilical.** Bowel sounds **BS+,** or **BS+ all 4Q,** or **BS+, no bruits heard.** Everyone in this test has bowel sounds! Write something like this depending on how many quadrants you listened to.
- Percussion: It is very unlikely you will have a patient with significant ascites. However, if you do need to document this, simply write: + **shifting dullness,** or **dullness in flanks to percussion.**
- Palpation: + **tender** [**epigastrium/periumbilical/RUQ,RLQ,LUQ,LLQ**], [**+/−**] **rebound.** For tenderness you must describe where the patient is simulating tenderness, and if there is rebound or not. To be more thorough, describe whether deep or light palpation elicits pain.

Another example of an abnormal abdomen exam:

ABD: + tender to epigastrium to deep palpation only. No rebound. Neg Murphy's. Tender RLQ to lite touch. Positive rebound. + obturator, psoas, and Rovsing's.

Neurological

Think about the entire neurological exam and write down the parts that you performed.

A complete normal cardiovascular exam may be documented as follows:

> **Neuro: A&O×3. CN 2-7, 9, 10, 12 NL. Sensation intact all 4 ext. To light touch. Position sense and vibration sense NL B/L lower ext. Motor 5/5 all 4 ext. DTR 2/4 brachial, patella, B/L. Gait–WNL. No Kernig or Brudzinski. Neck supple. Straight leg raise negative B/L. Romberg negative. Babinski–downgoing toes B/L.**

If abnormalities are found on the neuro exam, be as specific as possible.

Mental Status

If the patient only knows his/her name but not the place or date:

> **A & O × 1, or Alert and oriented to person only.**

Cranial Nerves

You can interpret the physical finding or just describe it. For instance, **Pt points tongue out to L.** This is the same as writing: **L 12th nerve palsy.**

Writing: **Entire R side of face is weak, pt cannot close R eye** is the same as **R peripheral 7th CN lesion.**

Sensation

Describe where the patient is experiencing numbness.

- **[Decreased/No] light touch below knee B/L; no position sense L toe, R WNL**
- **Numbness R ulnar nerve distribution.** (You could draw a picture or write: Numb 5th digit R hand.)

Motor

Motor function is traditionally graded on a 5-point scale:

0/5 = flaccid
1/5 = just a flicker of movement
2/5 = so weak that the patient cannot overcome gravity
3/5 = can overcome gravity
4/5 = somewhat weak
5/5 = normal

Some people also include 4–/5 and 4+/5 in the scale.

- **Motor: 3/5 RUE, other ext NL** describes someone with a weak R arm and the other three extremities normal.

You may also use regular language to describe the degree of weakness. For instance:

- **Motor: [Mild/Moderate/Severe] weakness RUE**
- **Motor: Pt with [dense paralysis/0/5] entire R side of body, L side WNL**

Reflexes

Reflexes are traditionally graded on a 4-point scale.

0/4 = no reflex
1/4 = decreased
2/4 = normal
3/4 = somewhat hyperreflexic
4/4 = very hyperreflexic

- **DTR: 1/4 brachial B/L** (decreased reflex brachial DTR both sides)
- **DTR: R brachial & patella 4/4, L 2/4** (a patient who is hyperreflexic on one side of the body)

Gait

- Gait: **Ataxic** if unsteady. **Pt unable to walk** is fine if patient cannot walk.
- Romberg: **Positive** if patient cannot perform the test and falls to one side.

Meningeal Signs

- **Meningeal signs: + stiff neck, + Kernig, + Brudzinski**

Straight Leg Raising

- **Straight leg raise: + R, neg on L** is how to chart the straight leg raise test.

Differential Diagnosis

One component of the Patient Note (and in advising the patient about your initial impressions) involves coming up with a Differential Diagnosis. This will also be asked of you for some patients on whom you have not done a physical exam. Guidelines for writing diagnoses include the following:

- Write the most likely diagnosis on the first line. You do get a little extra credit if you get the diagnosis correct on line #1.

- Try not to use abbreviations on your diagnosis.

- Be as specific as possible. Congestive heart failure is correct, but SOB is not. In that case, no credit will be given.

- Write diagnoses lower on the list only if they explain some of the patient's symptoms or physical findings.

- It is better to leave a couple of lines blank than to write down a diagnosis that has absolutely no support in the history and physical.

- Remember that "noncompliance with medicine" or "medication side effects" are legitimate diagnoses.

Unlike the Differential Diagnosis, the Diagnostic Workup gives no extra credit for putting the best test on the first line.

Diagnostic Workup

Another component of the Patient Note includes ordering the initial workup on the patient. This component of the Patient Note is also required for surrogate and telephone cases, unless otherwise specified. The best approach to writing the Diagnostic Workup is to follow a certain pattern; that way, you will not forget to document any important tests. Guidelines for writing the workup include the following:

- Make a habit of writing on the first line any prohibited physical exam maneuvers that the patient needs. For example, "rectal exam with hemoccult" or "complete physical exam."

- If you do not need to order any further physical exam maneuvers, go ahead and begin documenting diagnostic tests on the first line.

- Write on the first line any labs or x-rays that are needed.

- First, order the simple baseline tests that the patient needs now.

- There are no mandates or rules about what line should have blood tests or what line should have x-rays. It does makes sense, however, to group things together as you do in real life. "CBC, lytes, glu, Cr, BUN."

- You should assume that all of the tests will be done now, at one time, unless you write otherwise.

- It is incorrect to write diagnostic tests on the same line as the particular diagnosis.

- The tests you do order should help support or exclude the diagnosis you are considering. For instance, if your only diagnosis is "trauma to the foot," it would be wrong to order pulmonary angiography.

- There is no cost containment on this test. In other words, graders are not looking for the single best test.

- If no testing is indicated (a rare event, but possible), simply write in this section, "No tests indicated."

| SECTION TWO |

35 Complex Cases

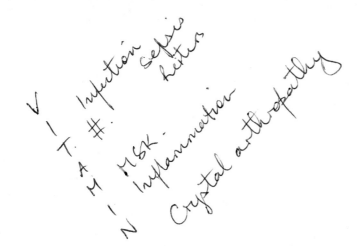

Case 1: **Ankle Pain**

DOORWAY INFORMATION

Opening Scenario

Mary Smith is a 21 y/o female who comes to the clinic complaining of ankle pain.

Vital Signs

- Temp: 38.3°C (101.0°F)
- BP: 120/80 mm Hg, right upper limb sitting
- HR: 80/min, regular
- RR: 20/min

Examinee Tasks

1. Obtain a focused history.
2. Perform a relevant physical examination. Do not perform rectal, pelvic, genitourinary, female breast, or corneal reflex examinations.
3. Discuss your initial diagnostic impression and your workup plan with the patient.
4. After leaving the room, complete your patient note on the given form.

BEFORE ENTERING THE ROOM

1. Cues: Write your mnemonics on your blue sheet. These will remind you of other questions to ask, and will ensure that you don't skip pertinent aspects of the history.

2. Clinical Reasoning: List several causes of ankle pain in the top right-hand corner of your blue sheet. Thinking about the diagnosis now allows you to do a more relevant history and focused physical. Consider the following conditions as part of your differential before you enter the room:

- Fracture
- Ligament injury
- Infection, e.g., Staph, gonococcal
- Deposition: crystals, gout

FROM THE STANDARDIZED PATIENT

History

HPI: Ms. Smith states that she twisted her right ankle last night when stepping off a curb. She felt a sudden popping sensation on the outside part of her right ankle. The pain is severe and sharp, and moves into her foot. She rates the pain as a 7/10 on the pain scale. Ms. Smith notices it is better when she elevates her leg and puts ice on the ankle. It hurts much worse when she walks on it, and she can walk only a couple of steps. She says her right foot and ankle had been bothering her for a few days prior to the injury. She also noticed some redness and swelling in her right ankle for the last week. She also scraped the skin over the lateral malleolus 1 week ago while walking barefoot. She has not noticed any fever. Before last week she never had any problems with her feet or ankles.

PMH: She has no allergies. She takes no medications. She has had no prior hospitalizations, trauma, major illness, or surgery.

Ob/Gyn: LMP: 1 week late. Her previous period was normal. She is G0P0. Her periods are always somewhat irregular. Normally she uses pads for 4–5 days. She has no urinary symptoms, discharge, or pelvic or abdominal pain. She is sexually active with two men in the last 6 months. She always uses condoms. She has never had a sexually transmitted disease.

Social Hx: She lives with her parents, and denies any tobacco, alcohol, or drug use.

Physical Exam

Upon entering the room you notice that the patient is in obvious discomfort. She is holding her right ankle and foot. There is redness about the ankle joint, centered on the lateral malleolus. She is alert and cooperative, and her speech is normal. The abdomen is soft and nontender without masses. Bowel sounds are normal.

Extremities: Inspection reveals normal L ankle. R ankle is red and swollen. No redness or streaking up the leg. There is also some purple discoloration at the lateral malleolus. Palpation shows a nontender L ankle and very tender R lateral malleolus.

Normal range of motion on the L ankle. The R ankle has very limited ROM because of pain. She will not co-operate with strength testing at the R ankle because of pain. There is normal ROM in both knees. Left ankle strength (motor) is 5/5. Sensation to light touch is intact bilaterally. Dorsalis pedis and posterior tibial pulses are equal 2/4 bilaterally. The Achilles reflex is normal in both ankles.

THE CLOSING

As with all cases, it is important to explain to your patient your clinical impression and discuss the next steps in working up her condition. It is important to provide some indication about the length of time she may be unable to walk, as this may affect her transportation and employment options. Be sure to answer any additional concerns she may have.

> **Doctor:** "Ms. Smith, I have finished my physical exam and would like to discuss what might be causing your ankle pain. You told me you stepped off the curb and had a popping feeling and sudden pain in your ankle. Is that correct?" *(Wait for response)*
>
> "You have also told me that the ankle has been red and swollen for a week. Is that right?" *(Wait for response)*
>
> "I believe you may have a broken ankle. However, I am also considering the possibility of an infection in your ankle because of your fever. So that we can treat you appropriately, I am going to take a blood test to

GRADING: STANDARDIZED PATIENT DATA-GATHERING CHECKLISTS

History Checklist

- ☑ **S**ite of pain
- ☑ **I**ntensity of pain
- ☑ **Q**uality of pain
- ☑ **O**nset of symptoms
- ☑ **R**adiation of pain
- ☑ **A**lleviating factors
- ☑ **A**ggravating factors
- ☑ **P**ast medical history
- ☑ **A**llergies
- ☑ **M**edicines
- ☑ **L**MP
- ☑ **S**exual history
- ☑ **A**sked about symptoms of STD

Physical Exam Checklist

- ☑ **I**nspect feet and ankles bilaterally
- ☑ **P**alpate feet and ankles bilaterally
- ☑ **I**nspect and palpate knees bilaterally
- ☑ **P**ulses: Check DP and PT pulses bilaterally
- ☑ **M**otor strength of ankles bilaterally
- ☑ **S**ensation: Check distal to ankle bilaterally
- ☑ **R**ange of Motion: Check ROM bilaterally
- ☑ **P**alpate lower abdomen

look for an infection, and an x-ray picture of your ankle to look for a broken bone. Also, because of the delay in your period, I would like you to have a pregnancy test. I will have the results back tomorrow and we will meet then to discuss the results and plan treatment. Do you have any questions at this stage?"

CHALLENGING QUESTIONS

Be prepared to answer the following types of challenging questions for this particular case:

- "Is it fractured or is it just broken?"
- "I'm part of a tennis team. When do you think I'll be able to play again?"

Answer: "A fracture and broken bone are the same thing. I will take a picture to find out if the bone is injured. When we meet again I will have the x-ray and will be better able to tell you when you can play tennis."

CASE DISCUSSION

Notes about the History-Taking

For this case, it is best not to offer to shake the patient's hand during your introduction. This patient is in obvious pain and is preoccupied with using her hands to splint her painful ankle. The most appropriate step when first entering the room is to attend to the patient's comfort and offer support. Offer her the drape and some assistance in finding a more comfortable position so that she can rest her leg on the exam table.

The initial history of stepping off a curb, twisting her ankle, and feeling a popping sensation is typical of an ankle sprain and/or fracture. However, it is important that you are able to recognize pertinent findings such as fever, which is listed in the doorway information and is not consistent with ankle sprain or fracture. In this case, the fever, the injury to the skin about the ankle, the red and swollen ankle for the week prior to the ankle

SAMPLE PATIENT NOTE

History: Include significant positives and negatives from history of present illness, past medical history, review of system(s), social history, and family history.

CC: *"My ankle hurts."*

HPI: *R ankle pain maximum at lateral malleolus*
            – Pain is severe, sharp, without radiation; 7/10 intensity
            – Began suddenly when stepping off a curb; twisted ankle and felt a "pop"
            – Also got abrasion to R lateral malleolus 1 week ago, now with redness and swelling
            – Denies fever or prior episodes of ankle problems

Meds: *None, NKDA*

PMH: *No hospitalizations, major illness, trauma, surgery*
            LMP "1 week late." GOPO.

SX: *Sexually active, two men in last 6 months. States always uses condom. No prior STDs. Denies dysuria, discharge, or abdominal pain.*

SH: *Lives with parents, denies tobacco, EtOH, or drug use*

Physical Exam: Indicate only pertinent positive and negative findings related to patient's chief complaint.

VS: *NL except for T = 101.0°F*

GA: *In mild distress 2nd ankle pain*

Abd: *Soft, nontender. No masses.*

R Ankle: *Swollen, red, tender over lateral malleolus. Some ecchymosis also present. Unable to check ROM, motor due to pain. No lymphangitis.*

L Ankle: *NL skin, nontender, Full NL dorsiflexion, plantar flexion, eversion, inversion. Strength 5/5.*

Ext: *2/4 DP, PT B/L. Light touch sensation intact both feet B/L.*

Differential Diagnosis: In order of likelihood (with 1 being the most likely), list up to five potential or possible diagnoses for this patient's presentation. (In many cases, fewer than five diagnoses are likely.)

1. *Fracture ankle*
2. *Sprain ankle*
3. *Cellulitis of ankle*
4. *Gonococcal arthritis*
5. *Pregnancy*

Diagnostic Workup: List immediate plans (up to five) for further diagnostic workup.

1. *Pelvic exam with GC, Chlamydia culture*
2. *Urine HCG*
3. *X-ray of R ankle if pregnancy test negative*
4. *CBC*
5. *Arthrocentesis with cell count, Gram stain culture, and crystal analysis*

injury, as well as multiple sexual partners, all suggest that another diagnosis is also possible. These additional clues allow you to list cellulitis and septic arthritis, as well gonococcal arthritis, in the Differential Diagnosis.

As with any patient with a pain in the body, SIQORAAA PAM should be asked. In the PMH it is very important to obtain gynecological and sexual history in any young adult with a possible inflamed joint.

Notes about the Physical Exam

The physical exam checklist highlights the importance of documenting the findings of both sides of any paired structures in the body. Had you documented physical exam findings on only one extremity, you would have missed about half of the physical exam checklist items. As a general rule, inspect and palpate at least one joint above and one joint below the site of injury. With a fall, injury is possible anywhere on the injured extremity and may be in more than one location. Specifically for the ankle, the lateral malleolus is most commonly injured from an inversion injury. Associated areas to palpate, because they are sometimes also injured, are both malleoli, the Achilles tendon, and the base of the 5th metatarsal, as well as the proximal fibula.

In this case the pain is so intense that the patient will not cooperate and move the ankle no matter how nicely you ask or how well you explain. In most cases the patient will cooperate with physical exam maneuvers when you show empathy and explain their importance. If you have made two attempts to get a patient to cooperate with a physical exam maneuver and the patient still refuses, recognize that this is part of the case and simply move on to your next step in the physical examination.

In the torso, the only related task for which you would have received credit is the examination of the abdomen. This is because of the consideration of STD and possible pelvic inflammatory disease as sequelae. While most cases on the test will have check-boxes on the physical exam for examination of the heart and lungs, a case that presents an isolated extremity injury may not. Had you listened to the heart and lungs and written it on your note, you would not have been penalized for the action; however, you would not have received additional points. As with all CS cases, it is important to remain focused on pertinent physical examination maneuvers because there is limited time allotted for completing the case.

Be sure to comment on any discolorations or skin markings you may observe, even if these markings are due to makeup (a technique used in order to simulate physical findings). Consider any diagnosis that includes inflammation and infection in any patient with red-powdered skin.

Getting a pregnancy test on every woman who is late on her period is an important step you should not overlook. Had this patient's period not been late, you would not have been expected to order an HCG prior to the x-ray.

X-rays of the lower extremity that can commonly be ordered are hip, femur, knee, tibia-fibula, ankle, foot, and calcaneus. You may order as many of the x-rays as are clinically relevant.

Comments about the Patient Note

All notes should contain a comment about the vital signs and general appearance. A common mistake on a case of an isolated extremity is to write only the physical exam of the injured extremity. It is essential to compare the good side to the bad, and include in your note the physical findings of the normal side as well.

Case 2: **Back Pain**

DOORWAY INFORMATION

Opening Scenario

James Jones is a 35 y/o male who comes to the clinic complaining of back pain.

Vital Signs

- Temp: 37.0°C (98.6°F)
- BP: 140/90 mm Hg, right upper limb sitting
- HR: 80/min, regular
- RR: 20/min

Examinee Tasks

1. Obtain a focused history.
2. Perform a relevant physical examination. Do not perform rectal, pelvic, genitourinary, female breast, or corneal reflex examinations.
3. Discuss your initial diagnostic impression and your workup plan with the patient.
4. After leaving the room, complete your patient note on the given form.

BEFORE ENTERING THE ROOM

1. Cues: Write your mnemonics on your blue sheet. These will remind you of other questions to ask, and will ensure that you don't skip pertinent aspects of the history. Since back pain is the chief complaint, you will already know that inspection and palpation of the back will be on the physical exam checklist and thus should be performed. If you have trouble remembering patient names, you can also write the name on your blue sheet before entering the room so you don't forget.

2. Clinical Reasoning: List several causes of back pain in the top right-hand corner of your blue sheet. Because there are different causes of back pain, you will first need to determine the site of the back pain (cervical, thoracic, or lumbar). For all levels of the spine there may be a fracture, infection, tumor, disk disease, or paraspinal muscle pain. However, not all pain in the back is coming from the spine and musculoskeletal system. Kidney, aorta, pancreas, stomach, duodenum, ovary, heart, and lung problems all can cause pain in the back at different levels. Knowing what organs cause pain in the back will be your cues for the organ systems you will ask about and examine. Don't forget to inspect the skin. A simple skin abscess can cause back pain, too.

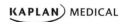

FROM THE STANDARDIZED PATIENT

History

HPI: Mr. Jones states that his back hurts. The pain is located 2 inches to the right of the midline at the level of his belt, and it feels about the size of a baseball. It is 3/10 pain if he is completely still. The pain increases to 7/10 on the pain scale with any movement or twisting. He had to call his neighbor to tie his shoes this morning, as he wasn't able to bend over without the sharp pain. It started a little bit last night after work but by morning it was really hard to get out of bed. He thought maybe he hurt it at work yesterday lifting something heavy. He felt a sudden twinge when picking up a car transmission by himself yesterday.

The patient took two aspirin right away and put some ice on his back as soon as he felt the pain yesterday. He was able to finish the workday. He felt a little better after the aspirin but not back to normal. "No work, no pay," Mr. Jones explains. The pain doesn't radiate. He denies any pain, numbness, or weakness in the legs. There has been no incontinence of stool or urine. Mr. Jones looked surprised when you asked about any numbness in the genitals. He states everything there is "100% fine." He has had no fevers.

PMH: He has had back pain once before, when he had a kidney stone 5 years ago. He states that pain was worse with the kidney stone 5 years ago because he could not find a comfortable position. Today the pain is bearable if he is completely still. He has no allergies. He takes no medications other than an occasional ASA for a headache. He was hospitalized once, at age 18 for appendicitis. No traumatic injuries other than a sprained ankle in high school once. Denies diabetes and hypertension.

Review of systems: No difficulties urinating. No blood in urine.

Family history: No one in the family with any acute or chronic back pain. "Come to think of it, I think my dad missed a few days of work once from a sore back."

Social Hx: Divorced, lives alone with two large dogs. Denies any tobacco, alcohol, or drug use. Works as an auto mechanic. His only stress is worrying about missing work and the mess the dogs are going to make if he doesn't get home soon.

Physical Exam

Upon entering the room you notice that patient is in obvious discomfort. He is standing up, perfectly still, at the side of the exam table, bent slightly forward at the waist. His right hand is holding his sore back and his left hand is on the exam table to steady himself. Mr. Jones is alert and cooperative verbally but doesn't want to sit down. His breathing is normal. Lungs are clear to auscultation. Respiratory excursion is normal. Heart sounds are normal without murmur or rub. Inspection of his back shows no bruising or erythema. Palpation of the spinous process in the cervical, thoracic, and lumbar area are nontender. Palpation of the right paraspinal muscles at about T11 is very tender and reproduces the pain. His gait is very slow, with small steps, as his back hurts. He has very limited ROM in the lumbar spine because of pain. There is minimal pain to palpation of the right CVA area as it is near the site from which most of his pain is emanating. The left CVA area is normal.

With great coaxing, the patient agrees to lie down on the exam table if you pull out the footstool and help him. The abdomen is soft, with bowel sounds present. No masses or tenderness. Extremities are without deformity or rash. Plantarflexion, dorsiflexion of the foot, and extension of the lower leg strength are normal and equal bilaterally. Patella and Achilles reflexes are intact, 2/4 bilaterally. Sensation to light touch is intact just above the kneecap, over the lateral lower leg, and over the lateral aspect of the foot bilaterally. Dorsalis pedis and posterior tibial pulses are normal bilaterally.

THE CLOSING

As with all cases, it's important to explain your clinical impression to the patient and discuss the next steps in working up his condition. It's also important to speak about how he can get some assistance with daily activities for a couple of days. Be sure to answer any additional concerns he may have.

Doctor: "Mr. Jones, I have finished my physical exam and would like to discuss what might be causing your back pain. First, let me make sure I understand correctly. Your back started hurting after you lifted something heavy at work yesterday, and by this morning the pain is a lot worse. Is that correct?" *(Pause and wait for patient to answer)*

"On your exam, you are most tender over the muscles of the lower back. There wasn't any pain when I pushed on the spine. Your exam of the nerves in the legs is normal, which is very important.

"I believe you most likely have a painful back strain. It sounds like this pain is different from when you had the kidney stone, but I would like to check a urine sample to be sure. This might take a couple of days to get better; you'll need your rest. Do you have anyone who can help with the dogs?" *(Pause for response)* "I will have the urine test back tomorrow and I'll give you a call to see how you are doing. Now, what questions can I answer for you?"

CHALLENGING QUESTIONS

Be prepared to answer the following type of challenging question for this case:

Mr. Jones: "I've got good health insurance, I want an MRI. Can you do it quick, Doc?"

Answer: "The MRI won't help you at this point, since you have no symptoms in your legs."

When a patient challenges you in this way, it is important to convey that the requested test will not help in diagnosis and management in this case. You may even be penalized for including tests that you know are not indicated. The communication skill is really to help the patient understand when an MRI is indicated.

GRADING: STANDARDIZED PATIENT DATA-GATHERING CHECKLISTS

History Checklist

- ☑ Site of pain
- ☑ Intensity of pain
- ☑ Quality of pain
- ☑ Onset of symptoms
- ☑ Radiation of pain
- ☑ Alleviating factors
- ☑ Aggravating factors
- ☑ Previous episodes of the chief complaint
- ☑ Allergies
- ☑ Medicines
- ☑ Hospitalizations, surgery, major illness, trauma
- ☑ R: Any hematuria
- ☑ S: Find out who patient lives with, as he may need some help for a couple of days

Physical Exam Checklist

- ☑ General appearance
- ☑ Inspect the cervical, thoracic, and lumbar posteriorly
- ☑ Palpate lower thoracic and lumbar spinous processes
- ☑ Range of motion of spine
- ☑ Motor strength L4, L5, S1 B/L
- ☑ Sensation L4, L5, S1
- ☑ Reflex: Achilles and patellar B/L
- ☑ Check pulses in feet B/L
- ☑ Palpate abdomen

SAMPLE PATIENT NOTE

History: Include significant positives and negatives from history of present illness, past medical history, review of system(s), social history, and family history.

CC:	Back pain
HPI:	Sharp pain in the R lower back, 3/10 intensity at rest, 7/10 with any movement. Began yesterday when lifting a "transmission." Somewhat relieve by OTC meds yesterday but pain much worse this morning. No radiation to legs. No weakness or numbness. No perineal paresthesia or incontinence. No blood in the urine.
PMH:	Hospitalized for appy at age 18 and had kidney stone 5 years ago. No trauma, DM, HTN. Pain with kidney stone was colicky
Meds:	None, NKDA
FH:	No chronic back pain in family
SH:	Lives alone with two dogs. No alcohol, drugs, or tobacco. Works as mechanic.

Physical Exam: Indicate only pertinent positive and negative findings related to patient's chief complaint.

VS:	WNL
GA:	In distress secondary to lower back pain. Pt standing still, slightly bent over in pain. Pt is holding his back with his hand.
Inspection Back:	WNL. No point tenderness in spinal processes cervical, thoracic, or lumbar. Mild R, CVA tenderness. Very tender R lumbar paraspinal muscle.
Abd:	Soft, BS+, no masses or tenderness
Neuro:	L4, L5, S1 Motor intact 5/5 lower ext B/L L4, L5, S1 Light touch sensation intact B/L Achilles, patellar reflex 2/4 BL
Pulse:	2/4 DP, PT B/L

Differential Diagnosis: In order of likelihood (with 1 being the most likely) list up to five potential or possible diagnoses for this patient's presentation. (In many cases, fewer than five diagnoses are likely.)

1. Musculoskeletal pain
2. Muscle strain
3. Nephrolithiasis
4.
5.

Diagnostic Workup: List immediate plans (up to five) for further diagnostic workup.

1. Rectal exam to check tone
2. U/A
3. IVP if microscopic hematuria
4.
5.

CASE DISCUSSION

Notes about the History-Taking

Both the Step 2 CS and Step 2 CK exams present to you cases that look less like textbook presentations and more like real life, where combinations of usually related problems are possible. To make matters more challenging, there are sometimes several different valid workups and approaches to any one unique patient. Being a first-year resident is very different from medical school days when each problem had one and only one correct answer. Because the Step 2 CS exam is designed to simulate realistic patient encounters, many of the cases will have several possible diagnoses and workup plans. So do not be alarmed if you cannot identify the diagnosis. You are not necessarily meant to!! There may be many right answers. Instead, concentrate on obtaining an accurate and relevant history and performing an appropriate, focused physical.

This man has a back strain by history and physical, a very common ailment. Certainly, starting by shaking Mr. Jones's hand is contraindicated. You don't want to cause him extra pain in the first minute you meet him. Some patients with back pain find that standing or lying flat provides some relief and is better than sitting. It is perfectly fine to take the history while the patient stands. Obviously, you cannot drape a standing patient. But you should help adjust the drape when the patient does eventually lie down.

Your introduction might go something like this:

> **Doctor:** "Hello. I'm Dr. First-Name Last-Name. I will be your physician today. I see you're in a lot of pain. Would you be more comfortable lying down? I can help."
>
> **Mr. Jones:** "I'd rather stand, Doc."
>
> **Doctor:** "Sure, that's fine. Tell me all about what happened."

Whenever you ask the patient a question, wait for the response. It would be wrong to start guiding the patient into bed before you have his permission. Note that in this situation you would not have to wash your hands if he wanted help getting into bed at the beginning of the interview. However, you will still wash your hands before you do the formal physical exam.

The fact that the pain began when the patient lifted something very heavy, and the fact that he wants to stand perfectly still, both indicate a musculoskeletal problem. Colicky pain from kidney stones frequently gives you a patient who can't sit still and is pacing about the room.

- Ask about hematuria for the less likely possibility of a kidney stone.
- Ask about pain, paresthesia, and weakness in the legs for the possibility of sciatica.
- Patients with bowel or bladder incontinence, decreased rectal tone, and paresthesias of the perineum may have cauda equina syndrome, sometimes caused by central disk herniation.

The family history was on this patient's checklist. The fact that Mr. Jones's father once hurt his back for a couple days is not a risk factor for our patient as back strain is such a common non-genetic ailment. The social history is important in any case where the illness is possibly affecting his ability to dress, eat, ambulate, toilet, and perform hygiene on his own.

DEATH is the mnemonic to assess disease states for ability to perform daily functions:

D = Dress
E = Eat
A = Ambulate
T = Toilet
H = Hygiene

KAPLAN) MEDICAL

Notes about the Physical Exam

Since the chief complaint is back pain, it's best to start with the back exam. That way, if you're short on time you can be sure you have completed an important step on the checklist. During palpation, be sure to palpate the midline and spinous processes separately from the CVA areas and the paraspinal areas. A meticulous physical can save a lot of unnecessary tests and, more importantly, gets you an accurate diagnosis. Detailed testing of the L4, L5, S1 nerve-root motor, sensory, and reflex will be on every checklist that possibly has sciatica as a potential diagnosis.

The abdominal exam cannot realistically be done in a standing position, so you will have to offer to assist Mr. Jones in lying flat. Make sure to prepare the bed by adjusting the footstep and footrest on the cart.

This is the perfect time for the patient to challenge and say he doesn't want to lie down. It might go something like this:

> **Doctor:** "Thank you, Mr. Jones. I am going to have you lie down briefly so I can check your belly."
>
> **Mr. Jones:** "Oh, Doc, I just can't."
>
> **Doctor:** "I'll help you, and I'll be as gentle and quick as I can. The more I know about your pain/problem, the better I'll be able to help."
>
> **Mr. Jones:** "Okay."

If the patient refuses to cooperate, just skip that exam and go on to something else. It is part of the script of the case. It is not proof that you have done anything incorrectly.

An abdominal exam is required for Mr. Jones because pancreatitis, abdominal aortic aneurysm, and a posterior penetrating ulcer all can cause back pain. There is such a low clinical suspicion for these entities that the physical is probably enough to exclude them for most practitioners without the need for additional testing.

Comments about the Patient Note

It's been recognized that doctors with many years of clinical experience find the Differential Diagnosis section more challenging than fourth-year medical students do. Attending physicians tend to think in terms of one or two diagnoses for the majority of patients. New doctors, less sure of their clinical acumen, feel more justified in broader differentials and workups

For the purpose of Step 2 CS, if you find yourself agonizing about whether a diagnosis or test is correct, go ahead and write it down. Err on the side of a little too broad a differential and an extra test if you are not sure. That being said, do not add diagnoses that have no basis in the history and physical; likewise, do not list tests that are irrelevant and dangerous just to fill up the blank lines. Some cases are designed so that no (or minimal) testing is needed.

Did you want to get a L/S spine film on Mr. Jones? He is young, without osteoporosis, and he did not fall or have direct trauma, such as being hit with a baseball bat. He has no fever, no drug use, no steroids, and no sciatica symptoms or neurological deficits. The yield of significant findings on x-ray in this population is very low.

In contrast to this, people with cervical spine pain over the spinous processes from the typical car accident should have plain films and CT scans of cervical spine. The cervical spine is much less robust and less well-protected than the lumbar spine when suddenly flexed or extended, and it is possible to have an injury that needs to be addressed in this situation.

IVP is an abbreviation for intravenous pyelogram. Do not use abbreviations in the differential diagnosis. You may use abbreviations in the diagnostic workup, however if you have time write out tests to avoid confusion.

Case 3: **Sore Throat**

DOORWAY INFORMATION

Opening Scenario

Pat Johnson is a 19 y/o female who comes to the clinic complaining of sore throat.

Vital Signs

- Temp: 38.0°C (100.4°F)
- BP: 130/84 mm Hg, right upper limb sitting
- HR: 90/min, regular
- RR: 16/min

Examinee Tasks

1. Obtain a focused history.
2. Perform a relevant physical examination. Do not perform rectal, pelvic, genitourinary, female breast, or corneal reflex examinations.
3. Discuss your initial diagnostic impression and your workup plan with the patient.
4. After leaving the room, complete your patient note on the given form.

BEFORE ENTERING THE ROOM

1. Cues: Write your mnemonics on your blue sheet. These will remind you of other questions to ask, and will ensure that you don't skip pertinent aspects of the history. Make a mental or written note that this patient has a fever. Any temperature 100.4°F (38.0°C) or greater is a fever.

2. Clinical Reasoning: List several causes of sore throat in the top right-hand corner of your blue sheet. Thinking about the diagnosis now allows you to do a more relevant history and focused physical. Consider the following conditions as part of your differential before you enter the room:

- Pharyngitis
- Upper respiratory infection
- Infection, e.g., bacterial (Strep), viral
- ~~Epiglottis~~ Epiglottitis
- Peritonsillar abscess

FROM THE STANDARDIZED PATIENT

History

HPI: Ms. Johnson has had a 4/10 intensity sore throat for 1 week. She complains of a scratchy feeling. The pain has not radiated to any other part of the body. She has felt feverish and sluggish for the past 3 weeks. She has not taken her temperature. She feels like she has no energy. Tylenol makes her feel better for a few hours. Nothing seems to make it worse. It has been difficult for her to go to ice hockey practice even though she is team captain. Ms. Johnson has no cough or sputum, no shortness of breath. She states she has had decreased appetite and lost 3–4 lb because it hurts when she swallows. She complains that her neck seems swollen. She has been sleeping more than usual. Her roommate was diagnosed with Strep throat last month.

PMH: She is allergic to penicillin. She was just a child when she first received it, but she remembers that it made her very short of breath. She takes no medications. She has had no prior hospitalizations, trauma, major illness, or surgery.

Ob/Gyn: LMP was 2 weeks ago and normal. She is not sexually active.

Social Hx: She lives in her college dormitory with her roommate. She does have a new boyfriend the last 6 weeks. She denies any tobacco, alcohol, or drug use.

Physical Exam

Upon entering the room you notice that patient is in no obvious discomfort. There is no rash or skin discoloration. Her head is normocephalic and atraumatic. Her sclera are clear and not jaundiced. Her pupils are equal, round, reactive to light. Tympanic membranes are normal. Nares are without congestion. Pharynx is red and inflamed. No exudates. Tonsils are enlarged. She has diffuse adenopathy, most prominent in the posterior cervical lymph nodes. Neck is supple. Her anterior neck hurts when the lymph glands are palpated. Lungs are clear to auscultation. Heart auscultation is normal. Her abdomen appears normal. She has tenderness in the abdomen just below the left costal margin upon palpation. Her spleen is not palpable. Bowel sounds are present. She is alert and oriented to person, place, and time. She is not sad; no feelings of guilt or hopelessness. Her gait is normal.

THE CLOSING

As with all cases, explain your clinical impression to the patient and discuss the next steps in working up her condition. It is important to provide some counseling about how her illness will affect her role as hockey captain. Be sure to answer any additional concerns she may have.

> **Doctor:** "Ms. Johnson, let me tell you what I'm thinking. First, let me make sure I understand you correctly. You have had a sore throat for a week, but have been feeling tired and low-energy for 3 weeks. Is that correct?" *(Pause for patient response, and if she corrects you, be sure to paraphrase again to prove you understand)*
>
> "On your physical exam I saw that your throat is very red, you have a little fever, and there is some tenderness in your tummy. I think you could have an infection in your throat."
>
> **Patient:** "I figured that. Could it be Strep?"
>
> **Doctor:** "Yes, it could. I'd like to take a throat swab to check. Also, I'd like to take a blood test to check for mono." *(All college students know what mono is, so likely no definition is needed)* "Then we will meet again and discuss the results. Until next visit, I'd like you to not play any hockey or any contact sports."

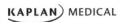

GRADING: STANDARDIZED PATIENT DATA-GATHERING CHECKLISTS

History Checklist

- ☑ Site of pain
- ☑ Intensity of pain
- ☑ Quality of pain
- ☑ Onset of symptoms
- ☑ Radiation of pain
- ☑ Alleviating factors
- ☑ Aggravating factors
- ☑ Associated symptoms
- ☑ Past medical history
- ☑ Allergies
- ☑ Medicines
- ☑ LMP
- ☑ Sexual history
- ☑ Exposure to other sick individuals

Physical Exam Checklist

- ☑ Inspect pharynx
- ☑ Inspect nares
- ☑ Inspect ears
- ☑ Inspect eyes
- ☑ Inspect the neck
- ☑ Palpate for cervical adenopathy
- ☑ Auscultate lungs
- ☑ Auscultate heart
- ☑ Palpate abdomen

CHALLENGING QUESTIONS

Patient: "Why can't I play hockey?"

Answer: "You might have some swelling in the tummy from the infection that makes it easy to get bleeding inside the belly from a minor fall. Just for a few weeks, hold off until you are better."

CASE DISCUSSION

Notes about the History-Taking

At the doorway you should begin thinking of a differential diagnosis for sore throat. Since this patient is in no distress, it is appropriate to shake hands with her as you introduce yourself.

In addition to the differentials listed in this case, you can also consider:

- Adult epiglottis, which causes a severe sore throat accompanied by a very hoarse voice
- Peritonsillar abscess, which presents with a severe sore throat and trismus. Trismus is the inability to open the mouth completely
- Upper respiratory infection
- Allergic rhinitis, the absence of coryza making it much less likely that the patient has this condition

Ms. Johnson's lack of energy or sluggish feeling preceding the sore throat is a clue that this is a mononucleosis case. Even though the patient complained of lack of energy, you do not need to consider major depression as a diagnosis because she has no additional symptoms of depression. The fact that the patient has a fever excludes the possibility of a simple unipolar major depression.

SAMPLE PATIENT NOTE

History: Include significant positives and negatives from history of present illness, past medical history, review of system(s), social history, and family history.

CC: Sore throat

HPI:
- Scratchy-feeling sore throat for 1 wk, front of neck feels swollen. 4/10 intensity, no radiation. Better with Tylenol, nothing makes it worse.
- Positive: 3 wks of feeling feverish, tired
  Negative: cough, coryza, SOB, or sputum
  Roommate recently treated for Strep throat

Meds: None. Allergic to PCN made her SOB, or (allergic to PCN-SOB).

PMH: No hospitalizations, major illness, trauma, surgery
LMP: 2 wks ago, NL

SX: Not sexually active

SHx: Lives in college dorm. Spends a lot of time with boyfriend. Denies tobacco, EtOH, or drug use.

Physical Exam: Indicate only pertinent positive and negative findings related to patient's chief complaint.

VS: NL except for T = 100.4°F

GA: NAD

HEENT: Pharynx red with swollen tonsils. Airway intact. TMs, nares WNL. PERRL.

Neck: Supple, diffusely tender cervical adenopathy

Lungs: Clear to auscultation

CV: S1, S2 NL, no murmur, rub, or gallop

Abd: Soft, with tenderness in the RUQ, no masses or rebound. Spleen not palpable.

Neuro: Alert and oriented. Gait NL. Not feeling sad or hopeless.

Differential Diagnosis: In order of likelihood (with 1 being the most likely) list up to five potential or possible diagnoses for this patient's presentation. (In many cases, fewer than five diagnoses are likely.)

1. Mononucleosis
2. Strep pharyngitis
3. Viral pharyngitis
4. Upper respiratory infection
5.

Diagnostic Workup: List immediate plans (up to five) for further diagnostic workup.

1. CBC
2. Mono spot
3. Throat culture
4. T. bili, ALT, AST
5.

Asking about exposure to Strep throat is an additional standard question frequently asked of patients who present with sore throat. The social history of living in a college dormitory, which typically has crowded conditions, can often be included in cases of other infectious diseases such as influenza, meningococcemia, or even TB.

Notes about the Physical Exam

The physical exam checklist highlights the importance of recognizing that a temperature of 100.4°F or greater represents a fever case. The focused physical exam concentrates on the organ systems involved. So for pharyngitis, a fairly complete HEENT exam is needed. Whenever you are considering an upper respiratory infection (URI), an exam for a lower respiratory tract infection (pneumonia) is also indicated. Since this patient has had no pulmonary symptoms (cough, sputum, or SOB, for instance), auscultation is sufficient. Had the patient also experienced positive pulmonary symptoms or abnormal lung auscultation, then the rest of the chest exam would have been indicated.

A patient may tell you about simulated physical findings when you start to examine an organ. Accept what she says and write it in your note in the History section. In this case, when you are checking for cervical adenopathy, the SP may comment.

> **Patient:** "Ouch, that's tender, Doctor."
>
> **Doctor:** "I'm sorry; can you show me where in the neck it is tender?" *(Patient points to cervical lymph nodes)*
>
> **Doctor:** "Have you noticed any swelling also?"
>
> **Patient:** "Yes, my neck seems swollen."
>
> **Doctor:** "Any problems breathing?"
>
> **Patient:** "No."

Be specific as possible in your diagnosis. In this case, the sample note listed only four possible differential diagnoses. It is acceptable to leave a line blank if you have fewer than five diagnostic possibilities.

Liver function tests (LFTs) were obtained because most patients with mononucleosis have some elevation in their liver enzymes. Ordering LFTs would be mandatory if she also mentioned skin yellowing, or if she had yellow makeup dabbed on her as a simulated physical finding. Finally, a throat culture was ordered in this case. A Strep screen would also have been correct.

Comments about the Patient Note

In this chart, the bullet style is used. This technique takes less time to write than traditional complete sentences. It relays the important information efficiently to the attending physician. Note that at the end of the HPI the associated symptoms are simply listed as "Positive," followed by a list of positive findings, and "Negative," followed by a list of negative findings. Pertinent negative findings that are relevant to the case are on the note checklist and are just as important as the positive findings. You could use the headings "−" and "+" as well.

In the Differential Diagnosis, it's good to be as specific as possible. In this case, listing the different types of pharyngitis, such as viral and Strep, is appropriate.

To generalize this concept: If it's an arthritis case, write down all the types of arthritis on the Differential Diagnosis. If it's an anemia case, write down all the types of anemia and you can quickly complete the Differential Diagnosis part of the note.

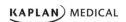

Case 4: **Car Accident**

BEFORE ENTERING THE ROOM

1. Cues: Write your mnemonics on your blue sheet. These will remind you of other questions to ask, and will ensure that you don't skip pertinent aspects of the history.

2. Clinical Reasoning: The challenge in this case is to obtain a history but to then focus most of your attention on the physical examination. The physical exam for acute trauma emphasizes inspection and palpation of all areas of the body. On a blunt trauma case you will need to inspect and palpate each section of the body to see if there are any "hidden" bruises or fractures. Rapidly palpate each extremity in two or three places with your open hand. If you are close to a simulated physical finding, the patient will grimace and then you can slow down and define the extent of the problem. Pay attention to all information on the doorway. In this case, you'll also need to determine why this patient's pulse is irregular.

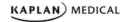

FROM THE STANDARDIZED PATIENT

History

HPI: Mr. Rodgers was not wearing his seat belt when his car was hit from behind 30 minutes ago. Mr. Rodgers says he was stopped at a red light when this happened. He doesn't really remember the accident, and the first thing he can recall afterward is waking up with a sore neck while the paramedics were knocking on the window. Mr. Rodgers quickly regained consciousness and then unlocked the door. He refused to have his neck immobilized and insisted on walking into the hospital. The neck pain is described as sharp, 5/10 intensity. He states that pain is worse when he tries to bend his neck, and better if he keeps perfectly still. He has no prior neck problems or any other injury, nor does he have any chest pain, shortness of breath, abdominal pain, or problems with his extremities.

PMH: Patient is allergic to strawberries. He was started on Coumadin and metoprolol 1 week ago after having new-onset palpitations for which he was diagnosed with atrial fibrillation. He had the palpitations about 3 days ago. He has never had any surgery or other trauma. He has had a history of hypertension for 20 years for which he takes Lisinopril.

SH: Mr. Rodgers has smoked one pack of cigarettes a day for the last 20 years. He has not had any alcohol for the past week, as he was advised to eliminate his daily glass of wine with dinner. He lives with his wife.

Physical Exam

The patient is alert and oriented to person, place, and time. He comes in walking normally, rubbing his neck. He has an obvious purple/blue ecchymosis to the forehead. The skin is intact. There is no deformity to the calvarium. PEERL. Pharynx and nares are normal. There is no hemotympanum. His neck is tender in the midline posteriorly as well as in both trapezius bilaterally. His chest is normal-appearing, and he has a normal respiratory excursion. Palpation of the chest wall reveals no tenderness or deformity. Radial pulses are 2/4 and equal bilaterally. Lungs are clear to auscultation. Heart tones are irregular without murmur. The abdomen is soft and nontender in all quadrants. No ecchymosis or abrasions present. There is no CVA tenderness.

His extremities are free of any trauma. He has no facial asymmetry, CN 9, 10, 12 are also intact. His motor strength is 5/5 all four extremities.

THE CLOSING

The closings seem more artificial the sicker the patient is portraying. Even had this been a multiple trauma case with life-threatening injuries, you would still do the closing. Remember, there is no treatment in Step 2 CS.

> **Doctor:** "Mr. Rodgers, I have completed your physical exam and I would like to tell you what I'm thinking. First of all, let me be sure I understand. You started Coumadin recently for abnormal heartbeat, and today you bumped your head and hurt your neck in a car accident. Is that correct?" *(Wait for the response)*
>
> "On your physical exam I see a bruise on your forehead, and your neck seems pretty sore. You most likely have a sprained neck, but I will ask you to have an x-ray to be sure. I will also take a picture of your head, and a blood test to check the Coumadin level. As soon as the x-ray is completed, I'll come and tell you the results. Do you have any questions?"

GRADING: STANDARDIZED PATIENT DATA-GATHERING CHECKLISTS

History Checklist

- ☑ **S**ymptom: Neck pain
- ☑ **I**ntensity
- ☑ **Q**uality
- ☑ **O**nset
- ☑ **R**adiation
- ☑ **A**lleviating factors
- ☑ **A**ggravating factors
- ☑ **A**ssociated symptoms: LOC, chest pain, SOB, weakness in extremities
- ☑ **A**llergies
- ☑ **M**edications
- ☑ **P**MH: Major illness—atrial fibrillation, HTN
- ☑ **S**ocial Hx: EtOH

Physical Checklist:

- ☑ **H**EENT: Pupils, TM, pharynx
- ☑ **H**EENT: Inspection and palpation of the head
- ☑ **H**EENT: Inspection and palpation of the spine
- ☑ **C**hest: Inspection and palpation of the chest
- ☑ **C**hest: Auscultation
- ☑ **A**bd: Inspection and palpation of the abdomen
- ☑ **E**xtremities: Inspection and palpation for any fracture
- ☑ **N**euro: Mental status
- ☑ **N**euro: Cranial nerves
- ☑ **N**euro: Motor strength
- ☑ **N**euro: Gait
- ☑ **C**V: Auscultation
- ☑ **C**V: Peripheral pulses

CHALLENGING QUESTIONS

Mr. Rodgers: "I should have taken my Coumadin a half-hour ago. May I take my own tablet? I have it with me."

Answer: "Please wait and let's get a picture of your head first. Then I'll know if you should take it or not."

Any patient who wants medication for any reason should always get the same response: You always need to do a history and physical, do a test, and then you'll know the correct medicine to give.

Mr. Rodgers: "Can you call my wife? She will think I was in accident when I don't show up on time."

Answer: "Yes, certainly. It will take a couple of minutes to finish examining you, and then I will call her."

CASE DISCUSSION

Notes about the History-Taking

This case is primarily designed to test your skills in handling a trauma patient. There are other elements in the history that in a normal office visit would require more thorough questioning. Though this patient is a smoker and has a history of hypertension, you will not be required to thoroughly question general health-maintenance issues. The possible neck injury and/or other possible injuries (fractures or bleeding) are the more important problems to address.

SAMPLE PATIENT NOTE

History: Include significant positives and negatives from history of present illness, past medical history, review of system(s), social history, and family history.

CC:	MVA (motor vehicle accident)
HPI:	Patient states he was rear-ended in the car 30 minutes ago while stopped at red light. No seat belt. Refused paramedic help and insisted on walking into hospital himself. Neck pain is sharp/burning feeling, 5/10 intensity. Radiates to both shoulders bilaterally. Better with rest. Hurts with any movement of the neck. Denies chest pain, SOB, Abd pain, or extremity pain. Denies any weakness in the extremities. Also states had brief LOC as he hit his head.
Allergies:	Strawberries
Medications:	Coumadin (1 wk), metoprolol (1 wk), lisinopril
PMH:	No prior trauma. Hospitalized for first presentation of sustained atrial fibrillation last week, and started on the medication. Hx of HTN as well. No surgical hx.
SH:	States drank 1 glass of wine per day but stopped on advice of cardiologist last week. Still smokes 1 pack of cigarettes/day. Lives at home with his wife.

Physical Exam: Indicate only pertinent positive and negative findings related to patient's chief complaint.

VS:	HR 110 and irreg, BP 160/90, T 37.0°C, RR 20
GA:	Awake, alert, mild distress, complaining of neck pain
HEENT:	Contusion and tenderness to forehead. No laceration. PERRL. TMs clear. Pharynx: clear, no other facial bone tenderness.
Cervical spine:	Tender in the midline and both trapezius bilaterally. No thoracic, lumbar, or CVA tenderness.
Chest:	No bruising, NL respiratory excursion. No chest wall tenderness. Lungs clear to A.
CV:	S1 S2 WNL no RMG, radial pulses strong and irregular, 2/4 B/L.
Abd:	Nontender
Ext:	No tenderness to palpation all 4 ext
Neuro:	Alert and oriented to person, place, and time. No facial asymmetry. Motor 5/5 all 4 ext. Gait intact.

Differential Diagnosis: In order of likelihood (with 1 being the most likely) list up to five potential or possible diagnoses for this patient's presentation. (In many cases, fewer than five diagnoses are likely.)

1. Acute cervical strain
2. Fracture of C-spine
3. Blunt head trauma
4. Subdural/epidural hematoma
5. Atrial fibrillation

Diagnostic Workup: List immediate plans (up to five) for further diagnostic workup.

1. CBC, INR
2. C-spine x-ray, CXR
3. CT of brain and C-spine
4. ECG
5. U/A

Notes about the Physical Exam

In this case, it would be incorrect (and potentially dangerous) to check the neck's range of motion prior to x-ray. In an ordinary emergency room setting you would provide immediate treatment with a cervical collar and c-spine immobilization. However, the Step 2 CS exam does not test your management and treatment skills; instead, you are tested on your clinical reasoning skills relating to the history and physical examination. Offer to help, hold the patient's head and neck still to prevent pain while the patient is lying down or changing position. Try not to move the neck throughout the entire encounter. Providing assistance to the SP during the encounter shows concern for the patient, and he will appreciate that you have helped to prevent the sharp pain that occurs when he moves his neck.

Note that in a case such as this you may find the patient to genuinely have an irregular pulse from chronic atrial fibrillation. Be sure to check the radial pulse for 3–5 seconds to determine if it is regular or not.

Comments about the Patient Note

You may document the loss of consciousness at the very beginning of the HPI. What's important is that you have documented *both* the neck pain and the loss of consciousness. Where exactly you document the LOC in the HPI narrative is less important.

Note: In a true clinical setting, the initial acute management of multisystem trauma integrates history, physical, and treatment. Advanced Trauma Life Support (ATLS) is a multiday class that has a different approach to the order of taking the history and physical from that presented here. If you are familiar with ATLS techniques, you may also use them in Step 2 CS—except for the treatment, which is not a component of the Step 2 CS exam. However, it is not necessary or advantageous to have taken ATLS training in order to pass Step 2 CS. Check the pulse on your SP. If it is irregular, write that in your physical exam.

Checking the INR on this patient, who is on Coumadin, is mandatory. Anyone with even a brief loss of consciousness needs a head CT to look for bleeding inside the skull. In this case, write Epidural and Subdural on one line of the diagnosis. Using two separate lines is equally correct.

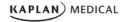

Case 5: **Left-Arm Weakness**

DOORWAY INFORMATION

Opening Scenario

Kenneth King is a 69 y/o male with left-arm weakness.

Vital Signs

- Temp: 37.0°C (98.6°F)
- BP: 160/100 mm Hg
- HR: 80/min, regular
- RR: 20/min

Examinee Tasks

1. Obtain a focused history.
2. Perform a relevant physical examination. Do not perform rectal, pelvic, genitourinary, female breast, or corneal reflex examinations.
3. Discuss your initial diagnostic impression and your workup plan with the patient.
4. After leaving the room, complete your patient note on the given form.

BEFORE ENTERING THE ROOM

1. Cues: Write your mnemonics on your blue sheet. These will remind you of other questions to ask, and will ensure that you don't skip pertinent aspects of the history.

2. Clinical Reasoning: Left-arm weakness can have many causes. Nervous system, vascular (blood flow), and musculoskeletal problems are all possible causes of weakness. A detailed examination of the arm, with close attention to motor strength, range of motion, and distal pulse, is an important part of this case. The weakness may also be coming from the spinal cord or nerve roots. Lastly, stroke is a common cause of weakness and should always be considered in an older patient. Be sure to include other questions about stroke in your history. Before you enter the room you will already be able to anticipate that a complete neurological exam will be needed in this patient.

Hint: A possible stroke may be embolic or thrombotic. Recognize that this patient's pulse is regular. This suggests an embolic stroke from atrial fibrillation is less likely.

FROM THE STANDARDIZED PATIENT

History

HPI: Mr. King tells you that about an hour ago he just recently started to have problems moving his left arm. He is right-handed. He was sitting at his computer typing when it started. These symptoms started 1 hour ago. When he got up and walked, he noticed that his left leg was dragging a bit.

The deficit came on pretty suddenly over the course of a couple of minutes. It now is getting neither better nor worse. Mr. King is getting worried that something bad is happening, as he could not put on and button his own jacket when he came over to see you. He took an aspirin tablet, but that doesn't seem to help. Nothing makes it worse. He has also noticed that he has trouble swallowing, and his face seems droopy. He almost choked while getting down the aspirin and a little water. He has no chest pain, headache, nausea, vomiting, or recent palpitations over the last few days.

He has never had anything this severe before, but last week his left arm got a little weak and numb but it only lasted several hours. Mr. King dismissed it as just being a little tired.

Allergies: None

Meds: HCTZ, lisinopril, ASA, Plavix, metoprolol, Lipitor

PMH: He was hospitalized for aortofemoral bypass surgery 1 year ago for claudication. He had a heart attack 2 years ago and had angioplasty with a stent performed. No diabetes or history of stroke. No trauma. Mr. King has a 5-year history of hypertension.

SH: He has been sleeping normally; is trying unsuccessfully to eat a low-cholesterol, low-fat diet; and has no problems urinating.

He lives with his wife of 48 years; she is disabled and he is responsible for taking care of all of her needs, including feeding and toileting. Mr. King stopped smoking years ago. He has one shot of whiskey every Sunday afternoon.

Physical Exam

Patient appears somewhat sloppily dressed, and his left shoelace is untied. He prefers to look to the right. He has some droopiness to the left-lower face. His forehead is wrinkled, and he can close his eyes when asked. He has normal carotid artery pulses and no bruits. His chest appears normal. His breathing is normal and his lungs are clear. He has normal regular heart tones. He is alert and oriented to person, place, and time. He has difficulty looking to the left. His pupils are equal, round, and reactive to light. The fundi show a normal red reflex. He has left temporal and right nasal visual field loss.

His motor strength is significantly weaker on the left side of the body than the right. His left arm is weaker than his left leg. He has decreased reflexes on the left patellar and brachial compared to the right. His gait is difficult because of the unilateral weakness. He has decreased sensation on the left side of the body.

THE CLOSING

> **Doctor:** "I have finished your exam and would like to be sure I understand you correctly. These symptoms of weakness started today, about an hour ago, and you had something similar but not as bad last week. Is that correct?" *(Wait for response)*

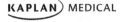

GRADING: STANDARDIZED PATIENT DATA-GATHERING CHECKLISTS

History Checklist

- ☑ **S**ymptom
- ☑ **I**ntensity: How is this affecting his life?
- ☑ **O**nset: When did it start?
- ☑ **O**nset: Course and duration
- ☑ **A**ggravating factors
- ☑ **A**lleviating factors
- ☑ **A**ssociated symptoms
- ☑ Previous episodes of chief complaint
- ☑ **A**llergies
- ☑ Medications
- ☑ **PMH**: Hospitalizations
- ☑ **PMH**: Major illness
- ☑ **PMH**: Surgery
- ☑ **PMH**: Trauma
- ☑ **SH**: Lives with and takes care of wife
- ☑ **SH**: Smoking and alcohol history

Physical Exam Checklist

- ☑ **H**EENT: Pupils
- ☑ **H**EENT: Visual fields
- ☑ **C**hest: Auscultate lungs
- ☑ **CV**: Heart tones, regular or irregular
- ☑ **CV**: Radial, dorsalis pedis, posterior tibial pulse
- ☑ **CV**: Carotid artery
- ☑ Neuro: Mental status—alert and oriented
- ☑ Neuro: Cranial nerves—note facial asymmetry (7th CN)
- ☑ Neuro: Motor strength (compare all four ext)
- ☑ Neuro: DTR
- ☑ Neuro: Sensory light touch
- ☑ Neuro: Gait

"On your exam, I see that your strength is decreased on one side. What you could have is a lack of blood going to your brain. I'd like you to have a picture of your head to find out why this is happening.

"I also want you to have a blood test to check how your blood is clotting. Then we'll meet again and I will have more information for you. At that point I can get you treatment. Do you have any questions?"

CHALLENGING QUESTIONS

Mr. King: "Someone has to take care of my wife while I am here. She is helpless on her own."

Answer: "Yes, I can have the visiting nurse (or social worker) make an emergency visit and help her now."

CASE DISCUSSION

Notes about the History-Taking

With some patients, like this one, you will need to show patience, speak slowly and clearly, and position yourself where you can be seen.

On the CS exam, you will not have patients that are mute, unresponsive, or pretending to have a Glasgow Coma Scale of 3. This type of case would prevent testing your SEP and CIS skills.

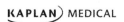

SAMPLE PATIENT NOTE

History: Include significant positives and negatives from history of present illness, past medical history, review of system(s), social history, and family history.

CC: Weakness LUE

HPI: R-handed patient began experiencing L arm and leg weakness 1 hour ago. Started suddenly. Not improving. Also has noticed problems with vision. Is having difficulty dressing himself. Took ASA without relief. Also noted trouble swallowing. Nothing makes it better. No headache, nausea, vomiting, or chest pain.

Allergies: None

Meds: ASA, Plavix, Lipitor, metoprolol, lisinopril, HCTZ

PMH: Last week had L arm numbness and weakness for several hours.
             Hospitalized for aortobifemoral bypass 1 yr ago. AMI 2 yrs ago with stent.
             No trauma, stroke, or DM. + HTN.

SH: Lives with wife who is bedridden. Mr. King is her primary caretaker. Stopped smoking years ago. Has one shot of whiskey every Sunday afternoon.

Physical Exam: Indicate only pertinent positive and negative findings related to patient's chief complaint.

VS: BP 160/110 mm Hg, HR 80/min and regular, RR 20/min, afebrile

GA: Pt appears in distress due to weakness. Shoe is untied on L.

HEENT: PEERL. Fundi: red reflex intact. Pt gaze is to the R with both eyes. Visual field L temporal & R nasal loss.

Chest: Lungs CTA

CV: S1 S2 WNL regular, no murmur. Carotid upstroke NL, no bruit. Radial 2/4 B/L. PT, DP 1/4 B/L, feet warm.

Neuro: Alert and oriented ×3
             L lower face droopy
             Motor RUE 5/5, RLE 5/5, LUE 2/5, LLE 3/5
             DTR: R brachial, patellar 2/4. L brachial, patellar 1/4.
             Sensory: Decrease light touch L side of body
             Gait: Difficult with leg weakness, no ataxia

Differential Diagnosis: In order of likelihood (with 1 being the most likely) list up to five potential or possible diagnoses for this patient's presentation. (In many cases, fewer than five diagnoses are likely.)

1. Acute ischemic cerebral vascular accident
2. Transient ischemic attack
3. Brain tumor
4. Cerebral hemorrhage
5. HTN

Diagnostic Workup: List immediate plans (up to five) for further diagnostic workup.

1. Head CT (noncontrast)
2. CBC, lytes, BUN, Cr, glucose, INR
3. EKG, CXR
4. Carotid duplex scanning
5.

Mr. King gives you the history that he has vascular disease. Since he has known peripheral vascular disease and known coronary artery disease, it is not surprising that he had a transient ischemic attack (TIA) last week and today is having either another TIA or a stroke. It is important to ask about headache, since headaches are more common in hemorrhagic stroke than ischemic stroke. You still need neuroimaging to confirm that a stroke is ischemic or hemorrhagic.

In real life this patient would be an extreme emergency, as he may be a candidate for thrombolytic therapy. However, for the Step 2 CS, treatment is not a component of the encounter. Simply collect your history and physical within your 15 minutes.

The family history does not seem relevant in this patient with known vascular disease. In Mr. King's case, the sexual history also can be skipped inasmuch as it will shed no light on the cause of his stroke. Save time here to concentrate on the neurological exam.

The social history that Mr. King is the sole caretaker of his wife presents an additional problem. You'll need to address this during the closing. It is appropriate to offer to send a social worker to check on the wife and make arrangements for her care while Mr. King is with you.

Notes about the Physical Exam

The physical exam in this case concentrates on the neurological exam. In this case, there should be some testing of mental status, cranial nerves, motor, sensation, reflexes, and cerebellar function. Certainly, checking the carotid artery, auscultation of the heart, and lungs will complete the checklist.

Comments about the Patient Note

While this man probably has a right middle cerebral artery stroke, the important thing for Step 2 CS is to recognize the need for a good neurological exam and CNS workup. Be as specific as possible if you recognize a stroke syndrome, but remember: the CS exam is designed primarily to evaluate whether you can collect the history and physical exam findings. It is acceptable if you write other, more general possibilities for the Differential Diagnosis.

In this case, it's important to note that the pulse is regular, since so many strokes are from atrial fibrillation.

Patients with middle cerebral arterty stroke tend to look toward the side of the brain that has the lesion, and tend to ignore the side of the body that is weak. (Notice that this patient had untied shoelaces on his left side.)

Similarly, you may also describe motor strength and DTRs in the patient note via the use of stick-figure diagrams, as discussed in Section I.

It is important to note that a CT scan was ordered in the workup plan. An MRI shows acute ischemia much sooner than CT, but a CT scan is more accurate in determining if an acute hemorrhage has occurred. It is also correct if you wish to also include an MRI. In a real patient setting this patient might be a candidate for thrombolytics. Don't forget to also check baseline tests that all patients get (e.g., CBC, electrolytes, etc.).

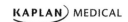

Case 6: **Positive Pregnancy Test**

S I Q O R A A A

P A M H R F O S S

DOORWAY INFORMATION

Opening Scenario

Mrs. Linda Williams is a 23 y/o female who has come to the clinic because a home pregnancy test is positive.

Vital Signs

- Temp: 37.0°C (98.6°F)
- BP: 110/70 mm Hg, right upper limb sitting
- HR: 72/min, regular
- RR: 16/min

Examinee Tasks

1. Obtain a focused history.
2. Perform a relevant physical examination. Do not perform rectal, pelvic, genitourinary, female breast, or corneal reflex examinations.
3. Discuss your initial diagnostic impression and your workup plan with the patient.
4. After leaving the room, complete your patient note on the given form.

BEFORE ENTERING THE ROOM

1. Cues: Write your mnemonics on your blue sheet. These will remind you of other questions to ask, and will ensure that you don't skip pertinent aspects of the history. A detailed sexual history and Ob/Gyn history will be needed.

2. Clinical Reasoning: Home pregnancy tests are accurate, so the diagnosis is likely to be pregnancy. Other causes of an elevated HCG, such as ovarian cancer, are extremely unlikely in a young woman. While you are outside of the room, it is important to begin thinking about common complications of pregnancy and what you should screen for during early stages of pregnancy, as well as how you will counsel this mother-to-be.

FROM THE STANDARDIZED PATIENT

History

As you enter the room, the patient is smiling broadly and says, "Hello, Doctor, nice to meet you."

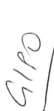

HPI: Mrs. Williams states she did a home pregnancy test 3 days ago and it was positive. This past week she noticed that her breasts are tender, and she felt a little nauseated without vomiting just this morning. She has no abdominal or back pain, and has had no vaginal bleeding since the end of her last period. She has no dysuria or frequency.

PMH: She has no allergies. She takes no medications. She has had no prior hospitalizations, trauma, major illness, or surgery. She remembers having chickenpox as a child, but is not sure about German measles. No history of hepatitis or skin turning yellow.

Immunizations: Had all the shots she needed to pass high school.

ROS: Mrs. Williams has no change in her normal sleep pattern and is on no special diet.

FH: There are no genetic diseases in the family, though her 75 y/o grandmother has diabetes. Her parents are healthy.

Sexual Hx: Mrs. Williams is sexually active with her husband. She has not had any other partners since they were married 3 years ago. They were using condoms for contraception but lately they have "forgotten" to use them most of the time. Mrs. Williams reports both she and her husband are happy and excited about the pregnancy. Five years ago, she was tested for a sexually transmitted disease and was positive for gonorrhea. She received treatment for it.

Gyn Hx: Her LMP began exactly 40 days ago. She had a normal period, which lasted 5 days. Her previous period was normal also. Menarche was at age 12 and she has had regular 29-day cycles for years.

OB Hx: She is now G1P0. She and her husband were thinking about having a baby but hadn't decided for sure when she found out she was pregnant.

Social Hx: She lives with her husband. She denies any tobacco or drug use, though when she goes out dancing with her husband once a week, she drinks about two alcoholic beverages. She works as a secretary. She denies any domestic violence and states that she and her husband are very much in love.

Physical Exam

She states she is 5 feet 4 inches, 130 lb.

HEENT: No jaundice. PERRL, pharynx clear.

The neck appears normal and there is no thyroidmegaly to palpation. The chest shows no chest wall deformity. There is no deformity to her spine on inspection. She has normal respiratory excursion. The lungs are clear to auscultation. Her heart has normal S1 S2, WNL; no rub, murmur, or gallop.

Patient's abdomen appears normal, as are bowel sounds. To palpation, her abdomen is nontender without masses or organomegaly. There is no suprapubic mass or tenderness. There is no swelling or edema in her legs. She is alert and in no distress. Her gait is normal.

THE CLOSING

Explain your clinical impression to the patient and discuss the next steps. For this case, the diagnosis is straight-forward and a lot of time will need to be spent counseling the patient. Be sure to answer any additional concerns she may have.

Doctor: "Mrs. Williams, I have finished my physical exam and would like to talk with you. I agree that most likely you are pregnant. I would like to collect another urine sample for a pregnancy test and do a pelvic exam to confirm the pregnancy. I would also like to do blood tests to check your general health and make sure there are no infections. These are standard tests for all pregnant women. Your physical exam is normal and I will be seeing you regularly throughout your pregnancy. Any questions so far?"

Mrs. Williams: "No."

Doctor: "The danger signs of pregnancy are bleeding and abdominal pain. Also, if you feel faint I want you to call me. I'm not expecting any problems based on what you told me, but you should know what to look for."

Mrs. Williams: "Yes, Doctor."

Doctor: "I want you to not drink any alcohol, and to limit your caffeine intake, all while you are pregnant. Is that all right with you?"

Mrs. Williams: "Of course. I stopped drinking as soon as I found out I was pregnant. I think I had four glasses of wine total when I was pregnant. Do you think I hurt the baby?"

Doctor: "No."

GRADING: STANDARDIZED PATIENT DATA-GATHERING CHECKLISTS

History Checklist

- ☑ Symptoms of pregnancy
- ☑ Ask about complications of pregnancy, bleeding, and abdominal pain
- ☑ Onset of symptoms
- ☑ Past medical history
- ☑ Allergies
- ☑ Medicines
- ☑ SH: Ask about diet
- ☑ Family hx: Ask about genetic diseases
- ☑ Sexual hx: Ask about contraception, planned pregnancy
- ☑ Sexual hx: Ask about any hx of STD
- ☑ Complete gynecological history
- ☑ Social hx: Ask about domestic violence
- ☑ Social hx: Ask about drugs, alcohol, smoking

Physical Exam Checklist

Height & Wt.

- ☑ Ask patient's height and weight
- ☑ Palpate the thyroid
- ☑ Inspect the chest and back
- ☑ Auscultate the chest
- ☑ Auscultate the heart
- ☑ Inspect the abdomen
- ☑ Auscultate the abdomen
- ☑ Palpate the abdomen and suprapubic area
- ☑ Inspect the legs

SAMPLE PATIENT NOTE

History: Include significant positives and negatives from history of present illness, past medical history, review of system(s), social history, and family history.

CC:	Positive home pregnancy test
HPI:	Tender breasts 1 week ago. + home pregnancy test. Felt nausea this A.M. No vomiting. Pt denies dysuria, frequency, abdominal pain, or vaginal bleeding.
Meds:	None, NKDA
PMH:	No hospitalizations, major illness, trauma, surgery. She recalls having varicella but not rubeola as a child. No history of hepatitis.
ROS:	On no special diet, no recent change in sleep
SX:	Sexually active, monogamous, stopped using condoms recently. Hx of Gonorrhea 5 years ago; treated.
Gyn:	LMP began 40 days ago. Regular periods for 5 days. 29-day cycle. Menarche age 12. No heavy bleeding.
SH:	Lives with husband, denies tobacco or drug use. EtOH: 2 drinks per week. Denies domestic violence.

Physical Exam: Indicate only pertinent positive and negative findings related to patient's chief complaint.

VS:	WNL. Reports 5 ft 4 in, 130 lb.
GA:	No distress, pt happy
HEENT:	PERRL, pharynx clear. No thyroidmegaly.
Chest:	No deformity, NL respiratory excursion, lungs clear to A*uscultation*
Back/Spine:	No deformity
CV:	S1 S2 NL; no murmur, rub, or gallop
Abd:	Soft, nontender. BS+. No masses all 4 quadrants and suprapubic.
Legs:	No swelling or tenderness. Neuro: alert, gait-NL.

Differential Diagnosis: In order of likelihood (with 1 being the most likely), list up to five potential or possible diagnoses for this patient's presentation. (In many cases, fewer than five diagnoses are likely.)

1. Pregnancy
2.
3.
4.
5.

Diagnostic Workup: List immediate plans (up to five) for further diagnostic workup.

1. Breast and pelvic exam, Pap smear, Gonorrhea, Chlamydia culture
2. CBC, blood type, and Rh
3. U/A, VCG, TSH
4. VDRL, HIV, rubella titer
5. Hepatitis B serology

CHALLENGING QUESTIONS

Mrs. Williams: "What else can I do to help the baby? And can I still go out dancing once a week? I really enjoy that."

Answer: "Eat a healthy diet with plenty of calcium and green leafy vegetables. And yes, go ahead and dance. You should still be physically active, and many women still remain active the entire pregnancy."

CASE DISCUSSION

Notes about the History-Taking

This scenario would be the perfect situation to initiate a handshake with the patient. She is smiling and happy, and begins conversing as soon as you enter the room. In the interest of time, it's best to limit small talk and get straight into her reasons for the visit.

The challenge in this case is not in determining the actual diagnosis but in obtaining the necessary family, Ob/Gyn, sexual, and social histories; asking focused questions about medical issues that may affect the pregnancy; and counseling her on the pregnancy. This patient has come in not just with a positive home pregnancy test but also describing the symptoms of early pregnancy. You will need to then follow the rest of the history and physical by asking questions that may alert you to complications or problems that suggest an abnormal pregnancy (such as a threatened abortion or ectopic pregnancy). Because your goal is to screen for likely problems that would appear in a first-trimester pregnancy, this case tests your ability to collect a fairly complete Ob/Gyn and sexual history.

Since the estimated date of confinement is calculated from the first day of the last period, it is essential that you take a detailed gynecological history and determine when her last period was.

As with other cases, you will need to ensure that when speaking with the patient you use lay terms for medical conditions, such as "chickenpox" or "measles." You will then document these in appropriate medical terms in the patient note ("varicella," "rubeola"). However, if you can't remember the medical terms it is acceptable to use the lay terms on your note as well. The attending physician who grades your note is familiar with both sets of terms.

In the sexual history, be sure to ask if this is a planned pregnancy, or "Is the baby coming at a good time for you and your husband?" This is a good way to gauge the patient's reaction and give her an opportunity to voice any concerns over the pregnancy. As with other cases, in the closing, always ask if the patient has any questions or concerns.

In some scenarios you will need to respond to a sudden change in the patient's tone of voice. This patient shifted tone when discussing her history of sexually transmitted diseases; she appeared sad and looked down at her feet when you asked about sexually transmitted diseases. The best approach is to discuss the topic as follows:

Doctor: "Have you ever been tested for any sexually transmitted disease?" (*Patient looks down at her feet and doesn't answer. She avoids eye contact.*)

Doctor: "You look sad all of a sudden. Can you tell me why?"

Mrs. Williams: "It's embarrassing, and if my husband ever found out ..." (*Her voice gets quiet*)

Doctor: "Remember, everything we talk about is confidential. The more I know about you and your medical history, the better I'll be able help you."

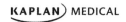

Mrs. Williams: *(Wiping away a tear)* "Before I met my husband, five years ago I got gonorrhea."

Doctor: "Thank you for telling me. I can see that this must have been difficult for you."

Notes about the Physical Exam

Vital signs: Unlike a real clinic, here you have no scale to take the patient's weight or tape measure to get the height. So in cases where it is important, you have to ask the patient for the height and weight and list it after the vital signs. Ask the patient for this information. Do not guess. Simply say "How tall are you?" (pause for a response), "How much do you weigh?" (pause for a response).

As with all case scenarios, begin the physical exam with the most important organ system. Certainly, the most important part of this physical exam is the pelvic exam. Since this is prohibited on the test you will simply list it in the Diagnostic Workup section. The next most important aspect of the physical is the abdominal exam. Of course, examining the heart and lungs and checking for any obvious or severe scoliosis is in order. This particular physical exam checklist also includes a thyroid examination. Checking for subclinical hypothyroidism is done because adequate thyroid hormone is needed for fetal brain development.

Comments about the Patient Note

There is only one diagnosis that seems credible at this time. It is perfectly correct in this case to leave the other diagnosis lines blank. The Diagnostic Workup in this case is not to make a diagnosis but to check for conditions that could harm the pregnancy, and to list an appropriate workup for a first-trimester pregnancy.

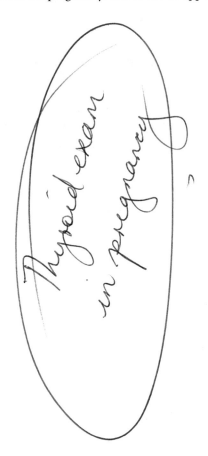

Case 7: **Pre-Employment Physical**

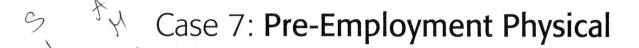

DOORWAY INFORMATION

Opening Scenario

Robert Davis is a 40 y/o male who needs a pre-employment physical.

Vital Signs

- Temp: 38.1°C (100.6°F)
- BP: 140/90 mm Hg, right upper limb sitting
- HR: 110/min, regular
- RR: 20/min

Examinee Tasks

1. Obtain a focused history.
2. Perform a relevant physical examination. Do not perform rectal, pelvic, genitourinary, female breast, or corneal reflex examinations.
3. Discuss your initial diagnostic impression and your workup plan with the patient.
4. After leaving the room, complete your patient note on the given form.

BEFORE ENTERING THE ROOM

1. Cues: Write your mnemonics on your blue sheet. These will remind you of other questions to ask, and will ensure that you don't skip pertinent aspects of the history. Consider thinking of diagnoses that cause fever, tachycardia, and elevated blood pressure.

2. Clinical Reasoning: Find out early in the interview what type of job the patient is applying for. You may find this patient a little nervous since his employment relies on this visit and on obtaining clearance from the physical exam you perform. Good eyesight and hearing, a normal neurological exam, and normal exams of the knees and spine are important for most jobs that involve physical labor. The PMH is also relevant because this may guide you to other issues that may need to be addressed in this visit.

In addition, this patient has a fever. Infection, infarction, hyperthyroidism, rheumatologic problems, drugs, and toxins are all possible explanations for his fever.

FROM THE STANDARDIZED PATIENT

History

HPI: Mr. Davis states that he just needs a note from you so he can get this job. He wants to be a taxi driver and he needs clearance from his physician saying he is fit for the job. He denies any other complaint such as cough, sputum, or dysuria. He didn't realize he had a fever or was shaky. He responds that he "gets like this sometimes but it always goes away." He thinks it might be nervousness, and suggests you not worry about it. He denies any weight loss, night sweats, joint problems, or difficulty with his hearing or eyesight.

PMH: Patient takes no medications. He has no known allergies. One hospitalization last month, when he fell and had a concussion. He just stayed overnight in the emergency room and was released the next morning. When you ask about surgery, he says he just needed some stitches on his head, no operations.

ROS: States he is on no special diet, his sleep pattern has not changed, and he has no problems urinating.

Family Hx: Mr. Davis states he has lost contact with his family and really doesn't know how they are doing. He doesn't know of any medical conditions in his family.

Social Hx: Lives alone, has shelter and food, but admits to some stress over finances. He has smoked tobacco regularly for the past 20 years (1.5 packs a day for 20 years). He also occasionally smokes "grass." He drinks a six-pack-plus of beer on Friday and Saturday nights, and sometimes during the week. Mr. Davis states he drinks "only beer, none of the hard stuff." He is CAGE-positive.

He frequently needs a drink in the morning to prevent the shakes. He suspects he should feel guilty, and he sometimes wakes up on the floor and isn't sure what happened. Last week it took him a long time to wake up, and he noticed that his tongue was bleeding. His pants were also wet from urine. Mr. Davis believes he "must have been punched in the mouth or something." He used to be very annoyed by his ex-wife criticizing his drinking, but she left last year.

CAGE Questionnaire:
- Have you ever felt you should **C**ut down on your drinking?
- Have people **A**nnoyed you by criticizing your drinking?
- Have you ever felt bad or **G**uilty about your drinking?
- Have you ever had a drink first thing in the morning to steady your nerves or to get rid of a hangover (**E**ye-opener)?

Physical Exam

Upon entering the room you notice that the patient is somewhat diaphoretic and tremulous. He isn't smiling and looks vaguely irritated. His speech is somewhat slow. His clothes are dirty and he has poor hygiene. He weighs 160 lb; his height is 5 feet 11 inches.

You see a healed scar over his forehead from last month. There is some tenderness still over the temple nearest the laceration. PERRL. Fundi shows the red reflex intact. His face has a spider angioma (Note: This is likely to be a simulated finding through the use of makeup). The pupils are equal, round, reactive to light. His cervical spine is not tender. His ribs are nontender. Lungs are clear. Heart tones are normal to auscultation. His abdomen is soft and nontender. His extremities show palmar erythema (Note: This is likely to be a simulated finding through the use of a little red makeup on the palms). There is no jaundice.

Patient is alert to person and place, but is fairly certain the year is 1995. Short-term memory is poor. He cannot repeat three words, nor can he spell the word *world* backward. He can name three objects. He does obey commands. His gait is ataxic. Extraocular movement appears intact, but he does have lateral nystagmus. Motor strength is normal on the left arm and leg, though he is noticeably weaker on the right arm and right leg.

THE CLOSING

As with all cases, it is important to explain your clinical impression to your patient and discuss the next steps in working up his condition. Explain why you cannot sign the note that clears him for employment, and be sure to answer any additional concerns he may have.

Doctor: "Mr. Davis, let me tell you what I am thinking. You told me you hit your head last month. Is that right?"

Mr. Davis: "Yes."

Doctor: "Also, you get shaky sometimes in the morning and take a drink to feel better. Is that correct?"

Mr. Davis: "Yes."

Doctor: "On your exam I found you having trouble walking. You also seem to have trouble remembering the date. The year is now 2007, not 1995."

Mr. Davis: "I just need a drink, Doc, and I'll be fine."

Doctor: "We have medicine that is better treatment than drinking. I also need to take a picture of your head, and blood tests to check your liver. Then we can talk about the rest of your treatment."

Mr. Davis: "I don't have no money for tests."

Doctor: "I will have our social worker come and talk to you to help you with that. Also, I'd like for you to meet our alcohol counselor. You need to stop drinking in order to improve your health. Do you have any other questions I can answer right now?"

CHALLENGING QUESTIONS

Be prepared to answer the following type of challenging questions for this case:

Mr. Davis: "You could just give me the note now and I'll be on my way. Also Doc, just to let you know, I have the cash on me to pay you."

Answer: "I cannot write that note today. I am concerned about your drinking and the falls you have had. I believe you may put yourself and others at risk if you drive a taxi in your current state of health. I would like you to see our alcohol counselor, and we will meet soon after you have the picture of your head. In fact, I'd like to arrange to take the picture now."

Apart from not providing the note, the key here is to remain nondefensive and nonjudgmental about the fact that an attempt was just made to bribe you. Just smile, and do what is in the patient's best interest.

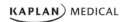

GRADING: STANDARDIZED PATIENT DATA-GATHERING CHECKLISTS

History Checklist

- ☑ Symptom: Find out what kind of job
- ☑ Review of symptoms
- ☑ PMH: Seizures, diabetes, blood pressure
- ☑ PMH: Hospitalizations and surgical history
- ☑ PMH: Trauma (head injury last month)
- ☑ Allergies
- ☑ Medicines
- ☑ Social Hx: Alcohol hx
- ☑ Social Hx: Marijuana use
- ☑ Social Hx: Injection drug use
- ☑ Social Hx: CAGE questions

Physical Exam Checklist

- ☑ Inspect HEENT, especially mouth and tongue
- ☑ Inspection: Skin—spider angioma and palmar erythema
- ☑ Palpate HEENT
- ☑ HEENT: Pupils
- ☑ HEENT: Visual acuity
- ☑ HEENT: Hearing
- ☑ Chest: Auscultation
- ☑ Cardiovascular: Auscultate heart
- ☑ Abdomen: palpation
- ☑ Neurological: Mental status
- ☑ Neuro: Motor strength
- ☑ Neuro: Gait

CASE DISCUSSION

Notes about the History-Taking

For this case, it may be appropriate to not offer a handshake. If the patient offered to shake your hand, he may lose his balance and begin to fall to the side. If this were to occur, you would be expected to catch him to prevent a fall.

For the average pre-employment case, find out a little about what the patient's job entails. Many jobs require checks of eyesight, hearing, height, weight, general flexibility, and cardiovascular fitness, with attention to knees and spine as well as little neurological (coordination, strength). An employer will not hire someone who is not oriented to person, place, or time. For the pre-employment case, you should ask:

> Doctor: "Besides coming in for the physical for your new job, do you have any other health concerns?"

If the patient says no, go directly to a complete PMH. Mr. Davis, however, is a complex case in that he is obviously quite ill, judging from his vital signs and initial appearance. As the doctor, you must shift his focus to the more acute health problems. Ask for associated symptoms for fever that relate to common conditions, e.g., pneumonia and UTI-type complaints.

By the time you complete the social history, it is evident that Mr. Davis may be suffering from alcohol withdrawal syndrome and/or possibly a seizure disorder. The history of head trauma should raise the possibility of intracranial bleeding. Never assume just because he was hospitalized for a day that everything is okay or that a subdural hematoma was ruled out.

Notes about the Physical Exam

The physical exam shows how important the general appearance is and the importance of your commenting on all of the simulated findings (e.g., makeup on the SP's skin). This case is centered around performing a good

SAMPLE PATIENT NOTE

History: Include significant positives and negatives from history of present illness, past medical history, review of system(s), social history, and family history.

CC: *Pt requests pre-employment physical clearance note*

HPI: *Pt denies complaints, wants physical exam to get job as taxi driver. However, presents with tremors, fever, and healing cuts on his tongue and forehead. States had concussion last month and "woke up" on floor with bloody tongue last week. He was not sure what happened.*
Denies cough, URI, sputum, or dysuria. + incontinence.

Meds: *None, NKDA*

PMH: *One hospitalization last month for head trauma, no surgery*

SH: *Lives alone. 20-pack-yr smoking, "occasional" marijuana. Binge drinking >6 drinks at a time.*
CAGE+, drinks frequently to stop shakes

Physical Exam: Indicate only pertinent positive and negative findings related to patient's chief complaint.

VS: *100.6°F, 140/90 mm Hg, 110/min, RR = 20/min. Skin: palmar erythema, spider angioma.*

GA: *Unkempt, dirty, tremulous*

HEENT: *Healing, still-tender laceration to forehead and tongue. PEERL EOMI, + nystagmus.*

Chest: *Clear to A, CV tachy, S1 S2 intact, no murmur, rub, and gallop*

Abd: *Soft, nontender, no organomegaly*

Neuro: *A + O × 2, states year is 1995. Poor memory and concentration. Pt obeys commands and language is intact. Motor weak on RUE, RLE 3/5, left side 5/5, gait ataxic.*

Differential Diagnosis: In order of likelihood (with 1 being the most likely), list up to five potential or possible diagnoses for this patient's presentation. (In many cases, fewer than five diagnoses are likely.)

Diagnostic Workup: List immediate plans (up to five) for further diagnostic workup.

1. Subdural hematoma	1. CBC, INR, lytes, glucose
2. Seizure	2. EtOH, drug screen
3. Alcohol withdrawal syndrome	3. CT brain
4. Wernicke encephalopathy	4. T. bili, AST, ALT
5. Alcoholic hepatitis	5. EEG

neurological exam with attention to the mental status. When a patient is not alert and oriented times three ("A + O × 3"), it is usually a good idea to complete the rest of the mental status. Quick testing of the motor strength of the four extremities reveals that this patient may have suffered a stroke.

Comments about the Patient Note

Certainly there are more than five correct possible diagnoses that explain his symptoms. Often there may be as many as 10 possible diagnoses that would be accepted as correct. Write down the ones that are most relevant to the history and physical you just completed. This doctor did not write down "alcohol intoxication"; however, if he had, it would be accepted as a reasonable diagnosis. It is important to realize that the patient probably would not be tremulous if he was currently self-medicated. Also, remember that alcohol intoxication does not cause focal neurological deficits. So it is not the most likely diagnosis.

Checking the CBC (which gives you a platelet count) and checking INR or PT/PTT is always correct for someone you suspect has intracranial bleeding. Finally, checking glucose (preferably a bedside test) on anyone with altered mental status is always correct.

Case 8: **Nosebleed**

DOORWAY INFORMATION

Opening Scenario

Kevin Green is a 45 y/o male with a nosebleed.

Vital Signs

- Temp: 36.8°C (98.2°F)
- BP: 110/80 mm Hg
- HR: 88/min, regular
- RR: 18/min

Examinee Tasks

1. Obtain a focused history.
2. Perform a relevant physical examination. Do not perform rectal, pelvic, genitourinary, female breast, or corneal reflex examinations.
3. Discuss your initial diagnostic impression and your workup plan with the patient.
4. After leaving the room, complete your patient note on the given form.

BEFORE ENTERING THE ROOM

1. Cues: Write your mnemonics on your blue sheet. These will remind you of other questions to ask, and will ensure that you don't skip pertinent aspects of the history.

2. Clinical Reasoning: With a bleeding case, always consider three things:

- Patient's hemodynamic status
- Patient's ability to clot
- Underlying disease that may cause bleeding

With someone who has blood loss, it's important to check the hemodynamic status. Is the patient tachycardic? Does the Doorway Information show that he has a low blood pressure or a narrow pulse pressure? Is he portraying diaphoresis by spraying his face with water before you enter the room? Does he have chest pain or shortness of breath, hypotension, confusion, syncope, or dizziness?

The other thing you know is that a detailed examination to look for the source and type of bleeding is needed. For example, what primary nose problems cause a bloody nose? Answer: Typically, dry air, nose-picking, and trauma. Less common causes include polyps, allergies, and upper respiratory infections. Asking about cocaine is also relevant.

Finally, anyone presenting with bleeding as the primary problem might have a bleeding disorder. Be sure to inquire into the family history for diseases such as hemophilia or Von Willebrand disease. Also, is the patient taking aspirin or Coumadin? Does he have bone marrow failure? Perhaps the patient has liver disease and a coagulopathy?

FROM THE STANDARDIZED PATIENT

History

HPI: Mr. Green has had a bloody nose off and on for the past 3 months, always in the left nostril. Sometimes it just drips a little; some days it doesn't bleed at all. On two occasions it bled so much that Mr. Green thought he might have to call 9-1-1. The nosebleeds started with a bad cold at the beginning of winter. The cold resolved, but the nosebleeds are continuing. It is now February in Chicago, and the air has been dry in the house for the last 3 months. He has no pain.

The patient has been treating himself by pushing tissues up his nose as a type of nasal packing. Sneezing and blowing his nose make it worse; nothing really seems to make it better. He has no nasal discharge (other than blood). He has had no trauma to the nose. He has also noticed that he has been bruising easily. He had never had problems with bleeding after dentistry. He has never had the current problem before.

Allergies: Cats, dogs

Meds: Tylenol (approx. 5 grams/day)

Be sure to ask how much Tylenol he is taking. Only if you ask why he takes Tylenol and how much he takes will you learn that he's taking about 5 grams of Tylenol a day.

PMH: Other than for multiple knee surgeries from college football, the patient has never been hospitalized. He is still a little bitter that his college injuries kept him from playing for a professional team. He has no history of diabetes, hypertension, or heart disease.

The patient's last doctor informed him that he has premature osteoarthritis of the knees as a result of so many football injuries. He switched from aspirin to Tylenol when the nosebleed first began because he knows aspirin is a blood thinner. He denies any recent trauma or injuries.

He sleeps through the night, unless it's a night when he wakes up with a nosebleed. He is on no special diet and usually eats junk food. He has had no problems urinating.

Family Hx: There is no family history of easy bruising.

Social Hx: He lives alone. He never leaves the house because he is on home-detention house arrest. He can leave only for medical appointments, and had to notify his parole officer that he was seeing you today. He smokes two packs of cigarettes a day and admits that a friend buys a gallon of bourbon for him each Sunday.

The SP will not admit that his friend buys him a gallon of bourbon each Sunday unless you make a statement of confidentiality during your transition to the social history.

You will need to build trust and emphasize confidentiality with this case. The patient denies using cocaine or recreational drugs, stating, "I never got into that shit!" He gets very annoyed when you ask him the CAGE questionnaire. He admits to drinking in the morning but argues that that isn't why he's here.

Physical Exam

This patient's general appearance is slightly disheveled. He smells of alcohol and has some bloodstained tissue protruding from his left nares. His speech is slightly louder than usual, and he tries to give you a big hello and a slap on the back. His gait is slightly wobbly and his speech is a little slurred. His face appears yellow (yellow powder on skin). His sclera are clear. (Note: The SP will not be able to simulate jaundiced sclera.) You will need to recognize that this is a jaundice case even though the patient will not be yellow all over.

> **Doctor:** "Your skin looks a little yellow."
>
> **Mr. Green:** "Yeah, yeah, my buddy has been telling me that. I think it's because I never go outside."
>
> **Doctor:** "I'll take a blood sample to find out why…"

Mr. Green's pupils are equal, round, and reactive to light. His extraocular movements are intact. His tympanic membranes are clear. There is no hemotympanum. His head is nontender to palpation. He removes the Kleenex from his nostril upon your request, and your examination of the nose reveals no mass or active bleeding. The nose is nontender. There is no perforation in the septum. His neck is supple.

His lungs are clear to auscultation and his heart tones are regular. You may see that he has some palmar erythema (simulated by red powder on the hands) and spider angiomata on the skin (spidery marks drawn with a red pen). His abdomen is soft, with mild tenderness to the right upper quadrant. There is no pain under the right costal margin when the patient takes a deep breath. Liver span is normal to percussion. His extremities show some edema, and there are multiple old scars on his knees. He is alert to person, place, and time. He cannot remember three objects for a minute. He cannot spell the word *world* backward. He may appear defensive over your questions and refuse to answer them, exclaiming that he is "not in school anymore!" There is no facial asymmetry and his cranial nerves are intact. His motor strength is normal bilaterally. His gait is best described as wobbly.

THE CLOSING

By now you realize your patient is probably very intoxicated. This does not change how you act toward him. Show Mr. Green the same courtesy you show patients who are not intoxicated.

> **Doctor:** "Mr. Green, I have finished your physical exam. You told me you have had the bloody nose off and on for 3 months."
>
> **Mr. Green:** "Yeah."
>
> **Doctor:** "You also have been using a lot of Tylenol, and have been drinking about a gallon of whiskey a week."
>
> **Mr. Green:** *(Somewhat defensively and loudly)* "So?"
>
> **Doctor:** "On your exam I noticed that your skin is yellow and you are tender over the liver. The bloody noses are likely to be linked to a possible liver problem."
>
> **Mr. Green:** "But I stopped taking aspirin!"

Doctor: "The Tylenol and bourbon are known to damage the liver. Tylenol is very toxic to the liver. I will need to take some blood tests to confirm this, but you need to stop taking both of these immediately to prevent further damage."

Mr. Green: "I'm not sure I can do that."

Doctor: "I know it's difficult. I will have my alcohol counselor come and talk with you. He will be able to help you through this."

Mr. Green: "Are you going to tell the police that I've been drinking? I stopped at a bar before coming to see you. If they test my alcohol level now, I'll be going to jail for sure!!"

Doctor: "No, I'm not going to call them. Remember, what we talk about is confidential."

Mr. Green: *(sloppily)* "You're not so bad, Doc!"

Doctor: "Thank you. I'll call you when I get the results of the tests. Do you have any questions for me?"

CHALLENGING QUESTIONS

Be prepared to answer the following type of challenging questions for this case:

Mr. Green: "Could you put me in the hospital? Anything would be better than being locked up at home all the time."

Answer: "I will call when I get your test results back. Then we can talk about the best treatment and where it should be done."

GRADING: STANDARDIZED PATIENT DATA-GATHERING CHECKLISTS

History Checklist

- ☑ Site/symptoms of nosebleed
- ☑ Intensity or quantity: How much has the nose been bleeding?
- ☑ Onset: When did it start?
- ☑ Onset: Course: How often?
- ☑ Onset: Duration of nosebleed
- ☑ Alleviating factors
- ☑ Aggravating factors
- ☑ Associated symptoms: Trauma, other easy bruising, no recent nasal surgery
- ☑ Allergies
- ☑ Medications: Critical to realize Tylenol is making his liver dysfunction worse
- ☑ PMH: Surgery
- ☑ PMH: Hospitalizations
- ☑ SH: Living conditions
- ☑ SH: Drug use
- ☑ SH: Smoking
- ☑ SH: Alcohol

Physical Exam Checklist

- ☑ General appearance: Skin—notice skin jaundice and stigmata of jaundice
- ☑ HEENT: Inspect nares
- ☑ HEENT: Palpate nares
- ☑ HEENT: Inspect ears
- ☑ HEENT: Inspect throat
- ☑ Chest: Auscultate lungs
- ☑ CV: Auscultate heart
- ☑ Abd: Inspect
- ☑ Abd: Auscultate
- ☑ Abd: Percuss
- ☑ Abd: Palpate
- ☑ Abd: Murphy's sign
- ☑ Neuro: Mental status
- ☑ Neuro: 7th, 3rd, 4th, 6th cranial nerves
- ☑ Neuro: Motor—all five extremities
- ☑ Neuro: Gait

SAMPLE PATIENT NOTE

History: Include significant positives and negatives from history of present illness, past medical history, review of system(s), social history, and family history.

CC: Epistaxis

HPI: 3 mo of intermittent nosebleed. Sometimes heavy. Treated with tissue placed in the nose. It started after a URI. Always the L nares. Sneezing makes it worse, nothing makes it better. Denies trauma or discharge. Pt has noticed easy bruising lately.

Allergies: Cats, dogs

Meds: Tylenol, (approx: 5 gm/d) for chronic knee pain. No aspirin or blood thinners.

PMH: No past history of nosebleeds or nasal surgery.
Hospitalizations—multiple orthopedic knee procedures in college.
+ osteoarthritis of knees. No DM/HTN. Heart disease.

FH: No familial bleeding disorders

SH: Lives alone, no cocaine or drug use, + smokes 2 ppd, + CAGE, 1 gal whiskey a week. Last drink was right before he came to the clinic.

Physical Exam: Indicate only pertinent positive and negative findings related to patient's chief complaint.

VS: WNL

GA: Pt smells of alcohol. Appears intoxicated and jaundiced. Palmar erythema, spider angiomata.

HEENT: Nares—no active bleeding, no discharge tenderness or perforation of septum.
TM—clear, pharynx clear.

Chest: Clear to Auscultation

CV: S1 S2 WNL, no MRG

Abd: Soft, BS+, mild tenderness without rebound RUQ. Neg Murphy's sign. Liver span NL to percussion.

Neuro: A + O × 3, memory poor, attention and concentration poor. No facial symmetry.
PERRL EOMI.
Motor 5/5 all four ext.
Gait—ataxic.

Differential Diagnosis: In order of likelihood (with 1 being the most likely), list up to five potential or possible diagnoses for this patient's presentation. (In many cases, fewer than five diagnoses are likely.)

1. Epistaxis from liver failure
2. Hepatic encephalopathy
3. Alcohol intoxication
4. Tylenol toxicity
5. Subdural hematoma

Diagnostic Workup: List immediate plans (up to five) for further diagnostic workup.

1. CBC, INR, lytes, glucose
2. T. Bili, AST, ALT, NH_3
3. Tylenol level, EtOH
4. CT head
5. Ultrasound RUQ

CASE DISCUSSION

Notes about the History-Taking

This case is a test of your ability to remain calm, cool, and professional during the challenges of dealing with a difficult patient. Mr. Green tells you he is under house arrest, he is obviously alcohol-intoxicated now, and he even curses throughout the encounter. The house arrest is not really part of the case and there is no need to find out what his offense was. (If you do inquire about the offense, you will learn that it was for killing a pedestrian with his car while driving under the influence of alcohol.)

This case is complex because you need to delve deeper into the situation than just looking at the patient's nose. Examining the underlying problems of liver failure caused by a toxic combination of alcohol and Tylenol is the key to the case.

Notes about the Physical Exam

In alcoholic patients, always suspect head trauma, even if patients don't present with any complaints of trauma or head pain. Looking in the ears for hemotympanum provides valuable information because bleeding can sometimes be found with basilar skull fracture. Looking at the nose for possible trauma or lesions is important. As with all patients with a history of alcohol or drug use, be sure to do a mental status exam. Be sure to tell the patient about the simulated findings you see (the yellow makeup for jaundice and the red marks for spider angiomata).

Comments about the Patient Note

In addition to the differential diagnoses listed, hypoglycemia may also be present in this patient; it is common in alcoholics with poor liver function.

In any situation where the mental status is not normal, always consider a subdural hematoma. The serum ammonia level (NH_3) may be useful in checking for hepatic encephalopathy. Patients with severe liver dysfunction may show hypoglycemia and/or elevated INR.

Case 9: **Sudden Abdominal Pain and Syncope**

BEFORE ENTERING THE ROOM

1. Cues: Write your mnemonics on your blue sheet. These will remind you of other questions to ask, and will ensure that you don't skip pertinent aspects of the history.

You will have noticed that this patient has *three abnormal vital signs*. Whatever has caused her to faint is still an active problem. In cases like this on the Step 2 CS, where the SP is portraying a very ill person with a life-threatening illness, you will need to pay very close attention to the doorway vital signs. When you enter the room the SPs may not really appear as ill as the cases they are portraying. You will also need to resist the temptation to treat SPs portraying critically ill patients. Remember, this exam is not testing you on your ability to treat a patient; rather, this exam tests your ability to take a focused history and physical as well as your communication and interpersonal skills and English proficiency. Despite alarming vital signs, you will need to maintain a calm and reassuring tone throughout the encounter.

2. Clinical Reasoning: What are the causes of syncope in a young patient?

- Vasovagal syncope is the first thing most people think of and the last thing ever tested on exams. If the patient had vasovagal syncope, you would expect bradycardia during the fainting spell, with the vital signs rapidly returning to normal.
- Subarachnoid hemorrhage causes syncope; however, it is not likely in this patient inasmuch as the patient does not have a bad sudden headache.
- Pulmonary embolism can cause syncope; however, this is not likely in the present case because the patient had no sudden onset of SOB and chest pain.
- Abdominal aortic aneurysm causes back pain and syncope. This patient, however, is too young for this condition.

Ms. Hall is hypotensive, has a narrow pulse pressure, and is tachycardic and tachypneic. Hypovolemia is certainly a possibility. Think of causes of hypovolemia and abdominal pain in a young woman and you will have the correct diagnosis.

FROM THE STANDARDIZED PATIENT

History

HPI: The patient states she got a bad left lower abdominal pain about 3 hours ago. It is 6/10 intensity and seemed to start instantly. The pain has not been getting any better or worse since it started. It feels really hot and sharp, and is continuous. It radiates up to her left shoulder. She thought going to the bathroom would make it better. Urinating and defecating did not help. She looked, and there was no blood in the toilet. She stood up from the toilet and felt very dizzy, with no power to stand up. She is pretty sure she fainted completely. She woke up on the floor, kind of sweaty. She denies any injury from the fall. At that point her husband drove her to see you at the hospital. She denies headache, shortness of breath, back pain, or dysuria. She feels nauseated. She denies vomiting or diarrhea. She has never had anything like this before.

Allergies: PCN, bee stings

Meds: Asthmacort, Ventolin inhaler, multivitamins

PMH: She was hospitalized 5 years ago for asthma attack. Her asthma is controlled with medications. She also had tubes put in her ears as a child for recurrent otitis. She has no history of trauma. She has been sleeping fine, with no special diet and no problems urinating.

Ob/Gyn: Upon questioning about her menstrual cycle, she suddenly appears sad and says she got her period 2 days ago. It is a little lighter than usual and a week later than her usual 28-day regular cycle. She is G0P0. She usually uses three to five pads on the first and heaviest day; however, this period she has had little more than spotting.

Sexual Hx: She is sexually active and does not use contraception. She stopped taking the Pill a couple months ago and she is trying to get pregnant. She tells you she is monogamous with her husband since their marriage 4 years ago. She never has had a sexually transmitted disease.

Social Hx: Ms. Hall lives with her husband and her cat and works as an editor. She does not smoke, drink, or use recreational drugs.

Physical Exam

She looks a little pale and is sweaty. Her mental status is normal but she is slightly anxious from her abdominal pain. Pharynx is normal. Lungs are clear to auscultation. Ms. Hall's heart tones are rapid. Her abdomen appears normal. Bowel sounds are present. She has marked tenderness to light palpation in the left lower quadrant. She has rebound tenderness. No mass is appreciated. There is no CVA tenderness. She is alert. If asked to walk she gets dizzy, has a lot of pain, and almost faints on you.

THE CLOSING

Despite this patient having peritonitis and impending hypovolemic shock, it is still necessary to go through the standard closing. As a transitional statement, tell the patient you are finished with the physical. Paraphrase the key historical points and describe a few key physical findings.

Tell the patient in lay terms what might be wrong and which tests will provide the answer. Be sure to inform her of when the results will be ready for the next doctor–patient contact. Counsel her about any behaviors that impact her health. Finally, ask if she has any questions.

> **Doctor:** "Ms. Hall, I have finished your physical exam. Thanks for cooperating. I can see you are in a lot of pain."
>
> **Ms. Hall:** "Just please don't shake the bed."
>
> **Doctor:** "Of course. You told me the pain came on suddenly 3 hours ago. Before that you felt fine and had no faint feeling."
>
> **Ms. Hall:** "That's correct."
>
> **Doctor:** "On your physical exam your heart rate is fast and you are very tender in the belly. I think this is most likely related to your period that is late. You could have a ruptured cyst. I want you to have a pregnancy test and an ultrasound wave picture of your tummy. Then we can know what is causing the pain for sure, and can plan treatment."

CHALLENGING QUESTIONS

> **Ms. Hall:** "Am I pregnant?"

Answer: "I'm concerned that with this much pain it could be a very abnormal pregnancy, a tubal pregnancy. Let me get this ultrasound for you quickly so we can find out."

CASE DISCUSSION

Notes about the History-Taking

You may find it a challenge to stick to the script for SPs portraying patients with life-threatening surgical problems. In real-life situations it is likely that you would be resuscitating and getting the operating team assembled while taking a history and physical. However, in the Step 2 CS exam you are being evaluated on your initial workup and diagnosis, and not on your treatment of or therapy for this patient's condition. Pain radiating to the shoulder suggests diaphragmatic irritation. Record the history of asthma. However, in this case the patient has currently no symptoms of asthma and it is not an active problem.

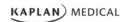

GRADING: STANDARDIZED PATIENT DATA-GATHERING CHECKLISTS

History Checklist

- ☑ Site of pain
- ☑ Intensity of pain
- ☑ Quality of pain
- ☑ Onset of pain
- ☑ Onset: Course and duration
- ☑ Radiation of pain
- ☑ Aggravating factors
- ☑ Alleviating factors
- ☑ Associated symptoms
- ☑ Previous episodes of the chief complaint
- ☑ Allergies
- ☑ Medications
- ☑ PMH: Hospitalizations
- ☑ PMH: Illness
- ☑ PMH: Surgery
- ☑ Ob/Gyn: LMP—complete gyn hx needed
- ☑ Ob/Gyn: complete OB hx needed
- ☑ SX: Sexually active, trying to get pregnant
- ☑ SHx: Lives with husband. No smoking, drugs, or alcohol.

Physical Exam Checklist

- ☑ General appearance
- ☑ Chest: Auscultate lungs
- ☑ CV: Auscultate heart
- ☑ CV: Check pulses
- ☑ Abd: Inspection
- ☑ Abd: Auscultation (before percussion)
- ☑ Abd: Percussion
- ☑ Abd: Palpation
- ☑ Abd: Check for rebound tenderness

Notes about the Physical Exam

A complete abdominal exam consisting of inspection, observation, percussion, and palpation is warranted. You would not do deep palpation because there is already pain on light palpation, though you would still go ahead and do the test for rebound tenderness. In fact, do rebound tenderness only if the patient is tender on either light or deep palpation. The rebound test is to see if the patient has peritonitis. The SP will be trained to have more pain "when you let go" in order to simulate a surgical abdomen.

Comments about the Patient Note

When the chief complaint is pain, it does not take long to chart the site, intensity, quality, and onset. You may also sketch the abdomen to indicate your findings. Differential diagnosis includes ruptured cysts that also can cause hemorrhage. The present case seems less likely to be an incomplete abortion because there is not much bleeding; however, it is possible. Renal colic seems even more unlikely. However, listing just about any diagnosis that can cause LLQ pain or vaginal bleeding would be appropriate. In this case a quantitative HCG is in order because it is useful in interpretation in conjunction with the ultrasound in some cases of ectopic pregnancy. Pregnancy test should be ordered on all cases of lower abdominal pain or any menstrual irregularity.

SAMPLE PATIENT NOTE

History: Include significant positives and negatives from history of present illness, past medical history, review of system(s), social history, and family history.

CC: Acute abdominal pain

HPI: Sudden onset 3 hrs ago, sharp/hot, 6/10 intensity LLQ pain. Pain is constant and radiates to L shoulder. Nothing makes it better. Standing up from toilet, had syncopal episode and was diaphoretic.
No vomiting, diarrhea, dysuria, or blood in urine or stool.

PMH: First episode. Allergies—PCN, bees. Meds—Ventolin, Asthmacort inhalers. Asthma. Only one hospitalization for asthma, 5 years ago.

Gyn: LMP now, 1 week late and just spotting, lighter than usual. Periods usually regular with 3–5 pads on heaviest day. GOPO. Has not done a home preg test.

SX: Active, no contraception, trying to conceive

SH: Lives with husband. No smoking, EtOH, or drugs.

Physical Exam: Indicate only pertinent positive and negative findings related to patient's chief complaint.

GA: In acute distress 2nd to pain. BO 80/70, HR 120, RR 24, afebrile.

Chest: Clear to auscultation

CV: Rapid heart tones

Abd: Appears NL, scaphoid. BS+, very tender LLQ. No mass felt. + rebound LLQ. No CVA tenderness.
Extremities: Too dizzy and lightheaded to walk.

Differential Diagnosis: In order of likelihood (with 1 being the most likely), list up to five potential or possible diagnoses for this patient's presentation. (In many cases, fewer than five diagnoses are likely.)

1. Ruptured ectopic pregnancy
2. Ovarian torsion
3. Ruptured ovarian cyst
4. Threatened/incomplete abortion
5. Renal colic

Diagnostic Workup: List immediate plans (up to five) for further diagnostic workup.

1. Complete pelvic and rectal exam
2. CBC, type, and Rh
3. U/A, UCG
4. Quantitative HCG
5. Pelvic ultrasound

Case 10: **Vaginal Bleeding**

DOORWAY INFORMATION

Opening Scenario

Carol Roberts is a 40 y/o with vaginal bleeding.

Vital Signs

- Temp: 37.1°C (98.8°F)
- BP: 150/100 mm Hg
- HR: 100/min
- RR: 20/min

Examinee Tasks

1. Obtain a focused history.
2. Perform a relevant physical examination. Do not perform rectal, pelvic, genitourinary, female breast, or corneal reflex examinations.
3. Discuss your initial diagnostic impression and your workup plan with the patient.
4. After leaving the room, complete your patient note on the given form.

BEFORE ENTERING THE ROOM

1. Cues: Looking at the chief complaint, realize that a good Ob/Gyn and sexual history will be needed. You already know that a complete abdominal exam is indicated and that a pelvic exam will have to be ordered in the Diagnostic Workup. Read all the information on the doorway. The tasks will be the same most of the time, but don't make any assumptions. *Read the Doorway Information!*

2. Clinical Reasoning: Tachycardia can commonly be caused by hypovolemia, anemia, fever, or pain. Vaginal bleeding in a 40 y/o woman will have a limited differential diagnosis, and you can fill out a preliminary Differential Diagnosis on your notepaper before entering the room. Your list should include:

- Menstruation
- Dysfunctional uterine bleeding
- Spontaneous miscarriage
- Infections such as cervicitis, vaginitis, endometritis

- Ectopic pregnancy can be found in 40 y/o women as well as in younger women
- Endometrial cancer (less likely but always a possibility)

FROM THE STANDARDIZED PATIENT

History

HPI: Ms. Roberts complains of really heavy periods lately. She states she has only had maybe two normal periods in the last 6 months. Normally her period lasts 3 to 5 days, but it is now lasting 8 to 10 days. She is using six to eight pads a day. There is no pain or cramps. She denies any fever or discharge. She states she is not having hot flashes.

Sometimes she gets a little irritable around her period, but not always. That has not changed in many years. She is just finishing her period for 10 days now. She made an appointment because she felt a little lightheaded when she stood up suddenly and ran for the bus yesterday. There was mild shortness of breath with running, though no chest pain, syncope, or palpitations. This is the first time she has experienced this. She states that she's never had an elevated blood pressure reading in the past.

Allergies: Amoxicillin

Meds/vitamins: She has not used birth control pills in 5 years.

PMH: She has been hospitalized for 2 C-sections only.

Ms. Roberts denies diabetes mellitus, hypertension, or heart disease.

She has had no changes in her sleep pattern. She has been trying to loose about 20 lb and has been on a low-calorie diet of 1200 calories per day. She is not a vegetarian. She has had no problems urinating.

Ob/Gyn: Her previous period was 4 weeks ago and also long and heavy. She started have periods at age 12. Ms. Roberts has been pregnant three times; she had two children and had one elective miscarriage when she was 16. She is now sexually active with three different partners in the last 6 months. (she has two different partners currently). She is sexually active with men only. She tries to have her partners always use a condom but sometimes they don't want to. She was tested for sexually transmitted diseases when her period was first irregular 6 months ago, by a different physician, and the results were negative. Ms. Roberts is divorced and has two college-age children that usually live at school. She works as the day manager of a small retail business. She smokes one pack of cigarettes per day and drinks two drinks maybe once a week, when on a date. She does not use any recreational drugs. She states she is well adapted to being single and an "empty-nester."

Physical Exam

The patient appears slightly pale (the SP may demonstrate that by having a little white makeup on her cheeks or forehead). You need to recognize this as anemia and can confirm it with the following conversation.

> **Doctor:** "I see you have a little white powder on your face."

> **Ms. Roberts:** "Oh, that, people have been telling me I look pale."

In this way the SP can give you the simulated physical finding of pallor, indicating anemia.

Ms. Roberts is awake and alert. Her pharynx is clear. Her thyroid is not enlarged. There is no jugular venous distention. Chest is clear to auscultation. Heart tones are regular. Her abdomen appears normal. Bowel sounds are normal. There are no masses or tenderness, specifically in the suprapubic and lower quadrants on both sides. There is no costovertebral angle tenderness. There is no cyanosis or edema to the extremities. Her gait is normal.

THE CLOSING

The key to this closing is to counsel Ms. Roberts on practicing safe sex. This needs to be done *without* a stern tone of voice. With the proper tone of voice, you will not appear judgmental. You simply need to tell her what type of sexual behavior will protect her health.

> **Doctor:** "Ms. Roberts, I'm ready to tell you what I am thinking. First, I want to make sure I understand. For the last 6 months you have been having periods that are lighter than normal."

> **Ms. Roberts:** "No, Doctor—heavier than normal."

> **Doctor:** "Excuse me, periods that are heavier than normal. And they have been lasting a lot longer also."

> **Ms. Roberts:** "That's correct."

> **Doctor:** "And yesterday you got a little lightheaded and short of breath."

> **Ms. Roberts:** "Yes."

> **Doctor:** "Well, I think you may be anemic from the heavy periods. That would explain all your symptoms and being pale too."

> **Ms. Roberts:** "What do we do about it?"

> **Doctor:** "I would like you to have a blood test to see how anemic you are. I will also need you to have a pregnancy test and tests to make sure you don't have an infection. I would like to take a picture of your chest and a heart tracing to be sure there are no other problems. I will call you with the results."

> **Ms. Roberts:** "All right."

> **Doctor:** "I can tell you now that I want you to practice safe sex every time. That means use a condom every time. It is still possible for you to get pregnant or contract a sexually transmitted disease."

> **Ms. Roberts:** "Okay."

> **Doctor:** "Do you have any questions?"

This doctor would not lose any points for paraphrasing the patient incorrectly because he corrected himself and eventually paraphrased the history correctly.

Paraphrasing is very important to do. The sample exchange above delicately addresses the patient's lifestyle of having two different sexual partners. At the same time, it provides a firm recommendation that safe sex be practiced all the time.

CHALLENGING QUESTIONS

> **Ms. Roberts:** "Should I go back on the Pill to regulate my periods?"

Answer: "I need to see the results of the blood tests to decide the best medicine for you. Can you come back in 3 days so we can discuss the results?"

GRADING: STANDARDIZED PATIENT DATA-GATHERING CHECKLISTS

History Checklist

- ☑ **S**ite/symptom
- ☑ **I**ntensity: Quantity of bleeding
- ☑ **O**nset: Duration
- ☑ **O**nset: Course
- ☑ **A**ssociated symptoms
- ☑ **PM**H: Surgery and hospitalizations
- ☑ **PM**H: Major illness
- ☑ **A**llergies
- ☑ **M**edications
- ☑ **O**b/Gyn: LMP, menarche
- ☑ **O**b/Gyn: Gravida, para status
- ☑ **SX**: Number of partners
- ☑ **SX**: Any history of STD and testing
- ☑ **SX**: Contraception
- ☑ **SH**x: Smoking
- ☑ **SH**x: Alcohol
- ☑ **SH**x: Drug use

Physical Exam Checklist

- ☑ **HE**ENT: Skin color
- ☑ **HE**ENT: Pharynx
- ☑ **CV**: Auscultate heart
- ☑ **CV**: JVD
- ☑ **CV**: Edema
- ☑ **Chest**: Auscultate lungs
- ☑ **Ab**d: Inspection
- ☑ **Ab**d: Auscultation
- ☑ **Ab**d: Percussion
- ☑ **Ab**d: Palpation
- ☑ **Ab**d: CVA tenderness

CASE DISCUSSION

Notes about the History-Taking

In this case, the gynecological history is of prime importance. This doctor chose to collect the information during the HPI, and even wrote most of the Gyn history in the HPI section. This is absolutely fine. Had you written the Gyn history in the PMH section as suggested by the SIQORAAA PAM HRFOSS mnemonic, this would have been correct as well.

Notes about the Physical Exam

Certainly some heart and lung exams are indicated because the patient was a little short of breath with exertion due to the anemia. Also, the chief complaint of vaginal bleeding indicates that a fairly complete abdominal exam is going to be on the checklist as well.

Be sure to comment on any makeup the SP is wearing that indicates a physical finding.

Comments about the Patient Note

The key here is getting the CBC and the pregnancy test. These are not the only correct workups; getting a pelvic ultrasound would also be acceptable. This doctor elected to be sure there was no heart disease by getting the CXR and ECG. This will always be a correct response in patients age 40 and over, especially if they are smokers with elevated BP readings and shortness of breath.

SAMPLE PATIENT NOTE

History: Include significant positives and negatives from history of present illness, past medical history, review of system(s), social history, and family history.

CC: Vaginal bleeding

HPI: Periods were normal until last 6 months of irregular painless heavy periods. Blood loss up to 8 pads/day. Periods can last 10 days. No fever, chills, dysuria, abdominal pain, or discharge. + dyspnea with exertion and some lightheadedness when stands up fast. Has never had irregular periods before.
Was tested ~5 mo ago for STD—negative.

PMH: Allergies—amox. Meds—vitamins, not on hormones for past 5 years.
Hospitalized for two C-sections. No trauma or other surg.
Denies DM, HTN, heart disease.

ROS: No change in her sleep pattern.
+ dieting 1200 cals/day. Not a vegetarian.

O: LMP ending now, started 10 days ago. Menarche age 12.

SX: + active 3 male partners in last 6 months. Does not always practice safe sex.

SH: Lives alone, states well adjusted to kids being in school. Smokes 1 ppd, EtoH 2 drinks "on a date." No recreational drugs.

Physical Exam: Indicate only pertinent positive and negative findings related to patient's chief complaint.

VS: NL except BP 150/100 and HR = 100 (pt states never had elevated BP before)

GA: Looks pale, NAD

HEENT: Pale, pharynx clear, no JVD

Chest: Clear to Auscultation

CVS: S1 S2 WNL, no GRM

Abd: Appears NL, BS+, no masses or tenderness all 4 Q, no suprapubic pain, no CVA pain

Ext: Normal, no cyanosis, or edema

Neuro: Alert, gait NL

Differential Diagnosis: In order of likelihood (with 1 being the most likely), list up to five potential or possible diagnoses for this patient's presentation. (In many cases, fewer than five diagnoses are likely.)

1. Dysfunctional uterine bleeding
2. Threatened abortion
3. Incomplete abortion
4. Cervicitis
5. Elevated BP reading

Diagnostic Workup: List immediate plans (up to five) diagnostic workup.

1. Complete GU exam, rectal and pelvic exam
2. Pap smear, Gonorrhea, Chlamydia culture
3. CBC, lytes, BUN, Cr
4. CXR, EKG
5. ß-HCG, pelvic ultrasound

In this case it will turn out that the patient has no heart disease yet, just anemia, making her short of breath with exertion.

Any diagnosis that causes vaginal bleeding will be a correct answer. So you could complete the Differential Diagnosis without ever seeing the patient! The purpose of the history and physical is to rank order the most likely diagnoses. You should have in your mind a list of causes of vaginal bleeding in young, middle-aged, and older women.

A single elevated BP reading does not make a diagnosis of hypertension. Serial readings are generally needed. "elevated BP reading" is appropriate for this case.

Case 11: **Vaginal Bleeding**

DOORWAY INFORMATION

Opening Scenario

Susan Walker is a 60 y/o female with vaginal bleeding.

Vital Signs

- Temp: 37.0°C (98.6°F)
- BP: 140/80 mm Hg
- HR: 80/min
- RR: 16/min

Examinee Tasks

1. Obtain a focused history.
2. Perform a relevant physical examination. Do not perform rectal, pelvic, genitourinary, female breast, or corneal reflex examinations.
3. Discuss your initial diagnostic impression and your workup plan with the patient.
4. After leaving the room, complete your patient note on the given form.

BEFORE ENTERING THE ROOM

1. Cues: Write your mnemonics on your blue sheet. These will remind you of other questions to ask, and will ensure that you don't skip pertinent aspects of the history. You already know that you will need a complete Ob/Gyn and sexual history. You can tell from the vital signs that this patient is hemodynamically stable. Her age is of critical importance in determination of a likely cause of her vaginal bleeding.

2. Clinical Reasoning: At age 60, the patient is 9 years past the average age of menopause. So it is likely that this is a case of postmenopausal bleeding. Of course, endometrial cancer is a likely cause of postmenopausal bleeding. Some risk factors for endometrial cancer are smoking, obesity, estrogen replacement, and nulliparity. Additional causes of vaginal bleeding include: cervical cancer, uterine polyps, hormone replacement therapy, and bleeding from the perineum, vagina, or cervix. Atrophic vaginitis and endometritis may also cause bleeding. Finally, vaginal bleeding is occasionally confused with rectal or urinary bleeding.

(Excess oestrogen)

Endometrial cancer : smoking, obesity, oestrogen, nulliparity

FROM THE STANDARDIZED PATIENT

History

HPI: Ms. Walker comes to you with a chief complaint of having a period after not having any periods for the past 9 years. It started last week. At first she noticed a little bit of blood on tissue when she urinated after sex. The next day she had bleeding with some clots, like the heaviest of periods she use to have when she was a younger woman. Last week she even had to go to the drugstore to get some pads; she told the checkout clerk they were for her granddaughter. She used about one pad an hour for 6 hours, and then the bleeding slowed. After that she had some spotting for 3 days. There has been no bleeding for the past 3 days. She figured she would keep the appointment with you because she had similar bleeding about 8 weeks ago. At that time she was not sexually active just prior to the onset of bleeding. Nothing seems to make the bleeding better. Other than sex once, nothing seems to make it worse. She has had no abdominal pain, fever, discharge, or dysuria. She has no shortness of breath, hemoptysis, or chest pain. She denies blood in urine or stool.

Allergies: ASA

Medications: Coumadin (taken regularly; her dose was increased 3 months ago), Diabeta, Lisinopril, occasional Tylenol. Last blood test 1 month ago to see how thin her blood is.

PMH: Hospitalizations: Gallbladder removed 20 years ago; right knee replacement 8 months ago; blood clot in right leg 5 months ago.

High blood sugar for last 10 years; high blood pressure for past 10 years. Denies trauma or any additional surgery.

ROS: Ms. Walker has not had any problems urinating, other than seeing blood last week. She is just now beginning to walk regularly after her knee replacement and has been going to physical therapy regularly.

Family Hx: There is no family history of cancer, diabetes, or hypertension.

Ob/Gyn: The patient has been pregnant three times and has had two children and one miscarriage. She started having periods at age 12 and stopped at age 51. She still complains of an occasional hot flash but is most bothered by vaginal dryness, making intercourse painful. She uses a condom regularly. She has been getting regular gynecological checkups every 2 years and had a normal mammogram while in the hospital for the blood clot.

Sexual Hx: She is sexually active with one male partner. She has never been tested for a sexually transmitted disease.

Social Hx: Ms. Walker lives alone but speaks with and sees her male friend everyday. She states she has been under stress because of her leg, but things are slowly getting better. She was a smoker for 20 years, and stopped smoking 5 months ago when she got the blood clot. No alcohol. She is finally weaned off the Vicodin tablets after the knee surgery. She says she understands how easy it is to get addicted to narcotics when you have chronic pain.

Physical Exam

Ms. Walker weighs 200 lb and is 5 feet 2 inches. She walks with a slight limp and a cane, but otherwise is in no acute distress. There is no visible ecchymosis or simulated skin findings on her skin.

HEENT: Inspection reveals no abnormalities.

Lungs are clear to auscultation. Inspection reveals no abnormalities.

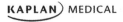

Heart tones are normal. Good pulses in the feet on both sides.

Her abdomen is obese, soft, and nontender without masses. There is no tenderness to percussion. Bowel sounds are normal. The old right subcostal scar is still visible. No CVA tenderness.

Extremities: Healing scar from knee replacement. No ecchymosis. Her right calf is still somewhat swollen. No redness or tenderness.

Neuro: Alert, walks with a cane.

THE CLOSING

The closing and the challenging questions in this case are to test your ability to discuss sexuality with the patient in a professional manner.

Doctor: "I'm finished with your physical exam and I'd like to go over the findings. You told me that you have had bleeding that was heavy for 1 day and spotting for the last 3 days. Is that correct?" *(Wait for response)*

"On your physical exam, your tummy exam is normal. By the way, it looks like your leg is healing from the blood clot.

"I think most likely the bleeding is from the combination of the Coumadin and dryness caused by menopause. I would like you to have some tests to make sure it is nothing else, then we will meet again to discuss treatment. Do you have any questions?"

CHALLENGING QUESTIONS

Ms. Walker: "Doctor, I'm really bothered by the dryness during sex. Is there anything I can do about it, like taking hormones?"

Answer: "Hormones would not be a good idea right now, with the healing blood clot and the bleeding. Have you tried a vaginal lubricant? I'll have my nurse bring you some samples."

There is no treatment on this test, so it would also be correct to give the standard answer about wanting to examine the patient and getting the test results before deciding on the best course of treatment.

In this particular case, your score might be higher if you recognize a contraindication to estrogen and tell the patient. You could recommend over-the-counter vaginal lubricants. This doctor couldn't think of any brand names offhand, so she cleverly decided that the patient could receive some samples from the nurse.

CASE DISCUSSION

Notes about the History-Taking

Each test day will include cases where you need to ask about personal information. USMLE is testing your communication and interpersonal skills; testing your ability to talk about personal information with the patient without appearing nervous, laughing, or losing your professional demeanor. Practice asking about the sexual history until you can ask the questions and discuss the symptoms with the same tone of voice you would ask about chest pain or any other symptom.

If the disease could be caused or exacerbated by sexual activity, it's always important to ask about.

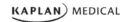

GRADING: STANDARDIZED PATIENT DATA-GATHERING CHECKLISTS

History Checklist

☑ **S**ymptom
☑ **I**ntensity: Quantify amount of bleeding
☑ **O**nset: When did it start?
☑ **O**nset: Description of course of bleeding
☑ **A**: What makes it better?
☑ **A**: What makes it worse?
☑ **A**: Ask about bleeding elsewhere, as patient on Coumadin
☑ **A**sk about signs of complications of blood clot (pulmonary embolism symptoms)
☑ **A**sk about discharge, fever, dysuria, pelvic or abdominal pain
☑ **P**: Pt does have previous experience with the chief complaint
☑ **A**: Allergies
☑ **M**edications: Anyone on Coumadin is likely to have complications from the drug
☑ **P**MH: List hospitalizations and surgery
☑ **O**b/Gyn: Gravida, Para scoring
☑ **O**b/Gyn: Menstrual history—menarche and menopause
☑ **O**b/Gyn: Menopausal symptoms
☑ **S**X: Need complete sexual history. No, you don't need to ask about contraception in a 60-y/o, but you still need to counsel about safe sex!!
☑ **S**Hx: Living arrangements, stress, and smoking will all be on the checklist

Physical Exam Checklist

☑ **G**eneral appearance
☑ **C**hest: Auscultate lungs
☑ **C**V: Auscultate heart
☑ **A**bdomen: Inspection
☑ **A**bdomen: Auscultation
☑ **A**bdomen: Percussion
☑ **A**bdomen: Palpation
☑ **E**xtremities: Inspection
☑ **E**xtremities: Palpation

Notes about the Physical Exam

In this case the most important organ system that you *are* authorized to examine is the abdomen. Do a complete abdomen exam in this patient. Also, inspect the leg at the site of the blood clot as this was a recent illness. As a general rule, examine areas of recent surgery and illness.

After a quick heart and lung exam, look over the entire skin surface for additional signs of bruising or bleeding, since the patient is on Coumadin. Patients on Coumadin need a rectal exam as well to look for gastrointestinal bleeding; however, a rectal exam is not permitted on this test, so order the rectal exam as a diagnostic workup.

SAMPLE PATIENT NOTE

History: Include significant positives and negatives from history of present illness, past medical history, review of system(s), social history, and family history.

CC: *"I had a period?"*

HPI: *Vaginal bleeding started after painful sex. Noticed some blood when urinating after intercourse. One day used 6 pads. Couple days of spotting after that. Now no bleeding. Nothing seems to make it better. Worse with sex. No SOB, chest pain, or hemoptysis. Denies hematuria, dysuria, blood in stool, or easy bruising. No fever, abdominal or pelvic pain. No discharge.*
NKDA.
Meds—lisinopril, DiaBeta, Tylenol, Coumadin. Coumadin dose increased 3 months ago. Good compliance, last INR 1 month ago.

PMH: *Has had similar episode of vaginal bleeding 2 months ago.*
+ cholecystectomy 20 yrs ago, R knee replacement 8 mo ago, DVT 5 months ago.
+ DM, HTN.

Ob/Gyn: *G3P2Ab1. Menarche age 12, menopause age 51. Occasional hot flash. + vaginal dryness.*

SX: *Active, one partner, uses condoms. Never tested for STD.*

SH: *Lives alone, regular physical therapy. Is able to walk and care for herself. No rec drugs or alcohol. Stopped smoking 5 mo ago. Previously a smoker for 20 yrs.*

Physical Exam: Indicate only pertinent positive and negative findings related to patient's chief complaint.

VS: *140/80 80 16 afebrile*

GA: *NAD*

Chest: *Clear to Auscutation*

CV: *S1 S2 NL, no S3 S4 murmur. NL peripheral pulses*

Abd: *Soft, BS+, nontender and without masses all 4 Q. Tympanic to percussion. CVA tenderness*

Ext: *R leg slightly swollen, nontender redness. L leg no swelling, tenderness or redness.*

Differential Diagnosis: In order of likelihood (with 1 being the most likely), list up to five potential or possible diagnoses for this patient's presentation. (In many cases, fewer than five diagnoses are likely.)

1. Bleeding from Coumadin
2. Atrophic vaginitis
3. Endometrial Cancer
4. Uterine polyp
5. Cervical Cancer

Diagnostic Workup: List immediate plans (up to five) for further diagnostic workup.

1. Complete GU, rectal, and pelvic exam
2. CBC, U/A, INR
3. Pelvic ultrasound
4. Pap smear
5. Endometrial biopsy

Comments about the Patient Note

The Doorway Information provided a good idea of the type of diagnoses to consider. Any of these top three diagnoses are likely. Don't spend a lot of time evaluating which one is more likely than another. Just make an educated decision and make sure you write down all of the likely diagnoses. Remember: This test is asking what is most likely—not what is most dangerous! In this case, knowing how frequently Coumadin complications occur, and the fact that the bleeding began after painful sex, suggests a combination of atrophic vaginitis and Coumadin-related bleeding (from a high INR). You will still be ordering all of the appropriate laboratory workups that evaluate for the common as well as the life-threatening problems.

Case 12: **Personal Problem**

DOORWAY INFORMATION

Opening Scenario

Charles Taylor is a 21 y/o male who comes to you with a personal problem.

Vital Signs

- Temp: 37.0°C (98.6°F)
- BP: 128/70 mm Hg, right upper limb sitting
- HR: 72/min, regular
- RR: 16/min

Examinee Tasks

1. Obtain a focused history.
2. Perform a relevant physical examination. Do not perform rectal, pelvic, genitourinary, female breast, or corneal reflex examinations.
3. Discuss your initial diagnostic impression and your workup plan with the patient.
4. After leaving the room, complete your patient note on the given form.

BEFORE ENTERING THE ROOM

1. Cues: Write your mnemonics on your blue sheet. These will remind you of other questions to ask, and will ensure that you don't skip pertinent aspects of the history.

2. Clinical Reasoning: "Personal problems" often turn out to be psychiatric illness, addiction problems, or some problem with the genitals or rectum. Whatever it is, expect the patient to be reticent about disclosing the topic until you gain his trust by showing empathy. You may need to tell him that your conversation is confidential long before getting to the sexual history, in order to gain his trust.

FROM THE STANDARDIZED PATIENT

History

HPI: Mr. Taylor tells you, somewhat reluctantly, that he has a penile discharge. He went to Fort Lauderdale over spring break. A couple of days after returning to his prestigious eastern university, the discharge began. He has burning with urination, nocturia, and frequency as well. The discharge is described as a yellow-greenish color. He states that he has never had anything like this before. He has had the discharge for several days and it is not getting better. He has no pain, other than the burning sensation in the penis. Nothing seems to make it better or worse. He denies fever, rash, joint pain, and sore throat. He has no pain in his abdomen, testes, or back.

PMH: He is allergic to PCN. He takes no prescription medications. He has had no prior hospitalizations, trauma, major illness, or surgery.

Sexual Hx: He was sexually active with multiple female partners while on spring break. He did not always use condoms. He has never been tested for HIV/AIDS or sexually transmitted diseases.

Social Hx: He lives in a college dormitory. He smokes marijuana once/month but no cigarettes. He drinks alcohol, three or four beers on weekends when he doesn't have to study. He states he typically has no stress, but he's now worried that he might have HIV.

Physical Exam

Upon entering the room you notice that the patient looks worried but is in no acute distress. His sclera are clear, and skin has no rash or icterus. Pharynx is clear and without exudates. There is no cervical adenopathy. Chest is clear to auscultation. Heart sounds are normal. Abdomen reveals no hepatosplenomegaly. Bowel sounds are present. There is no tenderness or masses in all four quadrants. There is no CVA tenderness. He has no erythema or tenderness to the wrists or knee joints.

THE CLOSING

As with all cases, it is important to explain your clinical impression to your patient and discuss the next steps in working up his condition. It is also important to answer any additional concerns he may have.

> **Doctor:** "Mr. Taylor, I'd like to tell you what I am thinking but first I want to review what you told me."

> **Mr. Taylor:** "Okay."

> **Doctor:** "To summarize, you have had a yellow-green discharge for the last several days."

> **Mr. Taylor:** "That's right."

> **Doctor:** "So far your exam is normal, but I will need to complete the exam and take a swab of the discharge. That way I can find out what type of infection you have and order medicine for you. You told me you are worried about HIV, so I will also order a blood test for you."

> **Mr. Taylor:** "Oh, okay, good."

> **Doctor:** "Until then I want you to not have sexual relations. Also, you need to contact your partners and tell them to come in and be treated. After you and your partners are treated I want you to practice safe sex. That means to use a condom every time."

Mr. Taylor: "Uh-huh…"

Doctor: "Do you have any other questions?"

Mr. Taylor: "No."

Doctor: "I'll be right back with the swab, and I should have the results in 48 hours."

It may seem more artificial not to treat the patient empirically, but there is no treatment included on Step 2 CS exam. Counseling about safe sex practices is key to this case and is essential.

CHALLENGING QUESTIONS

Be prepared to answer the following type of challenging questions for this case:

Mr. Taylor: "Can't you just give me a shot for everything and skip the tests?!"

Answer: "I need to find out exactly what kind of infection you have. Then I will know the correct medicine to provide you."

GRADING: STANDARDIZED PATIENT DATA-GATHERING CHECKLISTS

History Checklist

- ☑ Symptoms
- ☑ Intensity/quality of discharge
- ☑ Onset of symptoms
- ☑ Onset: Course
- ☑ Onset: Duration
- ☑ Alleviating factors
- ☑ Aggravating factors
- ☑ Associated symptoms
- ☑ Previous episodes of the chief complaint
- ☑ Past medical history
- ☑ Allergies: PCN allergy
- ☑ Medicines
- ☑ Sexual Hx: Condom use
- ☑ Sexual Hx: Number of partners in last 6 months
- ☑ Sexual Hx: Hx of STD in past?

Physical Exam Checklist

- ☑ General appearance
- ☑ HEENT: Inspect pharynx
- ☑ Skin: Any rash or jaundice?
- ☑ Chest: Auscultate the lungs
- ☑ CV: Auscultate the heart
- ☑ Abd: Palpation
- ☑ Abd: Check for CVA tenderness
- ☑ Joints: Inspect or palpate or do ROM to check for tenderness (wrist, hands, and knees)

SAMPLE PATIENT NOTE

History: Include significant positives and negatives from history of present illness, past medical history, review of system(s), social history, and family history.

CC: Penile discharge

HPI: Several days of greenish discharge from the penis. No prior episodes. + burning with urination. Nothing makes it better or worse.
No fever, back pain, rash or joint problems.

Meds: None, allergic to PCN

PMH: No hospitalizations, major illness, trauma, surgery

SX: Sexually active with multiple female partners recently. Does not always use condom.

SH: Lives in college dormitory. No cigarettes. Uses marijuana once/month. 3–4 "beers" on weekends.

Physical Exam: Indicate only pertinent positive and negative findings related to patient's chief complaint.

VS: WNL

GA: Looks worried

HEENT: Pharynx clear, no jaundice

Chest: Clear to Auscultation

CV: NL S1 S2. No rub, murmur, or gallop.

Abd: Soft, nontender. No masses or tenderness, no organomegaly. BS+, no CVA pain.

Ext: No rash. Major joints without tenderness, redness, or swelling.

Differential Diagnosis: In order of likelihood (with 1 being the most likely), list up to five potential or possible diagnoses for this patient's presentation. (In many cases, fewer than five diagnoses are likely.)

1. Gonorrhea
2. Chlamydia
3. Hepatitis B
4. HIV
5. Syphilis

Diagnostic Workup: List immediate plans (up to five) for further diagnostic workup.

1. Complete genital exam
2. U/A
3. Culture for gonorrhea
4. Culture for chlamydia
5. VDRL, HIV, Hep B serology

CASE DISCUSSION

Notes about the History-Taking

This patient would initially be very shy about telling you what is wrong. The interaction might go something like this:

Doctor: "How can I help you today?"

Mr. Taylor: "Well, it's kinda personal…"

Doctor: "You can tell me. I am here to help."

Mr. Taylor: "Are you going to tell my parents?"

Doctor: "No, everything we talk about is confidential."

Mr. Taylor: "I see. *(Pauses)* Well…I have this discharge…"

Of course, this is the case in which taking a complete sexual and social history is imperative. A patient who has one sexually transmitted disease may have contracted multiple diseases at the same time! So ask about associated symptoms that may indicate additional diseases. Also, ask about complications. For gonorrhea, be concerned about skin rash and septic joints from a disseminated gonorrhea infection.

Notes about the Physical Exam

The exam of the skin is important in sexually transmitted disease (STD) cases. There may be simulated physical findings for syphilis and disseminated gonorrhea. If the Doorway Information indicates that the patient has a fever, be sure to inspect a couple of major joints—such as wrist and knee—to look for any signs of septic arthritis.

If there are no complications from the STD, the Differential Diagnosis is simply every other STD that is possible, with the corresponding tests for the Diagnostic Workup.

Comments about the Patient Note

For the STD case, the Differential Diagnosis is frequently just complications of the infection. If no complications are present, the other likely possibility is that the patient has contracted more than one STD simultaneously. All you need to do is to have prepared in your mind a list of common STDs and the appropriate diagnostic workups—*before* test day.

In the Diagnostic Workup section of the Note, be sure to list the additional physical exam that in this test is forbidden. It is easy to forget that a genital urinary exam still needs to be performed.

Case 13: **Elevated Blood Pressure**

DOORWAY INFORMATION

Opening Scenario

Hy Pascal is a 55 y/o male who presents with a note that a health-fair nurse says his BP is elevated. He is here to have the BP rechecked.

Vital Signs

- Temp: 37.0°C (98.6°F)
- BP: 160/100 mm Hg
- HR: 80/min
- RR: 20/min

Examinee Tasks

1. Obtain a focused history.
2. Perform a relevant physical examination. Do not perform rectal, pelvic, genitourinary, female breast, or corneal reflex examinations.
3. Discuss your initial diagnostic impression and your workup plan with the patient.
4. After leaving the room, complete your patient note on the given form.

BEFORE ENTERING THE ROOM

1. Cues: This patient is here for a blood pressure check. It is traditional for a doctor to retake the BP himself while in the room. Of course, you will record on your patient note only what is listed the doorway (160/100 mm Hg). When developing differential diagnoses only think about the doorway vital signs!

2. Clinical Reasoning: For this case, think of symptoms and complications relating to hypertension (HTN). HTN is known as the "silent killer." Many experts feel that there are no symptoms, only complications that involve end-organ damage.

Heart failure, stroke, kidney failure, peripheral vascular disease, retinopathy, and angina are all more common in the hypertensive population. These complications of HTN give a good idea about what to ask regarding associated symptoms. For example, for heart failure ask about shortness of breath: "Do you ever wake up at night short of breath? Do you have any swelling in the ankles?"

FROM THE STANDARDIZED PATIENT

History

HPI: Last week, at a health fair, a nurse told Mr. Pascal that he had an elevated blood pressure reading. He recalls that it was 160/110 mm Hg. He states that he feels "fine" right now. He tells you that he has had "white coat syndrome" for at least 20 years: he just gets nervous around medical types, and knows that's the reason for his elevated blood pressure. He has never checked his blood pressure at home to confirm that his blood pressure does drop when there are no white coats around. He figured since one of his coworkers recently had a heart attack that maybe it is time to get checked. He tells you that he feels pretty good and never has had any chest pain. He is starting to "feel his age" as a senior citizen lately. He notices that when he runs for the commuter train he is really "winded," and it takes a good 15 minutes resting before he can catch his breath. Also, lately his shoes don't seem to fit so well—like his feet are a little bit bigger and swollen. Mr. Pascal mentions that he has heard that swelling could be related to salty foods, and admits that he does like to use extra salt.

These symptoms have come on gradually over the past 6 months and they really do not affect his life significantly. He says the swelling and the shortness of breath on exertion are mild. He also states that he's had a little runny nose and a cold for the past week.

He denies any palpitations, weakness on one side of the body, or change in vision.

No cough, sputum, or fever. No paroxysmal nocturnal dyspnea.

When asked about pain in the legs, he says, "Funny you should ask. I always seem to get a cramp in my left leg lately when I run to catch the train." That goes away with rest also.

Allergies: None

Medications: Recently he has been taking some pseudoephedrine for a URI.

PMH: Mr. Pascal had his gallbladder removed 5 years ago. (His blood pressure readings were elevated then, but it was assumed to be because he was in pain.) He has had no other hospitalizations or surgeries. He denies diabetes. He does not remember his last cholesterol reading. Mr. Pascal admits he has not seen a doctor since his gallbladder operation.

Social Hx: Mr. Pascal has not had any change in his sleep. His wife does report that he snores a lot and seems to choke in his sleep. Lately it seems that even though he sleeps 7 hours, he is tired in the morning and sometimes has a mild headache. His weight has increased 30 lb since the gallbladder operation, since eating fatty foods no longer hurts. He states that he has no problems urinating.

Family Hx: Mr. Pascal states his father died of heart disease at age 62.

Sexual Hx: He states that he is not sexually active and he thinks he has entered "male menopause." If questioned appropriately, he tells you that "the plumbing hasn't worked" for at least the last year.

He lives with his wife. His three children are older now. He stopped smoking 25 years ago. He does not use recreational drugs. He may have two or three drinks at a party once a month or so. He works in an office as buyer for an electrical supply company. He does not exercise at all. He is under no unusual stress.

Physical Exam

Mr. Pascal is in no acute distress. He weighs 220 lb. Height is 5 feet 9 inches. Pupils are equal, round, reactive to light. His fundi show no papilledema; the red reflex is intact. He has some coryza from his URI. Pharynx is clear. TMs are clear. No tenderness over the maxillae. It is difficult to see if there is any AV nicking or hemorrhage. Neck shows no thyroidmegaly. There are no carotid bruits. Carotid upstrokes are normal. Chest is clear to auscultation. Heart is regular with a possible gallop rhythm. His point of maximum impulse is displaced laterally and he has no jugular venous distension. His abdomen is obese. He is nontender in all four quadrants. There is a well-healed right subcostal scar. His legs have trace edema bilaterally. Distal pulse are intact and equal 2/4 B/L. Motor strength 5/5 all four extremities. His gait is normal.

THE CLOSING

Doctor: "I have finished your exam. Let me review. You told me you have had an elevated blood pressure reading and have been a little short of breath lately. Also you have been taking some cold medicine. Is that correct?"

Mr. Pascal: "Yes."

Doctor: "On your exam I found that you do have some leg swelling. This could be from elevated blood pressure. I want to do a blood test to check your heart as well as a picture of your chest. Then we'll meet again next week to discuss the results and plan treatment. Until then, please stop the cold medicine. It might be causing your high blood pressure reading. Do you have any questions?"

GRADING: STANDARDIZED PATIENT DATA-GATHERING CHECKLISTS

History Checklist

- ☑ Site/symptom: Ask if patient has any complaints other than elevated BP reading
- ☑ Site/symptom: Get history of SOB and edema
- ☑ Intensity: "Mild" does not affect his life
- ☑ O: History longstanding "white coat syndrome"
- ☑ Alleviating factors: SOB better when pt rests
- ☑ Aggravating factor: Exertion
- ☑ Associated symptoms: Find out about chest pain, palpitations, signs of stroke, kidney, retina or peripheral vascular disease
- ☑ Allergies
- ☑ Medication: Get hx of pseudofed use
- ☑ Past medical hx: Gallbladder operation
- ☑ Past medical hx: No DM
- ☑ ROS: Diet, change in weight, and sleep all important
- ☑ Family Hx: + family hx of heart disease
- ☑ Sx: + erectile dysfunction
- ☑ Social hx: Exercise, drugs, alcohol, smoking

Physical Exam Checklist

- ☑ General appearance
- ☑ HEENT: Pupils
- ☑ HEENT: Funduscopy
- ☑ HEENT: Ears, nose, throat
- ☑ HEENT: Carotid artery
- ☑ Chest: Lung auscultation
- ☑ CV: Heart auscultation
- ☑ CV: PMI, JVD
- ☑ CV: Peripheral edema and peripheral pulse
- ☑ Neuro: Motor strength all five extremities
- ☑ Neuro: Gait

CHALLENGING QUESTIONS

Mr. Pascal: "Do I have a bad heart?"

Answer: "It is possible that the blood pressure has caused the heart to be enlarged. I need to have you complete the tests to know. If you do have an enlarged heart, I have medicines available to treat you."

CASE DISCUSSION

Notes about the History-Taking

The chief complaint is an elevated blood pressure reading, so you will first need to find out the details and the onset of the elevated blood pressure. In this case you learn that the patient has not had a normal BP reading in possibly decades. It is good to ask the patient if he has any other symptoms he is concerned about. This case was designed for him to say "No." Your role as physician is to ask direct questions about the complications of hypertension. And as always, as the history unfolds there are many possible diagnoses that you can consider from the history.

ROS is usually relevant in these types of cases where the patient is coming for a checkup. The sexual history is also relevant in this case—erectile dysfunction is a symptom of his peripheral vascular disease.

Notes about the Physical Exam

Patients who are coming in for a checkup, as in this case, also need their height and weight documented. Simply ask the patient the height and weight. You will not be asked to calculate a Body Mass Index (BMI). However, by recording the weight you are showing you are concerned about the association between HTN and obesity.

In this type of situation in real life you have the patient sit quietly in a chair for 5 minutes before checking the blood pressure. Obviously, for the Step 2 CS test you are not going to do this—it would consume your entire time for doing a physical! The physical should be directed at looking for signs of end-organ damage. Therefore, the cardiovascular exam is most important.

Hint: Remember to write on your note the BP that was on the doorway. Disregard the SP's actual real-life blood pressure!

Comments about the Patient Note

In this case the patient came just for a blood pressure check, but there were plenty of other symptoms to un-cover and discuss in the HPI. This case is also complex in that there is not time enough to do all of SIQORAA on each of his symptoms. You simply need to get the list of symptoms and a few key features of each.

Most of the tests are to look for end organ damage. Certainly the CXR and BNP are to look for heart failure. Renal function tests will always be correct in this situation. Checking the lipid panel is standard on all adults coming for a periodic checkup. Checking for diabetes mellitus is also reasonable in this overweight, hypertensive patient.

The patient gives you past information about multiple elevated BP readings, making the diagnosis of HTN justified.

SAMPLE PATIENT NOTE

History: Include significant positives and negatives from history of present illness, past medical history, review of system(s), social history, and family history.

CC: Elevated BP at recent health fair

HPI: DOE × 6 mo. 15 minutes to catch his breath when runs for train. Gradual onset. Symptoms described as mild. Also with some pedal edema and pain in L leg with exertion. SOB and leg pain better with rest. No chest pain, focal deficits, change in vision. For past week has coryza. No fever, sputum, or cough. No PND.
Allergies—NKMA
Meds—Pseudoephedrine

PMH: Has history of "white coat syndrome" with elevated BP readings for 20 years. Hospital/surg—Cholecystectomy 5 yr ago. Denies DM. Unknown last cholesterol check. No regular heath care.

ROS: Snores, frequently tired in A.M. Wife reports pt "chokes" in his sleep.
+ 30-lb weight gain in 5 years. No problems urinating.

FH: Father died, heart, age 62

SX: Erectile dysfunction for past year

SH: Lives with wife, sedentary job, no exercise, no unusual stress. No smoking, drug use. EtOH—2–3 drinks/wk.

PE: 220 lb, 5'9"

Physical Exam: Indicate only pertinent positive and negative findings related to patient's chief complaint.

VS: NL except BP = 160/100. pt NAD. 220 lbs, 5'9" tall

HEENT: PERRL, fundi flat. TM, nares, pharynx clear. No thyroidmegaly. Carotid without bruits 2/4, B/L.

Chest: Lungs clear to Ausultation

Cor: S1 S2 NL. No murmur, possible gallop. −JVD, PMI slightly displaced laterally.

Abd: Obese, nontender

Ext: + pedal edema. DP, PT pulse 2/4 B/L.

Neuro: Alert. Motor 5/5 all 4 ext. Gait—NL.

Differential Diagnosis: In order of likelihood (with 1 being the most likely), list up to five potential or possible diagnoses for this patient's presentation. (In many cases, fewer than five diagnoses are likely.)

1. Hypertension
2. Congestive heart failure
3. Peripheral vascular disease
4. Elevated BP from medication
5. Sleep apnea

Diagnostic Workup: List immediate plans (up to five) for further diagnostic workup.

1. CXR, ECG, U/A
2. CBC, lytes, BUN, Cr, glucose
3. BNP, echocardiogram
4. Fasting total cholesterol, HDL, LDL, TG
5. Sleep study, arterial Doppler ultrasound, lower extremities

Case 14: **Medication Refill**

DOORWAY INFORMATION

Opening Scenario

Paul Thomas is a 49 y/o male who telephones to ask for a refill of his medication.

Vital Signs

No vital signs are given in this case since the patient is on the phone.

Examinee Tasks

1. Obtain a focused history.
2. Discuss your initial diagnostic impression and your workup plan with the patient.
3. After ending the call, complete your patient note on the given form.

BEFORE ENTERING THE ROOM

1. Cues: Read the Doorway Information carefully. Notice that this Doorway Information is a little bit different than most of the cases. There are no vital signs, as the patient is at home. Also, the tasks are a bit different. There is no physical exam listed in the "Examinee Tasks" section. You will not always be told in the doorway information that it is a phone case as you are in this example. Always be sure to knock on the door before you enter the patient's room. If it is a phone case, your score will not be lowered.

2. Clinical Reasoning: A drug refill case could be done on the phone, or the patient may present in person asking for a drug refill. A physical exam may or may not be required if the patient presents in person for a drug refill. If the patient is on the phone, no physical exam is possible for you to write on your note—at the closing, when you counsel the patient, you would simply ask the patient to come in for a physical exam. Be sure to order a "physical exam" as part of your Diagnostic Workup. Even without a physical exam, it is likely that in most cases you will tell these patients in your closing that you will refill their medications even before they come to see you. This is reasonable because we do not want our patients running out of their maintenance medications.

The occasions when you will *not* agree to refill medication are limited. One possibility is if the patient is telling you about a dangerous medical condition that cannot be managed on the phone and requires a physical exam. If this occurs it is important to tell the patient you need to see him for an exam to determine the best way to manage his condition. The advantage of the CS exam is that you may say you are always available. Tell the patient to come in immediately and you can see him. If he is too sick to travel on his own, simply tell him to call the ambulance ("Call 9-1-1") and you will meet him at the hospital.

It's possible that you may experience a patient scenario where you suspect the patient is seeking narcotics due to a prescription drug addiction. The key to this type of scenario is to maintain the same warm, professional composure as you would for any other case. Just like in a real-life setting, there is no reason to become defensive, and no reason to be nervous or become judgmental about the patient. If it's a phone case, tell the patient you need a physical exam and may be able to treat his pain more effectively if he sees you immediately. If the patient is in the room, use the same technique for any medication requests on Step 2 CS. For example, you may tell the patient that as soon as it's safe to do so, you will bring the pain medicine. Finally, some phone requests for narcotics are appropriate and should be filled without hesitation. For example, a known cancer patient is out of his or her pain medications, or sometimes the dog really *did* eat the narcotic prescription you just wrote before the patient could fill it.

Approach to the HPI on a Drug Refill Case: Do the same introduction as always. If the patient's chief complaint is that he needs more medication, find out if there are any other health concerns you can help with today.

Doctor: "How can I help you today?"

Mr. Thomas: "I need a refill of my blood pressure medicine."

Doctor: "Sure. Are you having any other concerns I can help with?"

If the patient has no other complaints, use the SIQORAA to find out the history of his hypertension. If he denies any complaints, ask symptom-based questions related to the disease for which he needs the medication.

For example, in a patient with hypertension:

S:	(Note: Many authorities believe that hypertension has no symptoms, only complications)
I:	How is hypertension affecting your life?
Quantity:	How high was your blood pressure?
Onset:	When did your hypertension start?
A:	What makes your blood pressure better?
A:	What makes your blood pressure worse?

Associated symptoms are the complications of the disease

When you get to associated symptoms, just ask about the complications of the disease. So for HTN, ask a few questions to see if the patient has any sign of heart disease or stroke.

If the patient has any additional symptoms, divide your History time between the most important additional symptoms and the history of hypertension that prompted the need for medications.

The medication history is a little more detailed in the drug refill case. For the medicine the patient wants refilled, get the name, dose, route, and number of times a day. For example, Lisinopril 20 mg PO q A.M. For other medications, obtaining just the drug name is sufficient. Remember: The test does not focus on your ability to prescribe treatment, and you will not be required to write a prescription on this test. Think about any drug interactions, and ask about any common side effects of medications. Also ask about compliance:

Mr. Thomas: "I need a refill of my nitroglycerin."

Doctor: "When did you last take it?"

Mr. Thomas: "Three months ago."

Doctor: "Why do you need it refilled now?"

Mr. Thomas: "Well, I haven't had any chest pain until this morning, but it's lasting for hours."

Doctor: "I want you to call 9-1-1 and go to the hospital; I will meet you there and I can examine you after we finish our phone call."

If you get a case like this, finish your full 15 minutes with the patient to get as much history as possible. It is somewhat artificial and unlike real life, where calling the paramedics immediately would be the right answer.

FROM THE STANDARDIZED PATIENT

History

HPI: Mr. Thomas called to get a refill of his Lisinopril 10 mg PO q d. When asked directly at the beginning of the interview, he denies any other health problems or current concerns. He has had hypertension for the past 10 years and it is not affecting his life in any way. He states that he checks the blood pressure now and then and the top number is usually 120 to 130 mm Hg. The bottom number goes from 70 to 84 mm Hg. Nothing seems to make his blood pressure better or worse. He has noticed some swelling in his legs for the past 2 months. He gets slightly short of breath when going up two flights of stairs at once. No chest pain or syncope. He has had a nonproductive dry cough lately. No sputum or fever.

Allergies: None. Lisinopril is his only medication.

PMH: He has never been hospitalized and has never had any bad accidents or surgery. Mr. Thomas has no history of diabetes, cancer, or heart disease.

Social Hx: Patient has noticed a 15-lb weight gain in the last year. He attributes this to his bad diet, as he frequently eats fast food for lunch. Now is 220 lb, 5 ft 10 in. He has no difficulty with urination. His sleep pattern has not changed. There is no family history of heart disease. He lives at home with his wife of 25 years. He works as an accountant and states that he is under stress only at tax time. He does not use alcohol, smoke, or use recreational drugs.

Physical Exam

There is no physical exam, as the patient is on the phone.

THE CLOSING

In this case the patient has a host of new symptoms that may necessitate a change in his medicines, and a physical exam is indicated.

Doctor: "Let me make sure I understand correctly. You told me you need a refill of your Lisinopril, you have had HTN for 10 years, and you have had some shortness of breath, swelling, and cough recently. Is that correct?"

Mr. Thomas: "Yes, that's right."

Doctor: "I'm concerned that you may have some fluid in your lungs. I'd like you to come into the office today so I can examine you and talk more with you.

"I'd also like to do pictures of your chest and heart, as well as a blood test to check your cholesterol. At the same time, I'd like to speak to you in person about your diet and exercise. Do you have any questions?"

In this sample exchange, the doctor wants to see Mr. Thomas in person before refilling his medicine. Had the scenario been slightly different and the patient really had no acute health problems, it would have been appropriate for you to refill the medicine prior to the physical exam. In that case you would explain to the patient that you'll refill the medication even prior to the patient making the appointment. For example:

> **Doctor:** "Let me make sure I understand correctly. You told me you need a refill of your Lisinopril, and you have had HTN for 10 years. Is this that correct? I will go ahead and refill your medicine today. Please also make an appointment for a physical exam. I would like to speak with you in person also about improving your diet and starting to walk for exercise. I'd also like to do picture of your chest and heart, as well as blood test to check your cholesterol and sugar. Do you have any questions?"

CHALLENGING QUESTIONS

> **Mr. Thomas:** "I really can't come in to see you. I have no health insurance—can't you just refill my pills? It's only $4 for a month's supply at Wal-Mart. If I do everything you say it will be a hundred times or a thousand times more!!!"

Answer: "I need to see you because you may need different or more medicine. I'll keep your concerns about cost in mind, however I'm going to recommend what is best for your health. I can have you speak with our counselor [social worker], who might be able to help get you health insurance."

Be sure not to promise that the counselor *will* be able to get the patient health insurance. Explain in lay terms why a visit and test are necessary. Have the patient talk to the social worker, if only to see if s/he can help.

GRADING: STANDARDIZED PATIENT DATA-GATHERING CHECKLISTS

History Checklist

- ☑ Symptom: Ask open-ended question to see if patient has any other problems besides needing refill
- ☑ Intensity: How is HTN affecting his life?
- ☑ Quantity: Does he check his blood pressure? What readings does he get?
- ☑ Onset: How long does he have HTN?
- ☑ Alleviating factors
- ☑ Aggravating factors
- ☑ Associated symptoms: Ask about symptoms of heart disease and stroke
- ☑ Allergies
- ☑ Medication: Get name, dose, route, number of times a day of medicine to refill
- ☑ Medication: Get names of all other meds patient takes
- ☑ PMH: Hospitalization, illness, trauma
- ☑ ROS: Weight
- ☑ SH: Diet, smoking, alcohol, sleep
- ☑ Sexual Hx

Physical Exam Checklist

None in this case—can't do physical exam over the phone.

SAMPLE PATIENT NOTE

History: Include significant positives and negatives from history of present illness, past medical history, review of system(s), social history, and family history.

HPI: Patient called on phone for refill of Lisinopril 10 mg PO q d. Patient initially denied any complaints.
HTN has not affected his life at all
HTN began 10 years ago
BP at home 120–130/70–84
States nothing makes HTN better or worse
No chest pain, extremity pain, weakness
Does have some swelling in legs and SOB on exertion for past 2 months. Patient also notices is coughing. No sputum or fever.
Allergies—None
Meds—Lisinopril 10 mg PO q d; is taking regularly

PMH: No hospitalizations, major trauma, or surgery. No Hx of DM, cancer, or heart disease. Weight has increased 15 lb in last year, 220 lb, 5'10". No change in sleep pattern. No problems urinating.

FH: Negative

SX: Pt is sexually active, one partner

SH: Married, lives with wife, works as an accountant. Under stress only at tax time. No exercise program. Pt states is on no special diet, eats fast food several times a week. No smoking, no alcohol or drug use.

Physical Exam: Indicate only pertinent positive and negative findings related to patient's chief complaint.

Differential Diagnosis: In order of likelihood (with 1 being the most likely), list up to five potential or possible diagnoses for this patient's presentation. (In many cases, fewer than five diagnoses are likely.)

1. Hypertension
2. Congestive heart failure
3. Renal insufficiency
4. Cough secondary to Lisinopril
5.

Diagnostic Workup: List immediate plans (up to five) for further diagnostic workup.

1. Physical exam stat
2. CBC, glucose, BUN, Cr, electrolytes
3. EKG, CXR, U/A
4. Fasting cholesterol, HDL, LDL, triglycerides
5. BNP, echocardiogram

CASE DISCUSSION

Notes about the History-Taking

Phone cases present unique challenges. Be sure during the introduction that you know with whom you are speaking. In a phone case you'll be able to take more notes, since there will be no eye contact to maintain with the patient—but that also means no nonverbal communication is possible. Speak slowly and clearly. You have more time for the history and counseling, as no physical exam is requested.

Notes about the Physical Exam

Leave this section blank on this particular case. USMLE knows you can't physically examine a patient who is fully clothed in regular street clothes (not in a patient gown when you enter) or who is only a voice on a telephone.

Don't worry if writing your history spills over into the portion of the note reserved for the physical—that's fine. The doctors grading your note will be able to figure it out!

Comments about the Patient Note

Asking a patient's height and weight on the phone is acceptable and could even be important in some phone cases. Notice how on this note it was just included in the history.

The Differential Diagnosis includes diseases that are known complications of hypertension for which the patient has suggestive symptoms. Don't forget that medication can sometimes be the source of a new problem. So it is acceptable to list "cough" as a possible side effect from the Lisinopril.

The Diagnostic Workup, of course, includes a physical exam. Renal function is always a correct test to order with HTN, as the kidney is a target organ. The U/A is indicated on most people with systemic disease. Because HTN, obesity, and DM often occur in the same patient, it is reasonable to check the glucose despite no specific questioning about diabetes in the history. It is also appropriate to order tests to look for signs of congestive heart failure. For example, B-type natriuretic peptide (BNP), echocardiogram, and a chest x-ray are all useful in looking for signs of congestive heart failure.

Case 15: **Menopause Drug Refill**

DOORWAY INFORMATION

Opening Scenario

Ruth Evans is a 53 y/o female who calls you on the phone for a refill of her estrogen tablets (Premarin™).

Vital Signs

There are no vital signs, as this is a phone case.

Examinee Tasks

1. Obtain a focused history.
2. Discuss your initial diagnostic impression and your workup plan with the patient.
3. After completing the call, complete your patient note on the given form.

BEFORE ENTERING THE ROOM

1. Cues: Write your mnemonics on your blue sheet. These will remind you of other questions to ask, and will ensure that you don't skip pertinent aspects of the history.

2. Clinical Reasoning: In this case, you are told that this is going to be a phone case. You will need to use the phone to speak with the patient. You will need a detailed medication history, and you need to find out the dose, route, and frequency of the medication. Checking compliance is critically important. Also, find out the names of any other medicines the patient is taking. As in all cases where the patient doesn't seem to have any pain or symptoms, you need to ask early on if the patient has any other health concerns you can help with.

For an asymptomatic patient, certainly focus the history around menopausal symptoms, the side effects of Hormone Replacement Therapy (HRT), and contraindications to the medication. Most frequent indications are for hot flashes, night sweats, and atrophic vaginitis. It is unlikely you will be asked to comment on the more controversial aspects of HRT.

Contraindications to using HRT include cancer of the uterus or breast; cardiovascular disease, including coronary artery disease, stroke, and blood clots; liver dysfunction; pregnancy; and, of course, allergy to the product.

Side effects include vaginal bleeding, headache, and vaginitis.

FROM THE STANDARDIZED PATIENT

History

HPI: Ms. Evans calls you because she ran out of her Premarin tablets 6 weeks ago. Unfortunately, the vaginal dryness and pain with intercourse has returned. Even worse, she hardly ever gets a good night's sleep because of hot flashes and night sweats. She feels a little more irritable during the day and it is beginning to affect her work and family life. She asks for a medication refill. She has no other complaints and otherwise feels fine. Nothing makes the symptoms better, including trying herbal cures (black cohosh). Nothing makes it worse. Ms. Evans has had no vaginal bleeding or discharge. She had no headaches or side effects from the Premarin.

Ms. Evans has no allergies. She was taking Premarin 0.3 mg by mouth every day for the past 6 years. She also takes calcium supplements and a multivitamin.

PMH: She was hospitalized at age 49 for a total abdominal hysterectomy and bilateral salpingo-oophorectomy for dysfunctional uterine bleeding. There was no cancer. She had a nondisplaced fracture of the wrist last winter. She has never had any blood clots, heart attack, stroke, or liver disease. Her last mammogram was 2 years ago and normal.

ROS: She is not sleeping well now due to the night sweats. Her weight is unchanged. She has noticed some frequency of urination lately. There is no dysuria, hematuria, or incontinence.

Family Hx: Her mother and sisters never had breast or uterine cancer.

Ob/Gyn: She has been pregnant twice and had two live births. Menarche was at age 12.

Sexual Hx: Ms. Evans is sexually active with her husband of 25 years.

Social Hx: Ms. Evans works as executive director of a social service agency. She does not feel generally stressed. She stopped smoking decades ago. No recreational drugs. Drinks one or two glasses of wine each week.

Physical Exam

There is no physical exam, as this is a phone case.

THE CLOSING

In this case, the diagnosis of menopausal symptoms seems rather obvious to both you and the patient, and is not mentioned in the closing listed below. A better alternative would have been to tell the patient the diagnosis in lay terms, just like every other case. Don't worry if you don't get everything absolutely perfect. Few patient encounters—in real life or on test day—are perfect.

This doctor did do an excellent job of answering the patient's chief complaint. She explained that she would refill the medication. This appears to be an exception to the no-treatment rule on Step 2 CS. It would have been a correct response as well if the doctor said she wanted to see what the test results showed prior to selecting the appropriate medicine. Remember: The Step 2 CS is testing your ability to speak and communicate comfortably with the patient.

Hormone Replacement Therapy still seems to be a very controversial topic. Don't worry about picking the "wrong answer." In areas of controversy either choice will be acceptable.

Doctor: "Thank you, Ms. Evans. Let me review what we talked about today. You told me you have stopped the Premarin for the past 6 weeks. Since then you have had night sweats, hot flashes, and dryness that causes pain with sex. Is that correct?"

Ms. Evans: "Yes."

Doctor: "I can go ahead and call in a prescription for you. In addition, I would like you to make an appointment for a physical exam."

Ms. Evans: "Okay."

Doctor: "It sounds like you are due for your yearly mammogram as well."

Ms. Evans: "Yes."

Doctor: "I would also like you to do an x-ray to look for weak bones. When we meet, we will go over the test results and plan treatment. Do you have any other questions?"

GRADING: STANDARDIZED PATIENT DATA-GATHERING CHECKLISTS

History Checklist

☑ **S**ymptoms: Elicit menopausal symptoms
☑ **I**ntensity: How is it affecting her life?
☑ **O**nset
☑ **A**ggravating factors
☑ **A**lleviating factors
☑ **A**ssociated symptoms: Can ask contraindications and side effects of estrogen here or when you get to PMH, asking about major illnesses
☑ **A**llergies
☑ **M**edications: Dose, route, frequency of drug requested
☑ **M**edications: Get names of all other medicines
☑ **M**edications: Ask about side effects
☑ **M**edications: Compliance
☑ **P**MH: Hospitalizations
☑ **P**MH: Surgery
☑ **P**MH: Major illness(es) that contraindicate pt receiving estrogen
☑ **R**OS: Urinary
☑ **F**H
☑ **O**b/Gyn: Any bleeding, discharge, dyspareunia
☑ **S**ocial Hx
☑ **S**exual Hx

Physical Exam Checklist

No physical exam checklist possible in phone cases

CHALLENGING QUESTIONS

> **Ms. Evans:** "Oh, that broken wrist was just because I slipped on the ice last winter. Do I really need a test for my bones?"

Answer: "Yes. It would still be wise to check what is called the bone density. It could be you need more than calcium tablets to protect the bones."

CASE DISCUSSION

Notes about the History-Taking

The patient wants a refill of her Hormone Replacement Therapy, so it is important to find out what symptoms, if any, she is having from menopause. Ask about complications of menopause during the associated symptoms. Also ask about contraindications to hormone replacement therapy. An Ob/Gyn history and sexual history will be on the checklists in this case.

Notes about the Physical Exam

In phone cases, no physical exam is possible.

Comments about the Patient Note

In this case the doctor wrote about a medication (black cohosh) during the HPI. It would have been equally correct to list this botanical in the "Medications" section, with a short explanation that it did not help as well. Either way, the doctor will get credit for asking about herbal medicine and looking for alleviating factors.

Some cases may not have an extensive Differential Diagnosis. The Diagnostic Workup will center on routine screening exams for menopausal women. Ms. Evans needs yearly mammography and is late. Any fracture needs evaluation for osteoporosis. DEXA stands for Dual Energy X-ray Absorptiometry. You can use either generic or trade names for medications.

SAMPLE PATIENT NOTE

History: Include significant positives and negatives from history of present illness, past medical history, review of system(s), social history, and family history.

CC: *Request for Premarin refill*

HPI: *Stopped Premarin 6 wks ago. Since then has had return of night sweats, hot flashes, and dyspareunia. Pt also has been having interrupted sleep. Pt has some frequency of urination without burning or hematuria. Nothing makes it better. No response to black cohosh supplements. Nothing makes it worse. Denies vaginal bleeding or discharge.*
Allergies—None
Meds—Premarin 0.3 mg PO q d

PMH: *TAH-BSO for DUB. No liver disease, blood clots, MI, or stroke. No DM, HTN. No hx of cancer. Fell and broke her wrist last winter.*

FH: *No family hx of breast or uterine cancer*

Ob/Gyn: *G2P2*

SX: *Sexually active, 1 partner*

SH: *Married. Does not feel stressed at work or home. Nonsmoker, no drugs, 1–2 glasses wine/wk.*

Physical Exam: Indicate only pertinent positive and negative findings related to patient's chief complaint.

No physical exam in phone cases.

Differential Diagnosis: In order of likelihood (with 1 being the most likely), list up to five potential or possible diagnoses for this patient's presentation. (In many cases, fewer than five diagnoses are likely.)

1. *Menopausal symptoms*
2. *Osteoporosis*
3.
4.
5.

Diagnostic Workup: List immediate plans (up to five) for further diagnostic workup.

1. *Physical exam, pelvic and rectal exam*
2. *U/A*
3. *Mammogram*
4. *Bone density test (DEXA)*
5.

Case 16: **Fever and Weight Loss**

DOORWAY INFORMATION

Opening Scenario

Scott Brown is a 29 y/o male who comes to the clinic with fever and weight loss.

Vital Signs

- Temp: 39.0°C (102.2°F)
- BP: 110/80 mm Hg
- HR: 110/min, regular
- RR: 24/min

Examinee Tasks

1. Obtain a focused history.
2. Perform a relevant physical examination. Do not perform rectal, pelvic, genitourinary, female breast, or corneal reflex examinations.
3. Discuss your initial diagnostic impression and your workup plan with the patient.
4. After leaving the room, complete your patient note on the given form.

BEFORE ENTERING THE ROOM

1. Cues: This patient has three abnormal vital signs (temperature, heart rate and respiratory rate). Write them on your scratch paper when you are standing outside the patient's room. This way you'll be ready to transcribe them onto the final note 15 minutes from now.

2. Clinical Reasoning: When two symptoms are given in the opening scenario, it is likely that the final diagnosis will explain both symptoms. It is much less likely that the patient will have two completely unrelated problems. Because weight loss takes some time to notice, this situation is probably not an acute febrile illness; it is more likely to be something chronic. Patient's vital signs indicate that he is tachypneic. This is a hint to perform a good chest exam and ask some pulmonary questions. Metabolic acidosis can also cause a compensatory tachypnea.

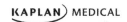

FROM THE STANDARDIZED PATIENT

History

HPI: Mr. Brown comes to you and tells you he has been sick for most of the past 6 months. It started at that time with fever, headache, malaise, and swollen glands. That lasted about 3 months. He went to a different clinic and a mono test was done, but that turned out negative. Then he started to get high fevers, cough, and shortness of breath with exertion. Three months ago, the SOB was only with exercise. He has stopped exercising completely and now gets dyspnea on exertion (DOE) going up one flight of stairs.

The cough is nonproductive. There is occasionally some mild chest discomfort with coughing. Nothing seems to make it better or worse. The chest discomfort changed about 2 weeks ago. He also complains that for the last 2 weeks he has had extreme pain with swallowing both solids and liquids. He has noticed some white, cheesy rash on his tongue and oral mucosa. Prior to this past 6 months, he was perfectly healthy.

Allergies: None

Meds: Tylenol and Motrin for fever without relief

PMH: Mr. Brown has never been hospitalized. He has had not surgery or trauma. He denies diabetes, hypertension, and heart disease. He denies any exposure to tuberculosis.

SH: He has been sleeping more than usual lately, has lost approximately 20 lb, and has a decreased appetite. He has been having some liquid brown stools. He has no problem urinating. He is sexually active, with four different sexual partners in the last year—all male. He has not practiced safe sex.

Mr. Brown lives alone. He is a social worker for the state child protective agency. He is upset that he has been missing so much work due to illness recently. He does not smoke, drink, or use any recreational drugs.

Physical Exam

Mr. Brown looks unhappy. He is 135 lb and is 5 feet 9 inches. He is holding a little cup, into which he spits occasionally because it hurts to swallow. Occasionally during the interview he has a dry, hacking cough.

Aside from looking thin, the patient has some obvious reddish lesions on the vermillion border of his lip, which indicate the simulated physical finding of herpes labialis.

His neck is supple. Lungs are clear to auscultation. Tactile fremitus, percussion, and auscultation are normal. His heart tones are fast without any murmur or gallop. When you check for cervical and supraclavicular adenopathy, he tells you that his glands are still swollen. His abdomen is soft and nontender. Bowel sounds are normal. Gait is normal. He is alert and does not seem confused.

THE CLOSING

Doctor: "I have finished your physical exam, Mr. Brown. Would you like to know what I'm thinking?"

Mr. Brown: "Yes, Doctor."

Doctor: "You told me you have not felt well in six months—first with fever, swollen glands, and weakness, then with shortness of breath and cough, and now with a lot of pain when you swallow."

Mr. Brown: "That's correct."

Doctor: "On your physical exam I find that you have a high fever and some fever blisters on your lip."

Mr. Brown: "Oh, so that's what those are."

Doctor: "Yes. This could be a problem with your immune system."

Mr. Brown: "You mean I have AIDS, don't you?"

Doctor: "Yes, it could be. But you need to have a blood test to be sure. I would also like to take a picture of your chest to look for pneumonia as well. I will also ask for a general blood test to make sure you are not dehydrated."

Mr. Brown: "Am I dying?"

Doctor: "What you have might be serious, but whatever we find, I'll be able to provide you with good treatment. I am very glad you came to see me today. I can help."

GRADING: STANDARDIZED PATIENT DATA-GATHERING CHECKLISTS

History Checklist

- ☑ **S**ymptoms: Fever, weight loss, swollen glands
- ☑ **S**ymptoms: SOB, cough (nonproductive), dysphagia
- ☑ **I**ntensity: How it is affecting his life—not able to work
- ☑ **O**nset: When did it start?
- ☑ **O**nset: Course
- ☑ **A**ggravating factors
- ☑ **A**lleviating factors
- ☑ **A**ssociated symptoms: If you realize this pt has HIV, ask about SX of AIDS
- ☑ **A**llergies
- ☑ **M**edications
- ☑ **P**MH: Hospitalizations
- ☑ **P**MH: Major illness, TB contacts
- ☑ **R**OS: Quantify weight loss
- ☑ **R**OS: GI—diarrhea
- ☑ **S**X: Sexually active
- ☑ **S**X: Multiple male partners
- ☑ **S**X: Unprotected sex
- ☑ **S**H: Works as social worker with children for state. Concerned that he has missed too much work.

Physical Exam Checklist

- ☑ **G**A: Height and weight
- ☑ **H**EENT: Observe lesions on lips
- ☑ **H**EENT: Inspect pharynx
- ☑ **H**EENT: Check for meningitis (supple neck)
- ☑ **H**EENT: Check for adenopathy
- ☑ **C**hest: Inspect chest
- ☑ **C**hest: Tactile fremitus
- ☑ **C**hest: Percussion
- ☑ **C**hest: Auscultation
- ☑ **C**V: Auscultation of heart
- ☑ **A**bd: Palpation
- ☑ **N**euro: Mental status alert
- ☑ **N**euro: Gait

CHALLENGING QUESTIONS

Mr. Brown: "Are you going to tell my employer? I work with children, you know."

Doctor: "What we discuss is confidential. I do want you to tell your sexual partners to come in and be tested. Will you be able to do that?"

Mr. Brown: "Yes."

Doctor: "Great. I'll have my nurse come in and take the blood sample now. Do you have time to do the picture of your chest now? The sooner we have the test results, the sooner we can start treatment."

Mr. Brown: "I guess so."

Doctor: "Fine. Do you have any other questions?"

Mr. Brown: "No."

Doctor: "So then I'll see you after the picture of your chest."

CASE DISCUSSION

Notes about the History-Taking

Pay close attention to any testing the patient states he previously had. In this case, Mr. Brown had a prior mono test that was negative. This is the Board's way of telling you that mononucleosis is a much less likely diagnosis and is not the cause of the patient's symptoms.

Notes about the Physical Exam

The sicker the case the SP is portraying, the harder it is to visualize. This patient is giving you historical symptoms strongly suggestive of pneumonia. However, the actor is not going to be able to simulate abnormal breath sounds. He probably will cough a couple of times during the exam to remind you he really has pneumonia-like signs and symptoms. Write on your note what you actually hear, feel, and percuss on the SP's chest. But don't be dissuaded from listing pneumonia on your diagnosis.

Comments about the Patient Note

Certainly, many types of HIV testing can be performed. These are not the only tests that would be accepted as correct answers. The same is true for the Differential Diagnosis list. For example, the diarrhea and decreased PO intake from the patient's esophagitis were never mentioned in the Differential Diagnosis. There may be 10 different diagnoses and 20 tests that would be considered acceptable. Always think in terms of the best initial tests that the patient needs. Do not worry about tests the patient may need later in his illness.

SAMPLE PATIENT NOTE

History: Include significant positives and negatives from history of present illness, past medical history, review of system(s), social history, and family history.

CC: Cough, fever, wt loss

HPI: 20-lb weight loss in 6 months. Illness began with fever, fatigue, and diffuse adenopathy. Three mo ago, started with nonproductive cough, SOB, DOE. Now with 2 weeks of oral sores, "cheesy" rash in mouth, and severe dysphagia. Pt spitting into cup to avoid swallowing. Pt has been missing a lot of work. Nothing seems to make it better or worse. Also has sores on lips, diarrhea lately. No syncope or confusion.

           Allergies: None

           Meds: Tylenol and Motrin for fever

PMH: Never hospitalized. No trauma or surgery. No TB, DM.

ROS: No trouble urinating

SX: Sexually active, multiple male partners. Doesn't always practice safe sex.

SH: Lives alone, works as social worker. No smoking, alcohol, IV, or rec drugs.

Physical Exam: Indicate only pertinent positive and negative findings related to patient's chief complaint.

VS: Temp: 102.2°F fever, pulx: 110, RR: 24, BP: 110/80

GA: Looks chronically ill

HEENT: 3–5-mm red lesions on vermillion border. Pharynx clear. Neck supple. No cervical, supraclavicular adenopathy.

Chest: Clear to A + P. Normal fremitus.

CV: Tachycardic. No obvious murmur, rub, or gallop.

Abd: Soft, nontender

Neuro: Pt alert, gait normal

Differential Diagnosis: In order of likelihood (with 1 being the most likely), list up to five potential or possible diagnoses for this patient's presentation. (In many cases, fewer than five diagnoses are likely.)

1. HIV/AIDS
2. Tuberculosis
3. Pneumocystis carinii pneumonia
4. Esophageal candidiasis
5. Herpes labialis

Diagnostic Workup: List immediate plans (up to five) for further diagnostic workup.

1. CXR, pulse Ox, sputum culture
2. Lytes, BUN, Cr, glucose, blood culture U/A
3. HIV-antibody (ELISA)
4. CD4, PPD
5. Upper endoscopy

Case 17: **Broken Nose**

DOORWAY INFORMATION

Opening Scenario

George Clark is a 19 y/o male who comes to the clinic complaining of a broken nose.

Vital Signs

- Temp: 37.0°C (98.6°F)
- BP: 130/82 mm Hg, right upper limb sitting
- HR: 74/min, regular
- RR: 16/min

Examinee Tasks

1. Obtain a focused history.
2. Perform a relevant physical examination. Do not perform rectal, pelvic, genitourinary, female breast, or corneal reflex examinations.
3. Discuss your initial diagnostic impression and your workup plan with the patient.
4. After leaving the room, complete your patient note on the given form.

BEFORE ENTERING THE ROOM

1. Cues: Write your mnemonics on your blue sheet (SIQORAAA and PAMHRFOSS). These mnemonics will remind you of other questions to ask, and will ensure that you don't skip pertinent aspects of the history.

2. Clinical Reasoning: Fracture of the nares is from trauma. You will have to find out the details of how this happened without being judgmental. Remember: If there is trauma to one part of the body, there may be trauma elsewhere. Trauma exams focus on inspection and palpation to uncover additional injuries.

FROM THE STANDARDIZED PATIENT

History

HPI: Mr. Clark comes in complaining of a black-and-blue nose. He thinks he was punched in the nose at a party last night but was really too drunk to remember. He thinks he got knocked out because he woke up in the morning on a couch with the bloody nose. He has a bit of a hangover and is complaining of a headache.

The patient's pain is about a 4 out of 10 on the pain scale. The pain is sharp and it does not move anywhere. Nothing else seems to hurt. It feels better if he applies ice on the face and worse if he tries to push on the nose, as when he wipes off the dried blood. He had a nosebleed earlier this morning when he blew his nose, but it stopped in a minute. There has been no change in vision and no weakness in arms or legs.

Patient does not feel confused. There has been no vomiting, nor has there been any chest, abdominal, back, or extremity pain. He does feel a little unsteady as he walks this morning. He was not incontinent of urine or stool last night and did not bite his tongue.

PMH: Mr. Clark has no allergies and takes Dilantin regularly. Mr. Clark was hospitalized for seizures last year. He has a seizure about every 6 months or so. No history of trauma, except for bumping his head when he has a seizure. No surgery. Mr. Clark has no history of diabetes or hypertension.

SH: Mr. Clark is on no special diet and does not take vitamins. There has been no change in his sleep pattern and he has no problems with urination. There was no blood in his urine this morning when he voided. Mr. Clark has smoked a pack of cigarettes a day since age 14. On the weekends, he drinks 6 to 12 cans a beer each Friday and Saturday night. On weekdays, he has just a couple of beers after work to unwind.

Patient is annoyed that his parents criticize his drinking. He does feel guilty about a couple of things he has done while intoxicated. Lately, he has just one beer in the morning to get the day started. He tells you he is "no drug addict" and does not use recreational drugs. He lives alone. His parents live upstairs in a two-bedroom flat. Over the past 6 months, he has spoken with them infrequently. Mr. Clark finished high school and now works as an apprentice electrician. He denies being sad, hopeless, or depressed. He states he is full of energy and ready for a good time.

Physical Exam

Patient has not washed up since the party and smells of stale beer and cigarettes. He is dirty and his shirt is torn. His nose is very tender and most likely broken. There is some dried blood on the philtrum, and because of the dried blood, there is limited air entry on the left. The rest of his face is nontender. There is no tenderness to the calvarium. His pupils are equal round and reactive to light. The fundi are flat. There is no hemotympanum. His teeth are intact. His neck is nontender.

Mr. Clark's chest has a normal appearance and normal respiratory excursion without pain to palpation. There is no pain to palpation of the spine and no costovertebral tenderness. There are no marks on his abdomen and it is nontender. There is full range of motion of his extremities. There are some bruises on the shoulders and lower legs. No bony tenderness. He is alert and oriented to person, place, and time. He has no facial asymmetry and his motor strength is equal, normal, and strong in all four extremities. His gait is ataxic.

THE CLOSING

Mr. Clark is somewhat confrontational from the start. He is testing you. If you keep a calm, professional demeanor while projecting your concern for his well-being, the patient will accept your direct diagnosis of alcoholism. If you appear angry, unsure of yourself, or judgmental, this conversation will escalate in a negative direction.

The counseling in this case can focus on the alcohol problem as well as the seizures. Seizure patients should be advised not to drive, to take showers instead of baths (to prevent drowning), to keep off ladders, and to avoid dangerous machinery.

Doctor: "Mr. Clark, I have finished your exam and I'd like to tell you what I'm thinking."

Mr. Clark: "Yeah, you're thinking I'm a failure!"

Doctor: "No, I think you have a broken nose and an alcohol problem."

Mr. Clark: "*I* knew that, and I haven't even gone to medical school!"

Doctor: "I want you to have a picture of your nose to see how bad it is. I also want to check a picture of your head, as it sounds like you passed out or were knocked out last night."

Mr. Clark: "To see if I have any brains?"

Doctor: "To make sure there was no brain injury. We also need to find out why you are so unsteady on your feet today. I'd like to do the tests now so we can begin any treatment immediately.

"Drinking alcohol and working with electricity is a dangerous combination. I would like for you to see our alcohol counselor. As far as having a possible seizure is concerned, I would like you to not drive a car until we know that the seizures are under control."

GRADING: STANDARDIZED PATIENT DATA-GATHERING CHECKLISTS

History Checklist

- ☑ Site: Trauma to nose
- ☑ Intensity: 4/10 pain
- ☑ Q: Sharp
- ☑ Onset: Last night
- ☑ R: No radiation
- ☑ A: Worse to the touch
- ☑ A: Better with ice
- ☑ Associated: +LOC
- ☑ PMH: Past history of seizures makes seizure or complication of seizure more likely
- ☑ ROS: Always a good idea to ask about hematuria in a possible trauma case
- ☑ Allergies
- ☑ Medications
- ☑ SH: Alcohol history, CAGE+, lives alone

Physical Exam Checklist

- ☑ General appearance

Inspection/Palpation:
- ☑ HEENT: Inspect and palpate
- ☑ Eyes: Fundi and pupils
- ☑ Ears: Inspect TMs
- ☑ Pharynx: Inspect tongue
- ☑ Neck: Check for c-spine fracture
- ☑ Chest: Inspect and palpate
- ☑ Abd: Inspect and palpate
- ☑ Back: Inspect and palpate
- ☑ Ext: Inspect and palpate

Neurological:
- ☑ Mental status
- ☑ CN VII
- ☑ Motor: All four extremities
- ☑ Gait

SAMPLE PATIENT NOTE

History: Include significant positives and negatives from history of present illness, past medical history, review of system(s), social history, and family history.

CC: Nose pain

HPI: Intoxicated last night + LOC. Possibly punched in nose, had epistaxis and sore, tender nose with no air entry L nostril. Pain is sharp, 4/10 intensity, and does not radiate. Denies any other pain in body or other injury. Pain worse with palpation, relieved with ice. Negative vomiting, confusion, incontinence, tongue biting. Positive ataxia, epistaxis.

PMH: NKMA, meds—Dilantin (good compliance)
Hospitalized for seizure in past. Has seizure about q 6 mo. No trauma other than when has seizure and hits head. Denies DM, HTN. No hx of surgery.

ROS: No change in sleep pattern, no special diet, denies hematuria

SH: Smokes 1 ppd, no recreational drugs. EtOH 6–12 beers each weekend night. Drinks in A.M. to "get the day started." CAGE+. Lives alone in apt with parents living upstairs—little contact. No sadness, hopelessness (but does feel guilty about drinking). Works as electrician, denies stress.

Physical Exam: Indicate only pertinent positive and negative findings related to patient's chief complaint.

VS: Vital signs NL, dirty clothes, nose ecchymotic with dried epistaxis

HEENT: Only nose is tender. Nontender to jaw, maxilla, and calvarium. PERRL. No hemotympanum. Pharynx and teeth intact, no tongue biting. Nose, decreased air entry on L.

Neck: Nontender, good ROM

Chest: No bruises, NL respiratory excursion, nontender to palpation

Back: No marks or tenderness to spine or CVA

Abd: Soft, nontender all 4 Q

Ext: Scattered bruises, nontender, full ROM

Neuro: A + O × 3, no facial asymmetry. Motor 5/5 all 4 ext, gait ataxic.

Differential Diagnosis: In order of likelihood (with 1 being the most likely), list up to five potential or possible diagnoses for this patient's presentation. (In many cases, fewer than five diagnoses are likely.)

1. Cerebral concussion
2. Fractured nares
3. Seizure disorder
4. Alcoholism
5. Dilantin toxicity

Diagnostic Workup: List immediate plans (up to five) for further diagnostic workup.

1. Head CT, plain brain
2. X-ray nasal bones
3. Dilantin level
4. CBC, INR
5. T. Bili, ALT, AST, EtOH

Mr. Clark: "Yeah, I lost my license from drinking anyway…"

Doctor: "Do you have any questions for me?"

CHALLENGING QUESTIONS

In the above conversation, the challenge is to not respond to the patient's sarcastic remarks or appear judgmental.

CASE DISCUSSION

Notes about the History-Taking

Eighteen years is the age of legal adulthood in most states. The SP probably will be a little older pretending to be a 19-year-old. Again, assume you have permission to do a history and physical on every SP you are given. The issues of adolescent history may be part of a case. In this particular case, however, there are plenty of other historical and physical findings to consider. If the patient said he remembered everything from last night and stated only that his nose was broken, you could focus your attention on the facial structures. In this particular case, he really doesn't know what happened. This is your clue to check over the entire body in general.

Notes about the Physical Exam

The physical exam of any possible trauma patient is centered about inspection and palpation of all the major areas of the body to find possible other injuries. If you find one area of tenderness, like the nose in this case, then slow down and palpate all the surrounding areas to determine the extent of injuries. With any head trauma, HEENT and neurological exams will be prominent. Do not forget to check the c-spine for tenderness to palpation. The CAGE questions can simply be charted "CAGE+" or "CAGE–," in order to save time.

Comments about the Patient Note

The first sentence from the patient gives you a clear indication of what this case is about. As with all cases, the pertinent negatives are very important in determining the cause. Mr. Clark may have had a seizure, an alcoholic blackout, and/or suffered trauma last night. To screen for seizure activity, ask about tongue biting and incontinence. Inspect the tongue as well.

His Differential Diagnosis includes blunt head trauma and seizure disorder, as well as possible side effects from Dilantin toxicity.

Workup for anyone with loss of consciousness and head trauma always includes neuroimaging. For acute trauma, CT is better than MRI because acute hemorrhage shows up better initially on CT.

Case 18: **Adolescent Weight Loss**

DOORWAY INFORMATION

Opening Scenario

Mr. Wright comes to the clinic to discuss his 16 y/o granddaughter, Amy, who is losing weight.

Vital Signs

N/A

Examinee Tasks

1. Obtain a focused history.
2. You will not be required to perform a physical examination in this case.
3. Discuss your initial diagnostic impression and your workup plan with the patient.
4. After leaving the room, complete your patient note on the given form.

BEFORE ENTERING THE ROOM

1. Cues: Assume that you have permission to treat all patients that are presented to you on Step 2 CS, and that you have permission to talk to family members. In this case, there are no vital signs because the patient is not present. Only a family member is available to describe what is happening with the patient. You will need a pediatric and adolescent history in place of the physical exam. The patient will have to be scheduled for a physical exam.

2. Clinical Reasoning: Causes of weight loss can include the following:

- Depression
- Anorexia nervosa
- Hyperthyroidism
- Drug use
- Cancer
- Diabetes

All of the above would be common possibilities. Having an idea of what causes common chief complaints makes it easier to ask relevant history and appropriate questions, especially during the associated symptoms. Getting some description of how much weight has been lost over what period of time will be important.

FROM THE GUARDIAN

History

HPI: Mr. Wright says he is Amy's grandfather and primary caretaker. Amy lives with him because her mother died last year after being hit by a drunk driver. Mr. Wright says Amy is a gymnast in high school and has a goal of being on the Olympic team. Mr. Wright says Amy seems to have recovered from the death of her mother, but she is not eating very much. She always says her coach wants her to keep her weight down. Mr. Wright estimates Amy has lost about 20 lb in the last 6 months. She is 5 feet 3 inches, and 105 lb. Sometimes she does go to the bathroom during dinner and comes back to the dinner table with red, blurry eyes. She denies vomiting. Amy complains of frequently feeling hot, as well as being sweaty a lot of the time. She drinks a lot of ice water to "cleanse her system."

Amy takes no medicine other that a multivitamin, and she has no allergies.

PMH: Amy has never been hospitalized and has had no surgery or trauma. She has never had any major illnesses.

ROS: Amy does seem to urinate frequently, however she has no burning or pain with urination. She is sleeping less than usual, now about 6 hours a night. She claims to be up doing homework. She has no constipation or diarrhea. She has two bowel movements a day. Mr. Wright does not know what happened to her father, who left 14 years ago. Amy's mother was healthy before the accident.

Ob/Gyn: Amy's periods have never been regular. Mr. Wright does think she had a period in the last few months but isn't sure. He doesn't think she is sexually active, as no boys call the house. Mr. Wright states Amy is a health enthusiast and would not smoke or use alcohol or drugs.

Amy is very concerned about her weight and looks, and feels she is still too fat to make the Olympic team. She realizes she must be strong also. Amy doesn't seem to enjoy the gymnastics team as much as she did a year ago. She still has periods of sadness over her mother's death 18 months ago. She has not been in contact with her friends outside of gymnastics. Her grades are slipping a little. Amy says classes are boring and she can't concentrate. Mr. Wright does not think that she ever has wanted to kill herself.

Physical Exam

There is no physical exam in this case, as the patient is not present.

THE CLOSING

Doctor: "Okay, Mr. Wright, I think I have the information I need. Is there anything else you would like to talk about?"

Mr. Wright: "No, I just want to see Amy doing better."

Doctor: "Yes. You told me she has lost 20 lb. Amy is still very concerned that she is too heavy to be a top gymnast?"

Mr. Wright: "That's correct."

Doctor: "Amy might have an eating disorder, or she might be depressed."

Mr. Wright: "That's what I thought when I researched her symptoms on the Internet."

Doctor: "There are other possibilities as well. We need to take a blood test to look at the minerals in her blood, and at her sugar and hormone levels. When can she come in for a physical exam?"

Mr. Wright: "Well, she's at school every day until 7 P.M. And I don't drive after dark."

Doctor: "How about this Saturday?"

Mr. Wright: "Sure."

Doctor: "Do you have any questions?"

CHALLENGING QUESTIONS

Mr. Wright: "Do you think Amy will need to be hospitalized?"

Answer: "I need to see Amy first and see the test results to know for sure what is best. Nothing you told me makes me think she needs to be in the hospital today, but I do need to examine her as soon as possible."

GRADING: STANDARDIZED PATIENT DATA-GATHERING CHECKLISTS

History Checklist

- ☑ **S**ymptom: How much weight has been lost?
- ☑ **I**ntensity: How is it affecting her life?
- ☑ **O**nset: When did the weight loss start?
- ☑ **A**lleviating factors
- ☑ **A**ggravating factors
- ☑ **A**ssociated symptoms: Ask about symptoms of diabetes, hyperthyroidism, and anorexia
- ☑ **P**revious episodes of the chief complaint
- ☑ **A**llergies
- ☑ **M**edication
- ☑ **P**MH: Hospitalizations, trauma, surgery
- ☑ **F**H: Death of mother
- ☑ **O**b/Gyn: LMP, regularity
- ☑ **S**exual Hx
- ☑ **S**ocial Hx: Lives with grandparents. No alcohol, smoking, or recreational drugs.

Adolescent Hx

- ☑ **B**ody image is poor
- ☑ **D**oing less well in school
- ☑ **F**ew friends, few activities outside of gymnastics
- ☑ **F**requently sad, not enjoying gymnastics.
- ☑ **N**o suicidal ideations.
- ☑ **C**oping strategies/Adjustment to deah of mother

SAMPLE PATIENT NOTE

History: Include significant positives and negatives from history of present illness, past medical history, review of system(s), social history, and family history.

CC: *Weight loss*

HPI: *20-lb weight loss in the last 6 mo. Now 5'3", 105 lb. Poor appetite. States wants to keep weight down for gymnastics team. Sometimes goes to bathroom during mealtime. Comes back to the table with red, watery eyes. She denies vomiting. Amy frequently feels hot; is frequently thirsty and drinks a lot of ice water.*

           NKMA; Meds: Multivitamin

PMH: *No hospitalizations, trauma, major illness, or surgery*

ROS: *Pt sleeping less than usual, about 6 hrs/night. No dysuria, hematuria. No constipation or diarrhea. Has 2 bowel movements/day.*

FH: *Amy's mother was healthy prior to her fatal car accident. No known hx for father.*

O: *LMP: Not sure, grandfather thinks maybe was a couple of months ago. Periods irregular.*

SX: *Grandfather does not think pt is sexually active*

SH: *Lives with grandparents after death of mother 18 mo ago. No alcohol, cigarettes, or recreational drugs. Poor body image, thinks she is still too heavy to make Olympic team. Does not seem to be enjoying gymnastics anymore, frequently sad. Has few friends, grades are dropping, and cannot concentrate. No known suicidal ideation.*

Physical Exam: Indicate only pertinent positive and negative findings related to patient's chief complaint.

There is no physical exam in this case.

Differential Diagnosis: In order of likelihood (with 1 being the most likely), list up to five potential or possible diagnoses for this patient's presentation. (In many cases, fewer than five diagnoses are likely.)

1. *Anorexia nervosa*
2. *Depression*
3. *Hyperthyroidism*
4. *Diabetes mellitus*
5. *Pregnancy*

Diagnostic Workup: List immediate plans (up to five) for further diagnostic workup.

1. *Physical exam*
2. *TSH*
3. *CBC, lytes, BUN, Cr, Glu*
4. *U/A, UCG*
5. *ß-hCG*

CASE DISCUSSION

Most of the Differential Diagnosis reflects possible organic causes of weight loss. Certainly diabetes, cancer, and hyperthyroidism are likely causes. Be sure to ask if the weight loss is intentional. Perhaps the patient is just dieting. Even if the cause of symptoms seem to be psychological, it is always correct to broaden your search for medical illnesses that might be causing psychiatric symptoms.

Notes about the History-Taking

Thinking about the common issues discussed in the adolescent history will also bring up possible diagnoses. Ask about self-esteem, depression, and eating disorders, as well as the social history. Finding out about what happened to Amy's parents is also important. In the closing you could mention sending Amy to a counselor, but it is essential to mention that you personally need to speak to and exam the patient.

Notes about the Physical Exam

There is no physical exam in this case.

Comments about the Patient Note

On the first line of the Diagnostic Workup, be sure to list that a physical exam is needed. Anyone with abnormal periods needs a pregnancy test to exclude pregnancy. Although SPs are not going to try to deceive you on your exam, pregnancy testing is one area where liberal testing frequently provides unexpected results.

SLEEP/SEX

INTEREST

GUILT

ENERGY

CONCENTRATION

APPETITE & WEIGHT

PSYCHOSIS & PSYCHOMOTOR

SUICIDE

Case 19: **Adolescent Depression**

DOORWAY INFORMATION

Opening Scenario

Mrs. Lewis comes to the clinic to discuss her 15 y/o daughter, Carol, who has seemed very unhappy recently.

Vital Signs

N/A

Examinee Tasks

1. Obtain a focused history.
2. You will not be required to perform a physical examination in this case.
3. Discuss your initial diagnostic impression and your workup plan with the patient.
4. After leaving the room, complete your patient note on the given form.

BEFORE ENTERING THE ROOM

1. Cues: This is another surrogate case. That means the parent or guardian is coming to speak to you about the patient. If you are given the patient's name but not the name of the surrogate, find out the name of the SP during the introduction so you know what to call her.

2. Clinical Reasoning: An adolescent history and social history will be required. You may already have a clue that this is a case about depression, based on the Doorway Information. You will need to ask about the following signs of depression.

The mnemonic for depression is SIGE CAPS:

S Sleep/Sexuality

> **Doctor:** "Has there been any change in how much you sleep?"

In any patient, too much sleep can be the result of depression, hypothyroidism, or drugs. Too little sleep can result from depression, bipolar disorder, hyperthyroidism, or drugs. Awaking early in the morning can be a sign of major depression.

> **Doctor:** "Has there been any change in your interest in sex?" (This question is for adult patients, not 15-year-olds.)

You will need to discuss confidentiality early in a suspected depression case. This way you will be able to gain the patient's confidence and then ask about sex. Patients with depression often lose interest in sex. Patients who have mania may be hypersexual compared to their baseline.

I Interest/Hope

> **Doctor:** "Have you lost interest in activities you enjoy? Do you feel hopeless?"

Patients with depression often lose interest in activities they used to find enjoyable.

G Guilt

> **Doctor:** "Do you feel guilty?"

E Energy

> **Doctor:** "How is your energy level?"

Patients with depression often exhibit psychomotor retardation. This is something you can observe and write in the Physical Exam notes under general appearance (GA). These people are often monotone, speak slowly, look sad, and take a little longer than usual to respond to verbal questions.

C Concentration

> **Doctor:** "Have you had any difficulties with concentration?"

Patients with depression have a hard time staying on task. You will test this with the Mini Mental Status exam (asking the patient to remember three words and to spell the word *world* backward). This diminished concentration is why depressed patients often fail in school and on the job.

A Appetite and Weight

> **Doctor:** "Has there been any change in your weight?"

Depression can cause weight loss or obesity. Eating disorders and obesity are common with depression.

P Psychosis/Psychomotor

> **Doctor:** "Sometimes when people are under a lot of stress, they hear things or see things that other people do not. Has this ever happened to you?"

Psychosis means hallucinations. This can be from depression, drugs, medical causes, or schizophrenia.

S Suicide

> **Doctor:** "Have you had any thoughts of harming or killing yourself?"

All depression checklists will make sure you ask this. Asking about suicidal intent *does not* cause suicide. If the patient answers "No" while making eye contact, you can take him at face value. If the patient becomes evasive, looks down or away, or won't answer at all, that is a positive response. Try responding with, "Tell me about it. I'm here to help."

FROM THE GUARDIAN

History

HPI: Mrs. Lewis has come to speak with you about her 15 y/o daughter Carol. She states that Carol is moody, cries frequently, and seems sad. She often says, "What's the use?" and storms off to her bedroom. She doesn't seem to enjoy anything or want to do anything. She has started sleeping 12 hours a day, compared to her usual 8 hours.

Mrs. Lewis asked Carol if she was thinking of suicide because she seemed so sad. Carol denied it but then wouldn't talk to her mother for 2 days. This has been going on for at least the past 3 months. It started rather suddenly, but the mother can't think of any precipitating factor. Nothing seems to make Carol better. Every time her mother tries to talk to her, it seems worse. Mrs. Lewis doesn't think her daughter is hearing any voices.

PMH: Carol has no allergies and takes no medication. Four months ago she went through a phase where she drank a lot of coffee to stay awake. She has had no medical or psychiatric hospitalizations, and no surgery, trauma, or major illness. She has never been depressed before. She has been eating less than usual at the dinner table and Mrs. Lewis says, "I think she may have lost some weight." Carol does not leave the table during dinner. Her body image is poor; she thinks she is ugly.

FH: There is a strong family history of depression. Mrs. Lewis states that she and all of her sisters have been depressed at some time in their lives. No history of bipolar disorder.

Ob/Gyn: Mrs. Lewis states that Carol does get her period but it is still somewhat irregular. She does not believe that Carol smokes, uses drugs, or is sexually active.

In fact, Carol has seemed to drift away from her friends and rarely leaves the house. Carol's grades are starting to slip, and she seems to have more absences for minor illness than usual. Carol lives with both of her parents and a younger brother.

Physical Exam

There is no physical exam in this case.

THE CLOSING

Doctor: "Mrs. Lewis, let me see if I can summarize what is going on with Carol."

Mrs. Lewis: "She's depressed?"

Doctor: "Right, she is often sad and tearful, sleeping more, missing some school, and feeling hopeless. She is just not enjoying life right now."

Mrs. Lewis: "That's right."

Doctor: "Of course, I'll need to do a physical exam as soon as possible, but I agree the most likely diagnosis is depression. I would like to check a blood test as well as look for other causes of depression."

CHALLENGING QUESTIONS

Mrs. Lewis: "What should I tell Carol about coming to the doctor? Should I say it's for a school physical?"

Answer: Honesty is the best policy. Whatever the cause, physical or emotional, explain that you can help.

Doctor: "I think you should tell her you are concerned and want the doctor to find out if anything is wrong."

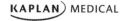

GRADING: STANDARDIZED PATIENT DATA-GATHERING CHECKLISTS

History Checklist

☑ **S:** Sleep/Sex
☑ **I:** Interest in activities
☑ **G:** Guilt
☑ **E:** Energy
☑ **C:** Concentration
☑ **A:** Appetite
☑ **P:** Psychomotor retardation/Psychosis
☑ **S:** Suicide

☑ **O**nset
☑ **A:** Nothing makes it better
☑ **A:** Nothing makes it worse
☑ **A**ssociated symptoms: SIGE CAPS and adolescent issues
☑ **A**ssociated: Recent stressor
☑ **A**llergies
☑ **M**edication
☑ **P**MH: Hospitalization, trauma, surgery
☑ **O**b/Gyn: LMP
☑ **S**X: Sexually active?
☑ **S**H: Alcohol, drugs

CASE DISCUSSION

Notes about the History-Taking

To organize your thoughts on this case you can collect the data you need in any order. It is correct to stick with the SAIQORAAA PAMHRFOSS format. You can ask about the signs of depression (SIGE CAPS) as the associated symptoms, or you may discuss them at the beginning or the history as symptoms. It would be equally correct to ask about SIGE CAPS if you did a formal adolescent history. If you have a plan on how you will approach this case as outlined above, you will not miss any of the important data.

Notes about the Physical Exam

There was no physical exam in this case.

Comments about the Patient Note

The Sample Note integrates most of the adolescent history into the standard History format. It would be equally correct to list the adolescent history as a separate heading.

Remember: Always consider pregnancy in a female of child-bearing age. That the patient also complained of mild nausea might also be a clue for pregnancy, though it is a rather subtle one.

SAMPLE PATIENT NOTE

History: Include significant positives and negatives from history of present illness, past medical history, review of system(s), social history, and family history.

CC: *15 y/o daughter with possible depression*

HPI: *Pt has 3 months of depressive symptoms and is frequently sad, tearful, with loss of interest in enjoyable activities. No precipitating factors identified. Has not been going out with friends and is starting to have more absences at school. No treatment so far. Nothing makes it better or worse.*
No suicidal ideations or hallucinations. + Feelings of hopelessness.

No meds, no allergies

PMH: *No past history of similar symptoms. No hospitalizations, trauma, or surgery.*

ROS: *Increase in sleep from 8 to 12 hours. Possible weight loss, + less appetite. Pt does not excuse herself from dinner table. Sometimes says she is nauseous.*

FH: *+ Depression. No bipolar disorder.*

SX: *Mother believes child is not sexually active. LMP irregular. Not sure when last period was.*

SH: *No smoking, drugs. Lives with both parents and younger brother.*

Physical Exam: Indicate only pertinent positive and negative findings related to patient's chief complaint.

There is no physical exam in this case.

Differential Diagnosis: In order of likelihood (with 1 being the most likely), list up to five potential or possible diagnoses for this patient's presentation. (In many cases, fewer than five diagnoses are likely.)

1. *Depression*
2. *Hypothyroidism*
3. *Pregnancy*
4.
5.

Diagnostic Workup: List immediate plans (up to five) for further diagnostic workup.

1. *Physical exam*
2. *CBC, glucose, TSH*
3. *ß-hCG*
4.
5.

Case 20: **Bed-Wetting in 7 y/o Child**

BEFORE ENTERING THE ROOM

1. Cues: From the Opening Scenario you cannot tell if this is a phone case or the mother came to speak to you in person. Knock on the door and enter as always. If it is a phone case you will not be graded lower for knocking.

2. Clinical Reasoning: You know that with pediatrics cases there will be no actual child SPs to examine.

Enuresis is a very common complaint in children. It is often not due to any medical or psychiatric illness, and most cases resolve spontaneously. As with any symptom, it is important to obtain the intensity, onset, and quantity, as well as any factors that make it better or worse. Ask about any recent stressors. When discussing associated symptoms, ask about dysuria, constipation, polyuria, polydipsia, and polyphagia.

While taking the past medical history, specifically ask about how the bed-wetting is affecting the child's self-esteem. Determine the parents' reaction to the bed-wetting, since emotional trauma inflicted by the parent(s) may be a larger problem than the dirty laundry. In place of the physical exam, a pediatric history will need to be completed. Counseling and teaching parents about enuresis during the closing will be a prominent component of this case. This is a great case to test your interpersonal and interviewing skills.

FROM THE GUARDIAN

History

HPI: Mrs. Jackson states that her son, Jason, has always been a bed-wetter. It has occurred since early childhood, and he's never been able to reliably stay dry through the night. Bed-wetting happens about once a week. It seems to happen more frequently when he stays with his grandparents. It is a bigger problem when he wets the bed at the grandparents' home because they criticize Jason about it. Mrs. Jackson has come to accept it and just knows she will frequently need to wash the sheets. The mattress is protected with a plastic cover that can be wiped down. Unfortunately, Mrs. Jackson has to travel on business frequently and the bed-wetting has become more of a source of conflict lately between the grandparents and grandchild. Not drinking fluids before bed sometimes prevents bed-wetting—but having a lot of liquids prior to bed doesn't always lead to bed-wetting. The Jacksons have tried having Jason urinate right before bed, and even setting the alarm clock for 2 A.M. so he can go to the bathroom. He has no dysuria, weight loss, or polydipsia. He has never fainted. Sometimes he needs to strain to have a bowel movement every 3 or 4 days.

PMH: Jason takes no prescription medications and has no allergies. He has never been hospitalized or had any surgery or trauma. His sleep pattern is normal and he does not snore. He sometimes complains of constipation or abdominal pain.

SH: Jason's father, who is currently deployed in Iraq, has a history of bed-wetting until he was 11 years old. There is increased stress at home worrying about Mr. Jackson. The grandparents never hit or scream at or act neglectful toward Jason, but Mrs. Jackson is aware of how their remarks about bed-wetting affect him.

Ped Hx: Mrs. Jackson tells you she received regular prenatal care during her pregnancy. She did not smoke or use drugs or alcohol. Jason was a full-term baby and delivered normally, no C-section. Jason weighed 7 lb 6 oz and was 21 inches at birth. He had no problems with jaundice, breathing, or eating, and she recalls they went home within 24 hours after his birth.

Jason was breast-fed, and weaned at age 8 months to milk and solid food. He now takes a pediatric vitamin every day and Mrs. Jackson states she tries to put nutritious food on the table. He eats a lot of cheese and frequently needs to strain when defecating. Jason started walking at age 1 year, and was toilet-trained by age 2.5 years (except for this bed-wetting problem). His immunizations are up to date. He gets regular pediatric checkups.

Physical Exam

There is no physical exam in this case.

THE CLOSING

> **Doctor:** "Mrs. Jackson, let me tell you what I am thinking, but first, let me make sure I have the facts correct."

> **Mrs. Jackson:** "Okay."

> **Doctor:** "Jason has been wetting the bed about once a week for his entire life. You are concerned that his grandparents—who take care of him sometimes—might hurt his self-esteem by criticizing him for bed-wetting."

> **Mrs. Jackson:** "That's right. They have been asking me repeatedly to come talk to you because they think something must be wrong with Jason."

> **Doctor:** "Well, as it sounds like you know, most cases of bed-wetting are just normal and the child eventually outgrows them."

Mrs. Jackson: "Yes, that's what my husband says and what I read online."

Doctor: "I would be happy to call your parents and speak with them if you think it will help."

Mrs. Jackson: "Oh, thank you, Doctor!"

Doctor: "I also want to see Jason for a physical exam, and I will check his urine. Right now, the other thing is to suggest that Jason eat more vegetables and fruit and a little less cheese. Sometimes constipation can make this problem worse. Do you have any questions for me?"

CHALLENGING QUESTIONS

Mrs. Jackson: "I've read there are some medicines that prevent bed-wetting. Can you give me a prescription?"

Answer: "I need to examine Jason and collect a urine sample to find out if any medicine is needed. Usually, bed-wetting is just a normal developmental stage and medicine is not needed, but I need to examine him to be sure. Can you bring him in tomorrow?"

GRADING: STANDARDIZED PATIENT DATA-GATHERING CHECKLISTS

History Checklist

- ☑ Symptom
- ☑ Intensity: How is this problem affecting you and your child?
- ☑ Q: Any burning, blood in urine? How frequently does Jason go during the day?
- ☑ O: When did it start? How often does it happen?
- ☑ Percipitating factor: What was going on in his life when it started?
- ☑ A: Does anything make it better?
- ☑ A: Does anything make it worse?
- ☑ A: Has Jason had any burning with urination? Fainting?
- ☑ ROS: Ask about sleep, bowel habits, weight change, fever
- ☑ PMH
- ☑ FH: Family history must be asked, since enuresis can be genetic
- ☑ SH: Who does the child live with?
- ☑ SH: What is parents' reaction to bed-wetting (stress at home)?

Pediatric/Adolescent History:

- ☑ Prenatal
- ☑ Birth
- ☑ Feeding
- ☑ Growth and development
- ☑ Routine care: Immunizations
- ☑ School performance
- ☑ Self-esteem/depression screen

SAMPLE PATIENT NOTE

History: Include significant positives and negatives from history of present illness, past medical history, review of system(s), social history, and family history.

CC: *7 y/o son with enuresis*

HPI: *Since toilet-trained at age 2.5 yrs, wets bed about once a week. Mother states grandparents sometimes "belittle" the child regarding enuresis. Mother has no other concerns regarding grandparents' care of child. Nothing reliably makes it better or worse. No dysuria, fainting, polyuria, or polydipsia. No fever. Has bowel movement every 3–4 days. Sometimes constipated.*

           Allergies: None

           Meds: Pediatric vitamins

PMH: *No hospitalizations, trauma, or surgery*

ROS: *Sleeps 9 hours a night, no snoring. No weight loss. Eats a lot of cheese. Has bowel movement q 3–4 d.*

FH: *Father wet bed until age 11*

SH: *Jason lives with mother. Father is a soldier in Iraq. Some increased stress. Mother does not punish child for bed-wetting.*

Ped Hx: *Full-term vaginal delivery. + Prenatal care. No drugs or alcohol. No complications in neonatal period. Toilet-trained at 2.5 yrs and walked at 12 months. Immunizations are up to date.*

Physical Exam: Indicate only pertinent positive and negative findings related to patient's chief complaint.

There is no physical exam in this case.

Differential Diagnosis: In order of likelihood (with 1 being the most likely), list up to five potential or possible diagnoses for this patient's presentation. (In many cases, fewer than five diagnoses are likely.)

1. *Primary nocturnal enuresis*
2. *Constipation*
3. *Cystitis*
4.
5.

Diagnostic Workup: List immediate plans (up to five) for further diagnostic workup.

1. *Schedule child for physical exam*
2. *U/A*
3.
4.
5.

CASE DISCUSSION

Notes about the History-Taking

All enuresis cases require a family history because primary nocturnal enuresis is genetic. Always ask about dietary history, since constipation is another cause of enuresis. Cystitis is also a common cause of enuresis, so be sure to ask about symptoms of a urinary tract infection. In this case, enuresis has been persistent rather than secondary or new-onset, making cystitis much less likely.

Other, less common subjects you may ask about include snoring, since sleep-disordered breathing is another cause of enuresis; and gait, which will help you identify a possible neurogenic bladder (for example, meningomyelocele can cause gait disturbance with a neurogenic bladder).

You'll want to ask about fainting because seizure from a neuro or cardiac cause can lead to incontinence. Thyroid disease and diabetes are two endocrine causes of enuresis.

Psychological stress may also be a cause in this case, and is more likely if the child's bed-wetting began only after his father went to war. It is important to take the social history, and also to understand the parents' response to bed-wetting.

Notes about the Physical Exam

There is no physical exam in this case. It is acceptable to write the pediatric history in the Physical Exam section if you find that you are out of space in the History section. The doctors grading your note will be able to figure this out.

Comments about the Patient Note

A physical exam and U/A are required on all cases of enuresis. Other tests may be ordered.

Besides the physical exam and bladder ultrasound, a voiding cystourethrogram may also be done. If the enuresis patient has difficulty walking, that may be a clue for neurogenic bladder. In this case do urodynamic studies of the bladder and MRI of the spine.

In this particular case, the bed-wetting is probably genetic and the patient has no problem with gait. Therefore, no MRI or urodynamic studies are indicated.

Case 21: **Shortness of Breath in 9 y/o Child**

DOORWAY INFORMATION

Opening Scenario

Mark Thompson is a 9 y/o male whose grandmother comes to the clinic because the child is coughing and short of breath.

Vital Signs

N/A

Examinee Tasks

1. Obtain a focused history.
2. You will not be required to perform a physical examination in this case.
3. Discuss your initial diagnostic impression and your workup plan with the patient.
4. After leaving the room, complete your patient note on the given form.

BEFORE ENTERING THE ROOM

1. Cues: Use the blue sheet to write down any information you want to remember. The patient's name can be jotted down if you have a hard time remembering it. For a 9-year-old child, the pediatric history will need to be taken in the time usually allotted for the physical exam. Find out the name of the grandmother during the introduction so you know what to call her. After you introduce yourself ask "What is your name please?" if the SP does not spontaneously volunteer her name.

2. Clinical Reasoning: Shortness of breath can be from an airway, pulmonary, or cardiac cause. Less common causes would be anemia or ASA poisoning. In fact, anything that gives a metabolic acidosis can make the patient short of breath. The history of cough suggests that a pharynx, airway, and pulmonary diagnosis is more likely. Remember: The Board is most likely to test common problems that patients present with, so pharyngitis, pneumonia, and asthma all go to the top of the list.

FROM THE GUARDIAN

History

HPI: This is a surrogate case, and Mrs. Thompson is in the exam room without the patient. She tells you that her grandson, Mark, has a cough that is dry, with no sputum. He seems to have had it most of the winter. In fact, every time he gets a cold he seems to be coughing and occasionally short-winded for months afterward. This has been going on for several years.

Mark only rarely complains of being short of breath, although he tries to get out of gym class whenever he can. He has stopped playing soccer. He frequently refuses to go outside and play with his friends. He has never turned blue, but sometimes feels like everything is tight in his chest. It gets better when he rests. He feels worse in the cold air in winter (they live in Chicago). Also, sometimes when he visits his aunt, who has multiple cats, he feels worse, has trouble breathing, and gets watery eyes. There is no fever. Mark has occasional sore throats. No sharp pain in the chest. No rash. It seems as if he has had these symptoms off and on for years.

Allergies: Aspirin

Medications: None

PMH: Mark has never been hospitalized. He had to go to the clinic and emergency department for bronchiolitis a couple of times when he was an infant. He has never had any trauma or surgery. No history of diabetes.

FH: The only family member who has lung problems is Mrs. Thompson, who has a touch of "emphysema." That is because she smokes. She tries not to smoke around Mark, as it makes his cough and breathing worse.

SH: Mark's weight has not changed lately. He has no special diet. Lately, he has been waking up tired and with a headache. Mrs. Thompson has noticed he snores a lot lately.

Mark lives with his grandmother. He has never known his father, and his mother died 18 months ago after a drug overdose. Mrs. Thompson states that they both miss Mark's mother.

Mark's mother smoked and drank alcohol during pregnancy. Mark was 4 weeks premature and was in the hospital for 1 week at birth. He had jaundice at birth that responded to being "under lights." He had no trouble breathing. Mark was bottle-fed, and showed normal growth and development. Immunizations are up to date. He started doing poorly in school after his mother's death.

The counselor at school wants him to get a tutor to help with his reading. Mark feels sad frequently. He never talks about harming himself but sometimes makes drawings depicting violent scenes.

Physical Exam

There is no physical exam in this case.

THE CLOSING

> **Doctor:** "Mrs. Thompson, thank you for coming to see me today. It seems we have two problems we need to help Mark with. First, we need to find out why he is always coughing and somewhat short of breath. Second, it sounds like Mark is still very sad over his mother's death and needs help coping. Do I have it right?"
>
> **Mrs. Thompson:** "Yes, Doctor."

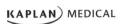

Doctor: "I think the breathing problem could be from infection but is more likely from asthma, based on what I know so far. Also, I'm concerned that Mark may be depressed. I would like to see Mark for a physical exam as soon as possible. I will take a picture of his chest and a breathing test. Also, I agree that a counselor is a good idea for Mark. I have a list of several excellent counselors that work with grieving children. Do you have any questions?"

In this closing, the caretaker says she is going to get spiritual help to handle the boy's depression. To deal with this challenge, you do not need to evaluate her beliefs. Remember: A good physician is nonjudgmental. Just stick to your conviction that a mental health counselor can help. Simply tell the patient that in addition to what she is already doing, you would like the child to see a counselor.

CHALLENGING QUESTIONS

Mrs. Thompson: "I have no health insurance and cannot pay for counseling. I take him to church every Sunday and get some help there."

Doctor: "In addition to church, I believe mental health counselors can help. I can have you speak with our social worker, who can help arrange for financial aid."

Mrs. Thompson: "Do you mean like welfare?"

Doctor: "Well, yes. I think we should do everything we can to help Mark."

Mrs. Thompson: "Okay. When you put it that way, I guess I'll have to swallow my pride and accept it."

GRADING: STANDARDIZED PATIENT DATA-GATHERING CHECKLISTS

History Checklist

- ☑ Symptom: Cough and shortness of breath
- ☑ Intensity: Not playing
- ☑ Onset: When did it start?
- ☑ Onset: Frequency (lasts for months after a URI)
- ☑ A: Better with rest
- ☑ A: Worse with exposure to cold, cats, smoke, exercise
- ☑ A: No fever, no sputum
- ☑ Allergies
- ☑ Medications
- ☑ Hospitalizations
- ☑ Trauma
- ☑ Surgery
- ☑ ROS: Sleep
- ☑ ROS: Diet
- ☑ FH: Family hx of asthma or lung problems
- ☑ SH: Lives with grandma, parents deceased

Pediatric/Adolescent History:

- ☑ Prenatal
- ☑ Birth
- ☑ Feeding
- ☑ Growth and development
- ☑ Routine care: Immunizations
- ☑ School performance
- ☑ Self-esteem/depression screen

SAMPLE PATIENT NOTE

History: Include significant positives and negatives from history of present illness, past medical history, review of system(s), social history, and family history.

CC: *9 y/o male with chronic cough and dyspnea*

HPI: *Dry, nonproductive cough and dyspnea for several years. Lasts for months at a time, occurring after a URI.*
- *Prevents him from playing sports*
- *Exertion, cold air, smoke, and cats make it worse*
- *Rest makes it better*
- *No fever, rash, or sore throat*
- *+ Chest "tight" feeling at times. Occasional sore throats.*

Allergies: Cats, aspirin

Meds: None

PMH: *Bronchiolitis as infant. No trauma or surgery.*

ROS: *Pt on no special diet. Sleep disturbed from "snoring."*

FH: *No family hx of asthma; grandma with emphysema*

SH: *Lives with grandmother. Mother died 18 months ago (drug overdose). Pt never knew father.*

Ped Hx: *Mother used alcohol and smoked during pregnancy. Pt was 4 weeks premature. No respiratory distress at birth. Did have jaundice. Normal growth and development. Immunizations are up to date.*

Pt has been depressed since death of mother. Has been doing poorly in school. Has not yet received counseling. Has not talked about harming himself but does occasionally draw violent pictures.

Physical Exam: Indicate only pertinent positive and negative findings related to patient's chief complaint.

There is no physical exam in this case.

Differential Diagnosis: In order of likelihood (with 1 being the most likely), list up to five potential or possible diagnoses for this patient's presentation. (In many cases, fewer than five diagnoses are likely.)

1. *Asthma*
2. *Pharyngitis/tonsillitis*
3. *Pneumonia*
4. *Depression*
5. *Grief reaction*

Diagnostic Workup: List immediate plans (up to five) for further diagnostic workup.

1. *Physical exam*
2. *Peak flow spirometry*
3. *CXR*
4. *Rapid strep*
5.

CASE DISCUSSION

Notes about the History-Taking

During the introduction, find out how the adult is related to the child. For the Step 2 CS, you are asked to assume that you have permission to talk about and treat all patients. A handshake would be appropriate, as Mrs. Thompson is in no distress.

A fairly complete HPI and PMH are needed. During the Family History you could ask directly about and history of asthma or lung disease.

The pediatric history is also important. Some typical adolescent issues surface in this case, such as school performance and depression. Feel free to combine some of the pediatric and adolescent histories as they seem relevant in cases that involve children.

Notes about the Physical Exam

There was no physical exam in this case.

Comments about the Patient Note

As much as possible, speak in lay terminology and write your notes in medical terminology. However, if you do not know the medical term for something, it is also correct to use lay terminology in your note. The physician grading the note knows both terms. As long as you are communicating in written form, you will get credit on the note and increase your ICE score.

In the Differential Diagnosis, list common possibilities. For Step 2 CS, get used to writing differentials and diagnostic workups on patients you have not even examined. In cases where there is no physical exam, the Differential Diagnosis must be construed completely from the history. Even in cases where you do a physical exam, the Differential Diagnosis is based mostly on the history, and the physical exam just confirms your suspicions.

Case 22: **Cancer Checkup**

DOORWAY INFORMATION

Opening Scenario

Nancy Young is a 50 y/o female who comes to the clinic for a checkup.

Vital Signs

- Temp: 36.9°C (98.3°F)
- BP: 122/80 mm Hg
- HR: 80/min
- RR: 16/min

Examinee Tasks

1. Obtain a focused history.
2. Perform a relevant physical examination. Do not perform rectal, pelvic, genitourinary, female breast, or corneal reflex examinations.
3. Discuss your initial diagnostic impression and your workup plan with the patient.
4. After leaving the room, complete your patient note on the given form.

BEFORE ENTERING THE ROOM

1. Cues: Upon first reading the Doorway Information, you will see that this is someone coming for a health maintenance visit. For this sort of case, history and physical and tests need to be directed toward finding preventable causes of death. The most common causes of death relate to the cardiovascular system and cancers. For this reason, most of your effort will be spent reviewing cardiovascular risk factors and cancer screening. You will also need to ask about other specific symptoms and address any specific concerns the patient may have.

2. Clinical Reasoning: To prevent cancer and cardiovascular disease, you must ask about tobacco use and recreational drugs. You will likely need to instruct the patient to limit alcohol intake, and to control hypertension, diabetes, and obesity. You will have to ask the patient's height and weight. For cardiovascular diseases, a few screening questions about dyspnea and pain should suffice. The physical will have to be directed toward the cardiovascular exam. Lab tests will need to include possibly a baseline ECG, certainly a lipid panel. Check renal function, and screen for diabetes. Have low threshold to send the patient for stress testing.

For cancer screening cases, the history may also include the general symptoms of fever, fatigue, pain, and weight loss. More specific signs that the lay public knows because of the efforts of the American Cancer Society are listed here.

- Change in bowel habits or bladder function
- Sores that do not heal
- Unusual bleeding or discharge
- Thickening or lump in breast or other parts of the body
- Indigestion or trouble swallowing
- Recent change in a wart or mole
- Nagging cough or hoarseness

Reprinted by the permission of the American Cancer Society, Inc. from *www.cancer.org*. All rights reserved.

The physical exam will be directed toward looking at the skin, oral pharynx, thyroid, and checking for swollen lymph glands.

FROM THE STANDARDIZED PATIENT

History

HPI: Mrs. Young has made an appointment for a checkup. She recently had her 50th birthday and realizes she needs to start taking care of herself. She has avoided going to the doctor for many years. She feels fine but is concerned about her health since so many of her family and friends have had heart disease and cancer. Upon questioning, there is no specific symptom troubling her now.

> **Doctor:** "Thank you for coming in for a checkup. It is so much easier to treat problems if you find them early. Is there anything that's troubling you?"
>
> **Mrs. Young:** "No, I just want to do any screening tests I need, and the peace of mind from being examined."
>
> **Doctor:** "Certainly."

Mrs. Young has had no cough, hoarseness, shortness of breath, or chest pain. She has no leg swelling. She has had no change in her weight and no fatigue or fevers. She has no problems urinating and has not had any blood in her stool or change in her bowel habits. She has no trouble swallowing. She has not noticed any change in her skin or any new lumps or bumps. She does not do self breast exams.

Allergies: Ragweed and pollen

Meds: Multivitamin, vitamin C, fish oil, garlic, and glucosamine. She takes all this just because she thinks it will help her live to an old age.

She has been hospitalized only twice briefly, for childbirth. She has had no trauma other than a broken wrist as a child when she fell off the monkey bars. No surgery. No history of diabetes or hypertension. She has never had her cholesterol checked.

There has been no change in her sleep pattern (8 hours). She tries to eat fresh fruits and vegetables, and has given up fast food. She still has an extra-large double-espresso coffee every morning.

Her father died at age 65 of colon cancer and her mother died at age 64 of heart disease. The mother smoked heavily and had diabetes for 25 years.

LMP: One week ago, normal. No hot flashes or moodiness. G2P2.

Sexual Hx: Sexually active with her husband of 30 years. She uses a diaphragm for contraception.

SH: Stopped smoking 20 years ago, 10-pack-year total. 1 glass of wine on special occasions. She works as the manager of a health club and still exercises three times a week. She is married, has two children in college, and thinks she is dealing with being an empty-nester pretty well.

Physical Exam

Mrs. Young is 5 feet 2 inches and weighs 130 lb. She is smiling and is in no acute distress. There are no suspicious lesions on her skin. Her pupils are equal round and reactive to light. Her mouth, tongue, and pharynx are normal. Palpation of the thyroid reveals no abnormalities. There is normal anterior and posterior cervical chain as well as normal supraclavicular and axillary lymph nodes. No jugular venous distension. Carotid upstrokes are normal and without bruits. The lungs are clear to auscultation.

Heart tones are normal. The point of maximum impulse is not displaced. The abdomen is soft and nontender, without masses. The extremities appear normal. Distal radial and tibial pulses are normal. Good range of motion at knees, shoulder, and wrists, without any redness or deformity. Her gait is normal.

THE CLOSING

Doctor: "Mrs. Young, I have finished your physical exam. Why don't I help you to sit up so that you are comfortable."

Mrs. Young: "All right." [assist patient into sitting position]

Doctor: "Let me review what you have told me. You are here for a checkup. You feel fine and take no prescription medicine."

Mrs. Young: "That's right."

Doctor: "Your weight, blood pressure, and heart rate are normal. In fact, I find no problems on your physical exam. Your exam is normal."

Mrs. Young: *(Smiling)* "I feel better already!"

Doctor: "I would like you to have the standard health screening tests."

Mrs. Young: "Like what?"

Doctor: "We should check your blood for cholesterol. I also recommend a Pap smear, a mammogram, and a colonoscopy. Do you have any questions?"

CHALLENGING QUESTIONS

Mrs. Young: "Now I'm a little nervous."

Doctor: "How so?"

Mrs. Young: "Colonoscopy is how they found my father's colon cancer."

Doctor: "Colonoscopy is good because it can find easily treatable polyps long before they turn cancerous."

Mrs. Young: *(Sighs)* "Okay, let's do it as soon as possible."

Doctor: "Great. I will call you with the results immediately so you won't be worried."

Mrs. Young: "Thank you, Doctor."

GRADING: STANDARDIZED PATIENT DATA-GATHERING CHECKLISTS

History Checklist

- ☑ HPI: Ask if the patient has any symptoms at all
- ☑ Associated symptoms: Screening questions for cardiovascular disease
- ☑ Associated symptoms: Screening questions for cancer
- ☑ Allergies
- ☑ Medications
- ☑ PMH: Hospitalizations
- ☑ PMH: Major illness
- ☑ PMH: Trauma and surgery
- ☑ ROS: Sleep
- ☑ ROS: GI
- ☑ ROS: Urinary
- ☑ FH: Find out if hx of heart disease or cancer
- ☑ Ob/Gyn: LMP; Gravida, Para
- ☑ Ob/Gyn: Any unusual bleeding. Menopausal symptoms.
- ☑ SX: ask general questions about sexual activity.
- ☑ SH: Drugs, alcohol, and tobacco products (think oral cancer from chewing tobacco)
- ☑ SH: Diet and exercise
- ☑ SH: Home life/work life/stress

Physical Exam Checklist

- ☑ GA: Height, weight, vital signs
- ☑ Skin: Can make separate heading or talk about inspection of each part of the body
- ☑ HEENT: Pharynx
- ☑ HEENT: Thyroid
- ☑ HEENT: Adenopathy
- ☑ CV: Auscultate heart
- ☑ CV: JVD
- ☑ CV: PMI
- ☑ CV: Carotid, radial, DP, PT pulse
- ☑ Chest: Auscultate
- ☑ Abd: Inspect and palpate
- ☑ Ext: ROM few major joints
- ☑ Neuro: Gait

CASE DISCUSSION

Notes about the History-Taking

This is one of the healthiest SPs you'll ever meet. The key is to write in the HPI that the patient has no chief complaint; she is here only for a periodic health exam. There is nothing on which to do SIQORAA. The associated symptoms are simply the screening questions for cancer and asking about a few cardiovascular symptoms. This patient probably takes more vitamins and supplements than she needs. Generally, you should tell her to stop only if you see a contraindication.

Notes about the Physical Exam

As in many Step 2 CS cases, this physical exam highlights the skin. This physician chooses to list skin as a separate organ system to highlight the fact he is looking for skin cancers. Be sure to document the presence or absence of any abdominal masses as well.

SAMPLE PATIENT NOTE

History: Include significant positives and negatives from history of present illness, past medical history, review of system(s), social history, and family history.

CC: Checkup

HPI: Mrs. Young (age 50) has no complaints. States has not seen a doctor in years and needs a checkup. She has no chest pains or SOB. Neg dysphagia, cough, hoarseness, weight loss, bowel or urine problems. No masses or skin changes.

Allergies: Ragweed and pollen

Meds: OTC garlic, vitamins, glucosamine, fish oil, Vit C

PMH: Hospitalized only for childbirth. Fractured arm as child. No surgeries.

DM: HTN or heart disease. Has not had cholesterol checked.

ROS: No change in sleep pattern. Diet: Has recently stopped eating fast food. Tries to eat five fruits and vegetables/day.

FH: Parents deceased. Dad; colon Ca age 65. Mom; heart, DM, age 64, smoker.

ObGyn: LMP 1 wk ago, NL. G2P2. No menopausal symptoms. No abnormal bleeding.

SX: Active, uses diaphragm, one partner

SH: Lives with husband, works as health club manager. Exercises regularly. Not feeling stressed. No rec drugs or tobacco. No significant use of EtOH.

Physical Exam: Indicate only pertinent positive and negative findings related to patient's chief complaint.

VS: WNL. Reports 5'2", 130 lb.

GA: NAD

Skin: No abnormal moles or skin changes

HEENT: PERRL. Pharynx: Clear. Nares: Clear. No increased cervical, supraclavicular, or axillary adenopathy.

Thyroid: WNL. Carotid upstroke NL without bruit.

Chest: Clear to Auscultation

CV: S1, S2 WNL, no S3, S4, or murmur. No JVD, PMI not displaced. Radial, DP, PT pulse 2/4 B/L.

Abd: Soft, nontender, no masses

Ext: NL, no edema. Full ROM shoulder, wrists, and knees without redness or deformity.

Gait: WNL

Differential Diagnosis: In order of likelihood (with 1 being the most likely), list up to five potential or possible diagnoses for this patient's presentation. (In many cases, fewer than five diagnoses are likely.)

1. Periodic health exam
2. Hx of environmental allergies
3.
4.
5.

Diagnostic Workup: List immediate plans (up to five) for further diagnostic workup.

1. Breast and pelvic exam, stool for occult blood
2. Pap smear
3. Mammography
4. Colonoscopy
5. CBC, BUN, Cr, glucose tolerance, chol, HDL, LDL, TG

Comments about the Patient Note

There really isn't much to diagnose in this patient. It is fine to leave the remainder of the diagnosis lines blank if nothing is appropriate.

Mrs. Young's workup first includes the physical exam that are forbidden on the test: specifically, you are not allowed to perform female breast exam, pelvic exam or rectal exam. She also needs a fecal occult blood test (FOBT).

Screening exams are for people who are completely asymptomatic. Yearly mammography can start at age 40. Annual Pap smears should begin no later than age 21, or sooner if the woman is sexually active. Regular colonoscopy screening should start at age 50 unless patient is in a high-risk group.

Had this been a male patient, you should have recommended annual prostate-specific antigen (PSA) testing, which should begin at age 50. A complete GU, rectal, and testicle exam would be indicated as well.

Case 23: **Health Fair Referral**

DOORWAY INFORMATION

Opening Scenario

Larry Mitchell is a 52 y/o male who comes from a health fair with a note from the nurse.

Vital Signs

Health fair note has documented the following:
- BP: 150/90 mm Hg
- Cholesterol: 220 mg/dl
- Glucose: 90 mg/dl

Vital signs at your office:
- Temp: 37.0°C (98.6°F)
- BP: 148/88 mm Hg
- HR: 90/min
- RR 16/min

Examinee Tasks

1. Obtain a focused history.
2. Perform a relevant physical examination. Do not perform rectal, pelvic, genitourinary, female breast, or corneal reflex examinations.
3. Discuss your initial diagnostic impression and your workup plan with the patient.
4. After leaving the room, complete your patient note on the given form.

BEFORE ENTERING THE ROOM

1. Cues: This patient had his blood pressure checked, and gave a drop of blood each to check his total cholesterol and blood sugar. Health fairs are usually done at work, at churches, or even at shopping malls. There is no doctor on site at these fairs, so all patients are asked to follow up with a physician.

2. Clinical Reasoning: You will have noticed prior to meeting the patient that he has elevated total cholesterol (>200 mg/dl) and elevated blood pressure documented at the health fair and at your office. You will have to ask this patient if he has any acute or chronic health complaints you can help him with. If he has any additional symptoms besides what was listed on the health fair note, focus on the symptoms he tells you about. If he has no symptoms or additional chief complaints, focus solely on asking about complications of hyperlipidemia and hypertension. This patient has now had two readings of elevated blood pressure. Most likely, you will find complications of hypertension and/or hyperlipidemia and you will need to address these complications in the HPI and ROS. This may also be a case of new-onset hypertension.

FROM THE STANDARDIZED PATIENT

History

HPI: Mr. Mitchell went to the health fair because he felt he should "get checked out." He occasionally gets pain in his upper abdomen and at times underneath the right rib cage. The pain can be from 1/10 to 4/10 and lasts anywhere from a few minutes to a few hours. It feels like a "hot" pain, and it started about 3 months ago. Now the pain occurs a few times a week and seems to be getting worse in intensity and duration. It sometimes moves to his back just at the right shoulder blade. He notices it more after eating fatty foods. It seems better when he takes some Tylenol or ibuprofen. He has no chest pain, SOB, vomiting, diarrhea, dysuria, or rash.

The pain does not get worse when he walks, and bending over exacerbates the pain. He also had a low-grade fever last week but he didn't measure his temperature. There has been no black or red bowel movement and no other change in his bowel movement pattern.

He takes no medicine regularly and has no allergies.

PMH: Patient has never experienced this before, and has not seen a doctor since he was released from the U.S. Army 30 years ago. He was hospitalized once for appendicitis 35 years ago. He has had no trauma or other surgery. He denies any history of DM, HTN, or heart disease.

Family Hx: Patient's parents both smoked heavily and died in their early 70s from heart disease and cancer.

SHx: He has not had any change in his sleep pattern, his weight has been slowly increasing each year, and he has no problem urinating. He is sexually active when he has a girlfriend. He is single at the moment.

Social Hx: He is divorced and sells cars for a living. He stopped smoking 20 years ago. Never used recreational drugs. Has two beers about three times a week. He does not get annoyed at those who criticize his drinking and does not feel guilty. He doesn't drink in the morning and has not tried to cut back.

Physical Exam

Mr. Mitchell is 6 feet 2 inches and 240 lb. He is in no distress. He last had the upper abdominal pain for most of the night after a pepperoni pizza for dinner 2 nights ago, but now the pain is now gone. His skin has normal color and there is no makeup on him to indicate that he is jaundiced. His pharynx is clear. Carotid upstrokes are normal without bruits. His lungs are clear. There is no jugular venous distention. Heart tones are normal. Abdomen is obese. He had mild epigastric tenderness. There is no rebound. Murphy's sign is negative.

The patient is alert. There is no pain when the RUQ is palpated and the patient inhales. His bowel sounds are normal and there is normal tympany to all four quadrants with percussion. There is no back tenderness. Extremities reveal no edema, nor does he feel weakness in any of them. His gait is normal.

THE CLOSING

Doctor: "Mr. Mitchell, I'd like to tell you what I am thinking. First, let me make sure I understand. You have an elevated blood pressure reading and a high cholesterol. You have also had a stomachache that has been getting worse over the past 3 months. Is that correct?"

Mr. Mitchell: "Yes."

Doctor: "On your physical exam, I find that your blood pressure reading is a little high. You also are tender in your belly. I think this pain in your belly might be from infection or from acid in the stomach. I'd like you to have blood tests today to find out the cause. It really does not sound like your heart, but I will take a heart test as well as a more complete cholesterol test to make sure there is no heart problem. We will meet again to discuss the results and plan treatment. Do you have any questions?"

Mr. Mitchell: "Do I have high blood pressure?"

GRADING: STANDARDIZED PATIENT DATA-GATHERING CHECKLISTS

History Checklist

- ☑ Site of pain
- ☑ Intensity: Pain scale 1–10
- ☑ Quality: What does it feel like?
- ☑ Onset: When did it start?
- ☑ Onset (course): Is it getting better or worse?
- ☑ Onset (duration): How long does it last?
- ☑ Radiation
- ☑ Aggravating factors
- ☑ Alleviating factors
- ☑ Associated symptoms (CV): Chest pain, SOB
- ☑ Associated symptoms (neuro): Change in vision, weakness, headaches?
- ☑ Associated symptoms (general): Vomiting, diarrhea, blood in stool?
- ☑ Allergies: None
- ☑ Medications: Occasional Tylenol or ibuprofen
- ☑ PMH: Hospitalizations and surgeries
- ☑ ROS: Sleep, weight change, urinary pattern
- ☑ FH: Parents deceased from cancer and heart disease
- ☑ SH: Lives alone, salesman
- ☑ SH: Drinks alcohol, Neg CAGE questionnaire
- ☑ Sexual Hx: Sexually active

Physical Exam Checklist

- ☑ GA: NAD
- ☑ HEENT: Sclera clear, pupil reflexes
- ☑ HEENT: Check for JVD
- ☑ Chest: Auscultate at least four locations on chest
- ☑ CV: Auscultate in four cardiac areas
- ☑ CV: Peripheral pulses (radial and tibial) and carotid artery pulses
- ☑ CV: No peripheral edema
- ☑ Abd: Inspect
- ☑ Abd: Auscultate
- ☑ Abd: Palpate
- ☑ Abd: Percuss
- ☑ Abd: Murphy's sign

Doctor: "Your blood pressure is higher than average today. But I would like to take one more reading on your next visit before we make that diagnosis. Certainly, losing 10 to 20 pounds will help. I do encourage you to avoid fatty foods and high sugar foods as this will lower your weight and your blood pressure."

Although the doctor in this exchange failed to counsel the patient initially about the diet, she would have received full credit for counseling because she responded nicely to the patient's question and did provide counseling before the encounter ended.

CHALLENGING QUESTIONS

Following is an example of how you should counsel patients about weight loss.

Mr. Mitchell: "I find it difficult to lose weight and have tried different diets over the years. Is there something else I can do?"

Answer: "Yes, I know that it can be difficult to lose weight. Increasing fruits and vegetables in your diet and being more active is an important first step. Also, be careful to avoid high-fat and high-sugar foods. I'll have you speak with our nutrition expert, who can help to plan out a diet and exercise program with you."

CASE DISCUSSION

Notes about the History-Taking

At the doorway we found that Mr. Mitchell wanted to follow up on some lab reports he received at a health fair. You should still ask whether the patient has had any other chief complaints, to ensure that you do not miss any initial complaints that he may have experienced.

Mr. Mitchell: "Doctor, here's the test results from the health fair." (*The SP hands you a slip of paper with the values*)

Doctor: "Thank you, I'd be happy to review these with you. Also, I would like to know if you have any other health problems."

Mr. Mitchell: "Why, yes, I have been having pain in my stomach."

Doctor: "Tell me about that."

Because Mr. Mitchell has pain in the stomach, run through your SIQORAAA mnemonic.

If Mr. Mitchell had explained that he was completely asymptomatic and that he just got the tests done and wants to know what to do about them, you can skip SIQORAA and go directly to the associated symptoms and review of symptoms. The associated symptoms for HTN and hypercholesterolemia are the complications of the disease. In other words, ask about symptoms relating to the cardiovascular system and nervous system (risk of stroke). This man has gallbladder disease, which is more common with those that are overweight and have high cholesterol.

Notes about the Physical Exam

This man has a series of various symptoms that may have a series of different causes when you first elicit the history. You should think to yourself, are these symptoms related to the cardiovascular system (heart)? Are they related to the gastrointestinal system (gallbladder, esophagitis, gastrointestinal ulcer)? These are all possibilities. Don't worry if the diagnosis does not jump out at you. This is a common way that patients present on the Step 2

SAMPLE PATIENT NOTE

History: Include significant positives and negatives from history of present illness, past medical history, review of system(s), social history, and family history.

CC: Abdominal pain

HPI: Epigastric and RUQ pain. 1/10 increasing to 4/10 pain described as hot. Started 3 mo ago, getting more frequent, and lasting longer. No pain now. Pain all night after pizza.

Made worse by fatty foods and sometimes when bends over. Better with Tylenol and ibuprofen. No SOB, chest pain, nausea, vomiting, diarrhea, dysuria, or rash. No blood in stool. No changes in vision. No headaches. + Mild fever the other day. Recently had BP 150/90, chol 220, glu 90.

Allergies: None

Medications: No regular medications

PMH: Appendectomy 35 yrs ago. No trauma, no h/o DM, HTN, heart disease.

ROS: Slowly gaining weight over years. No change in sleep pattern, no problem urinating.

FH: Parents died from heart disease and cancer

SH: Divorced, lives alone, works as car salesman. Stopped smoking 20 years ago. No drugs. 2 alcoholic beverages 3/wk. (CAGE neg)

Physical Exam: Indicate only pertinent positive and negative findings related to patient's chief complaint.

VS: 148/88, the rest are NL

GA: NAD. 6'2", 240 lb.

HEENT: Sclera NL, pharynx clear. NL carotid upstrokes. No JVD.

CV: S1, S2 WNL. No S3, S4. No RMG.

Chest: Clear to Auscultation

Abd: Appears NL; BS+, + mild epigastric tenderness to palpation. NL percussion. Neg Murphy's.

Ext: NL, no edema, no cyanosis

Neuro: Alert oriented x 3, gait-NL

Differential Diagnosis: In order of likelihood (with 1 being the most likely), list up to five potential or possible diagnoses for this patient's presentation. (In many cases, fewer than five diagnoses are likely.)

1. Biliary colic
2. Peptic ulcer/Esophagitis
3. Coronary artery disease
4. Hypertension
5. Hyperlipidemia

Diagnostic Workup: List immediate plans (up to five) for further diagnostic workup.

1. Rectal with FOBT
2. ECG, troponin, BUN, Cr
3. T. Bili, AST, ALT, alk phos
4. Ultrasound of gallbladder
5. Fasting T. Chol, HDL, LDL, TG

CS exam, and your primary role is not to identify the correct diagnosis. Instead, you are being assessed on your ability to complete a relevant history and physical to elucidate a relevant and likely differential diagnosis.

Your workup plan will help to determine the likely diagnosis based on the information you have found. Remember to include the most common and most likely differential diagnoses and avoid including obscure or unusual conditions. In this type of complex case, you are being tested on your ability to remain calm and professional when the diagnosis is not "textbook."

Comments about the Patient Note

In this note, the carotid artery exam and the neck vein exam were noted under HEENT instead of the cardiovascular exam. This is also acceptable, and you will not be penalized for this.

There are many possibilities for correct tests to order on this patient. Certainly, upper endoscopy would also be considered correct. The Sample Patient Note listed here concentrated on writing down the initial tests for this patient. Had the chief complaint been vomiting blood, then an upper endoscopy certainly would have been included in the initial diagnostic workup plan.

It is important to note that CBC was missed in writing up this patient note and should have been included. CBC is a standard test that is needed on any patient with a fever, where you may be considering infection, or in patients you think may have blood loss (i.e., from an ulcer).

Current recommendations for a lipid panel are fasting total cholesterol, HDL, LDL, and serum triglycerides.

Case 24: **Crying Baby**

BEFORE ENTERING THE ROOM

1. Cues: Based on the Doorway Information, you will know that this is a telephone encounter. Enter the room as always, and remember the ground rules for phone cases as reproduced from the USMLE:

- Do not dial any numbers.
- Push the speaker button by the yellow dot on the phone to be connected to the patient caregiver or patient.
- You will be permitted to make only one phone call.
- Do not touch any buttons on the phone until you are ready to end the call—touching any buttons may disconnect you.
- You will not be allowed to call back after the call is disconnected.

For more information on telephone encounters, refer to the *USMLE Step 2 CS Content Description and General Information Booklet* at www.usmle.org.

2. Clinical Reasoning: A pediatric history will be required in this encounter. Babies cry when they are too hot, too cold, hungry, bored, or overstimulated. Colic is another common cause. However, if the baby is in pain, the

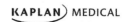

only form of communication available to the infant is to cry. It is important to remember that not all infants with infection will have fever at this age.

FROM THE MOTHER

History

HPI: Mrs. Moore calls at 6 A.M. and says the baby has been up crying for the past hour. She has changed Elizabeth, burped her, and swaddled her—all without success. Elizabeth stops crying only when Mrs. Moore holds the child to her chest, rocking her gently and singing. The child has been sleeping 4 hours straight during the day but is up every 2 hours at night. This began when Elizabeth was just 2 weeks old. She has a crying spell almost every day. She raises her legs and cries most days. She stops crying after being rocked gently, and sometimes she cries for an hour when left alone before falling asleep. Between crying spells, she seems fine. She never cries for more than 2 hours at a time. She is breastfeeding every 2–4 hours normally. She has never been given formula. She has a strong suck. Mrs. Moore checked a rectal temperature and it was normal. The child has no rash. There is no vomiting or diarrhea. Elizabeth seems to be gaining weight. Nothing in particular makes the crying worse.

Elizabeth has no allergies and takes no medications.

PMH: Mom had prenatal care and did not smoke or use alcohol or drugs. Full-term pregnancy; uncomplicated vaginal delivery. No respiratory problems, no jaundice, no fever in neonatal period. No hospitalizations (other than being born), no trauma, illness, or surgery.

ROS: Diapers are regularly wet. Elizabeth has a yellow-green, seedy stool after almost every feeding.

FHx: Both Mrs. Moore and her husband were reportedly "colicky" babies as infants.

SHx: Elizabeth lives with both of her parents. Mr. Moore left home a week ago for Iraq, and Mrs. Moore has not had any help in the past week. She does feel stressed but is not worried about harming the baby. She has read and understands that she should never "shake" the baby.

Physical Exam

There is no physical exam in this case.

THE CLOSING

As with all cases, it is important to explain your clinical impression to your patient, and to discuss the next steps in working up her condition.

> **Doctor:** "Mrs. Moore, I think I understand what is happening with Elizabeth, but I want to double-check. You told me Elizabeth has had crying episodes for the past 2 weeks. Sometimes she seems to cry even when she is fed, warm, and dry. She has no fever and seems fine in between crying."

> **Mrs. Moore:** "That's right."

> **Doctor:** "Some babies cry more than others; sometimes it is called colic. It is just a stage that babies usually grow out of in a couple of months. To make sure, I would like to see you and Elizabeth today. I will need to do a physical exam on Elizabeth. What time would you like to come to the office today?"

> **Mrs. Moore:** "I'm up already—how about 7 A.M.?"

> **Doctor:** "Umm, sure, that's fine. Do you have any other questions we should talk about before then?"

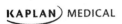

GRADING: STANDARDIZED PATIENT DATA-GATHERING CHECKLISTS

History Checklist

- ☑ **S**ymptom of crying
- ☑ **I**ntensity/quantity of crying
- ☑ **O**nset of symptoms
- ☑ **A**lleviating factors
- ☑ **A**ggravating factors
- ☑ **A**ssociated symptoms: Fever, feeding, any problems breathing, rash, diarrhea, vomiting (and anything else that might indicate this is not colic)
- ☑ **P**ast medical history
- ☑ **A**llergies
- ☑ **M**edicines
- ☑ **S**Hx: Who lives in family, any additional stressors in the home
- ☑ **S**Hx: How are parents coping with stress. Ask about harm to baby.

Pediatric History Checklist

There is no physical exam checklist in this case.

- ☑ **P**renatal Hx
- ☑ **B**irth Hx
- ☑ **N**eonatal Hx
- ☑ **F**eeding Hx
- ☑ **G**rowth and development
- ☑ **R**outine care—immunizations and checkups

CHALLENGING QUESTIONS

Mrs. Moore: "Can you give Elizabeth medicine to make her stop crying? How about Benadryl? I can get that without a prescription."

Answer: "Please don't give her any medicine right now. I need to examine Elizabeth to see if she needs any medicine."

CASE DISCUSSION

Notes about the History-Taking

Since this is a phone case and there is no physical exam, you have the advantage of using the entire 15 minutes to obtain the history. The disadvantage is that you do not have the chance to experience all the nonverbal communication that normally transpires between patient and doctor.

Do your standard introduction and be on your best phone behavior. Be sure to find out who you are talking to. If you are not talking to the patient but rather to a surrogate, make sure to get the patient's name.

Try to refer to the baby by name instead of saying "the baby" or "your baby." Never refer to the infant as "it." For example, you should never say, "Does it sleep through the night?"

SAMPLE PATIENT NOTE

History: Include significant positives and negatives from history of present illness, past medical history, review of system(s), social history, and family history.

CC: *Baby is crying*

HPI: *Mother of 4-week-old female calls clinic because of crying spells that occur almost every day for the past 2 weeks. Cries for up to one hour sometimes. Sometimes inconsolable. Has been nursing every 2–4 hours normally. Wets the diaper normally. Sometimes crying stops with rocking or swaddling the baby. Nothing in particular makes it worse. No fever, rash, vomiting, diarrhea, trouble breathing.*

Allergies: NKMA

Medications: None

PMH: *No hospitalizations other than at birth. Mother received prenatal care and did not use alcohol or smoke. Vaginal full-term delivery. No cyanosis or jaundice. Normal weight gain.*

SH: *Mr. Moore left for Iraq 1 week ago. Mom states not at risk to harm child.*

Physical Exam: Indicate only pertinent positive and negative findings related to patient's chief complaint.

There is no physical exam in this case.

Differential Diagnosis: In order of likelihood (with 1 being the most likely), list up to five potential or possible diagnoses for this patient's presentation. (In many cases, fewer than five diagnoses are likely.)	**Diagnostic Workup:** List immediate plans (up to five) for further diagnostic workup.
1. *Colic*	1. *Physical exam today*
2.	2. *No other tests now*
3.	3.
4.	4.
5.	5.

The neonate case need not be nerve-wracking. The associated symptoms for infants follow the few activities that babies do at this age (feed, sleep, make stools, and urinate). In addition to fever and rash, ask about breathing problems, feeding, urinating, defecating, and alertness/crying.

The social history is important here: Find out who lives in the home, who helps to care for the child, and how the family handles the stress of caring for a newborn. If you find a parent who is having difficulty and has been tempted to shake the baby, it's very important to provide initial guidance. Let the parent know that you would like to put her in touch with a counselor (social worker) immediately. You can also provide some advice on obtaining help with the baby so the primary caretaker can get some sleep and some rest.

In this case, the patient's mother indicates that she has a significant stressor in her life: Her husband has just been deployed to Iraq. It is important that you use a transition statement and reinforce confidentiality so that you can discuss some sensitive topics relating to this stressor, such as the effect of the stress on the family. Be sure to convey a sense of trust and a nonjudgmental attitude.

Doctor: "I'm going to ask you some personal questions. Everything we talk about is confidential."

Mrs. Moore: "Okay."

Doctor: "Who lives in your household?"

Mrs. Moore: "Now, just Elizabeth and me. My husband shipped out to Iraq last week."

* * * * *

Doctor: "Sometimes mothers under stress can be worried they might harm the baby. Does this ever happen to you?"

Mrs. Moore: "No, Doctor."

Doctor: "Do you ever shake Elizabeth?"

Mrs. Moore: "Oh, no! Do you think I'm going to hurt Elizabeth?"

Doctor: "Not at all. I ask these questions of all parents. Occasionally, when there is a problem, I can be of help. If you ever feel that you may need this help, please contact me."

Notes about the Physical Exam

There was no physical exam in this case.

Comments about the Patient Note

This case highlighted a child that is crying for approx 1 hour who has had this problem almost every day for 2 weeks. Had this case been slightly different (with, perhaps, an infant crying inconsolably for hours), then myriad additional diagnoses and tests would have been needed. Infection most commonly, but otitis, pneumonia, and UTI would also need to be considered. Infants with an acute abdomen from any cause can have prolonged consolable crying greater than 2 hours. Sometimes an inconsolable infant turns out to be something more simple, such as a corneal abrasion, a hair stuck in the eye, or even a hair tourniquet. In this particular case the doctor listed only one diagnosis. Any of these additional diagnoses could have been listed as well. It can happen that the USMLE designs a case where only one diagnosis is likely, but this will be uncommon.

The pediatric history in this case was easily combined with the past medical history. If you wish to make a separate heading of Ped Hx to list this information, that would be fine also.

Case 25: **Mental Status Changes**

BEFORE ENTERING THE ROOM

1. Cues: Write your mnemonics on your blue sheet. These will remind you of other questions to ask, and will ensure that you don't skip pertinent aspects of the history. No physical is possible in this case since the patient is not here. Many fathers and sons have the same name. Junior (David Jr.) is the son; Senior (David Sr.) is the father.

2. Clinical Reasoning: Based on the Doorway Information, you can anticipate that this case involves an elderly patient who requires mental status evaluation. Never assume that the problem is just "old age." Alzheimer's disease, depression, stroke, and thyroid disease, as well as cardiovascular and metabolic problems, may be the cause of this patient's symptoms. In addition, side effects of medications are a huge problem in the elderly, so it will be important to ensure that a detailed medication history is taken (dosages not required).

FROM THE STANDARDIZED PATIENT

History

HPI: David Jr. is the son of the patient. He tells you that David Sr. moved in with him last year after having lived alone for 20 years. David Sr. had always been fiercely independent, but 2 to 3 years ago he became increasingly forgetful. On one occasion, he left the stove on. Twice, he got lost taking a walk around the neighborhood he had known for 20 years. Bank officials had started to call David Jr. to tell him that David Sr. was bouncing checks even though he had enough money in other accounts.

A year ago David Sr. had a stroke, but the weakness in the left side of his body resolved completely. After that, he agreed to move in with his son. The son states that his father seems "slowed down" in recent months. David Sr. frequently has crying spells, and sometimes says he would be better off dead. He has lost his interest in reading. He is starting to need help bathing, and even eating. He hasn't been able to pour his own coffee for several months. He cannot get dressed and has been in pajamas for the last 2 weeks. He has been complaining of arthritis of the knees, and seems even more confused since taking a painkiller the last few weeks. Nothing seems to make any of his symptoms better. He talks a lot lately about his platoon when he was in France in 1944.

Allergies: PCN

Medications: Lisinopril, ASA, Vicodin PRN for knee arthritis

PMH: Hospitalized—for stroke 1 year ago. Illness—HTN for 10 years controlled with Lisinopril; osteoarthritis. No trauma. Surgery—appendicitis at age 23, transurethral resection of the prostate (TURP) at age 68. No recent surgery.

Review of Symptoms: No trouble urinating. Sleeps about 4 hours during the day. Has trouble sleeping at night.

Diet: States nothing tastes good; complains of constipation.

SHx: Has not smoked in last 30 years. Drinks 1 oz whiskey every evening to sleep. Worked as a journalist for 30 years. In retirement, taught underprivileged children to read. David Jr. tells you that he is using up all his vacation and sick time at work to stay home and care for his father.

Physical Exam

There is no physical exam in this case.

THE CLOSING

As with all cases, it is important to explain your clinical impression to your patient and discuss the next steps in working up the condition. It is perfectly acceptable to tell the son what you are thinking. The exam asks you to assume for Step 2 CS that you have permission to talk to families.

> **Doctor:** "Mr. Miller, let me summarize what we you've told me and make sure I understand. Your father has been declining in his mental abilities for over a year now. In particular his memory and mood. He came to live with you after having a stroke which resolved. More recently his memory and mood is even worse, and now he cannot wash and eat by himself."

David Jr.: "That's a good summary. Does Dad have Alzheimer's?"

Doctor: "It could be. But there are many other possibilities as well that we need to check. Part of his symptoms could be from the Vicodin. I need to examine your father. Could you bring him in tomorrow?"

David Jr.: "Yes."

Doctor: "I will need to take a blood sample and have an x-ray taken. I'll make arrangements now so we can do the tests he needs tomorrow. Do you have any questions?"

CHALLENGING QUESTIONS

David Jr.: "Will my dad need a nursing home?"

Answer: "Thank you for bringing that up. I'd like to fully evaluate your dad tomorrow to determine what help he needs."

David Jr.: "I'd like my father to stay home but I work outside the house and I don't want to leave him alone."

Answer: "I will have our social worker call you. She may be able to arrange for some in-home help for your father. Are you able to take care of him tonight, or should we make other arrangements today?"

The topic of how the caretaker is dealing with the stress of caring for the elderly parent ideally should be brought up by the doctor. Many cases have these built in "second chances" for the doctor if you do not discuss a topic you should.

GRADING: STANDARDIZED PATIENT DATA-GATHERING CHECKLISTS

History Checklist

☑ Site/symptoms
☑ Intensity of symptoms
☑ Onset of symptoms
☑ Alleviating factors
☑ Aggravating factors
☑ Associated symptoms: DEATH questions (see page 28 in section 1)
☑ Past medical history: Hospitalizations
☑ Past medical history: Major illnesses
☑ Past medical history: Trauma
☑ Past medical history: Surgery
☑ Allergies: PCN
☑ Medicine: Vicodin, Lisinopril, ASA
☑ ROS: Sleep, GI, diet is needed
☑ SHx: Alcohol, smoking
☑ SHx: Living situation
☑ SHx: Stress—how is Jr. coping?

Physical Exam Checklist

There is no physical exam in this case.

SAMPLE PATIENT NOTE

History: Include significant positives and negatives from history of present illness, past medical history, review of system(s), social history, and family history.

CC: *Patient is unable to care for himself.*

HPI: *History is from the son, David Miller Jr. Pt, David Miller Sr., 90 years old has been increasingly forgetful and unable to self-care. Started 2–3 years ago with forgetfulness and unable to do his own banking. For last year has lived with his son but is increasingly "slowed down." Episodes of crying. Has lost interest in reading, despite being a former journalist. In past months has increasing difficulty in preparing meals, eating, and hygiene. Pt has been worse since taking Vicodin recently for osteoarthritis.*

   Allergies: NKDA

   Medications: Lisinopril, Vicodin, ASA

ROS: *No change in urination. + constipation. Food no longer tastes good. Sleeps 4 hr/day. Reversal of day/night sleep cycle.*

PMH: *Hospitalizations for stroke 1 year ago, major illness, HTN. No trauma. Previous appendectomy at age 23. TURP at age 68.*

SH: *Lives with son, denies tobacco for past 30 years. Pt has 1 oz whiskey every evening. Stress: Son states will need help with his father next week.*

Physical Exam: Indicate only pertinent positive and negative findings related to patient's chief complaint.

There is no physical exam in this case.

Differential Diagnosis: In order of likelihood (with 1 being the most likely), list up to five potential or possible diagnoses for this patient's presentation. (In many cases, fewer than five diagnoses are likely.)

1. *Possible medication reaction*
2. *Depression*
3. *Subdural hematoma (possible unwitnessed trauma)*
4. *Multi-infarct dementia: Alzheimer's*
5. *Hypothyroidism*

Diagnostic Workup: List immediate plans (up to five) for further diagnostic workup.

1. *Physical exam*
2. *CBC, lytes, BUN, Cr, glucose*
3. *CT scan of brain: MRI of brain*
4. *TSH*
5. *B12, folate level*

CASE DISCUSSION

Notes about the History-Taking

This is a surrogate case. That means the patient is not present and a concerned family member wants to talk to the doctor. On Step 2 CS, these types of cases often involve pediatrics and geriatrics. Certainly, go ahead and shake hands with the surrogate. As there is no physical exam to perform, sit down and have a nice conversation with the surrogate. In fact, with no physical exam you will have more time to talk and get a detailed history. This is fortunate in the case of dementia, as there is a vast differential and not much can be skipped in the history. Get a detailed history about the onset. Find out the course and duration of symptoms. For the intensity, ask the DEATH questions. [Dressing, Eating, Ambulating, Toileting, Hygiene]

Notes about the Physical Exam

There is no physical exam in this case.

Comments about the Patient Note

As there is no physical exam, you have time to write a detailed chronology of events and ensure that all of the details from the history are documented. The workup for dementia that's listed here is fairly standard and you can use it for any older person with confusion or mental status changes.

Case 26: **Diabetic Checkup**

DOORWAY INFORMATION

Opening Scenario

Daniel Sugar is a 50 y/o diabetic male here for his regular 6-month checkup.

Vital Signs

- Temp: 37.0°C (98.6°F)
- BP: 130/80 mm Hg
- HR: 80/min
- RR: 24/min

Examinee Tasks

1. Obtain a focused history.
2. Perform a relevant physical examination. Do not perform rectal, pelvic, genitourinary, female breast, or corneal reflex examinations.
3. Discuss your initial diagnostic impression and your workup plan with the patient.
4. After leaving the room, complete your patient note on the given form.

BEFORE ENTERING THE ROOM

1. Cues: In this case, you're told that the patient has diabetes. Consider asking the symptoms of the disease (in this case polyuria, polydipsia, polyphagia) when you ask about the patient's symptoms. Most likely the patient will have poorly controlled DM or have complications from the disease.

2. Clinical Reasoning: The patient is here for a periodic health exam or checkup. Early in the interview, find out if he is having any concerns that need to be addressed in this visit. If there are any other health concerns, focus on them also. If there are no other chief complains, use your SIQORAAA mnemonic to find out all about his DM in general. When you get to associated symptoms ask about the complications of diabetes. The physical exam will concentrate on any problems you uncover in the history. You can expect that long-time diabetics will have difficulties with their eyes, kidneys, and cardiovascular systems, as well as peripheral neuropathy.

FROM THE STANDARDIZED PATIENT

History

HPI: Mr. Sugar states that he is here for his semiannual checkup. He also states that he needs more insulin syringes. He feels fine and really has no complaints to talk about. He states he has no polyuria, polydipsia, or polyphagia. He tests his bloodwork twice a day; his blood has been running between 70 and 120 mg/dl. Other than the hassle of watching what he eats, he claims that the diabetes is not affecting his life. Once last month he was on a hike and got a little sweaty. He had no chest pain, shortness of breath, or syncope. He sat down for a while and ate a granola bar. Mr. Sugar does mention that he was really tired for a week after that hike. This happened 2 weeks ago and it had never happened before.

The patient has been diabetic for the past 20 years. His sugars have been easier to control in the past decade since he lost a lot of weight: from 220 lb, he got down to 170 lb. He denies any change in his vision. He reports no change in sensation in his extremities. He feels he needs to further improve his physical conditioning, and would like a medically supervised physical fitness program.

PMH: Mr. Sugar has no allergies. He uses Humulin 70/30 and Lovastatin. History of high cholesterol. His medication doses have not changed in the last 6 months. Was hospitalized for gallbladder removal 5 years ago. Also had a cellulitis of the lower leg for which he was hospitalized for 2 days this last year. No history of trauma.

ROS: Mr. Sugar has no difficulties urinating, and his sleep pattern and weight are unchanged from his last visit 6 months ago.

PMH: Does not know his family's medical history, as he was adopted at an early age. Has no information about his biological parents.

SHx: Is not currently sexually active. He was divorced 2 years ago and lives alone, but calls his brother every day. He does not smoke or use recreational drugs. He drinks one or two alcoholic beverages on most weekends. He works as a librarian. He states he is under no unusual stress.

Physical Exam

Mr. Sugar's visual acuity is 20/30 OU. His pupils are equally round and reactive to light. His fundi are flat without hemorrhage. Pharynx is clear without exudates. Neck shows no jugular venous distension. Has no carotid bruit. Carotid upstrokes are normal and equal bilaterally. His lungs are clear to auscultation. Heart tones are normal and the point of maximum impulse is not displaced. Abdomen is soft and reveals a well-healed surgical scar in the right upper quadrant. He has normal radial pulses.

The dorsalis pedis and posterior tibial pulse seem decreased symmetrically compared to the upper extremities. There is no pedal edema, and the site of his former skin infection appears well-healed with chronic scarring of the skin over the leg. He is alert. His gait is normal. His muscle strength is equal and strong in all 4 extremities. He has decreased sensation below the knee to light touch as well as sharp sensation, and has decreased vibration sense below the knees bilaterally. Feet have intact skin and are without redness or tenderness.

THE CLOSING

Doctor: "Mr. Sugar, I have finished your physical exam. Let me make sure I understand you correctly. You had one episode where you got sweaty walking and felt tired for an entire week afterward. Is that correct?"

Mr. Sugar: "Yes."

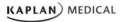

Doctor: "On your exam I see that your leg has healed nicely. You still have some numbness in the feet, however I think the numbness may be from the diabetes. I would like you to have a test to check how well the nerves are working in your legs. In addition, I'd like to check your blood for cholesterol and check the kidneys. I'll call you when I get the test results back. Do you have any questions?"

CHALLENGING QUESTIONS

Mr. Sugar: "I'd like to get in better shape so I can go mountain-climbing. Can I start running up little hills now to start training?"

Answer: "I'm glad you want to be in top shape. Before you begin a new exercise program, let me do a heart test to be sure it's safe to begin strenuous activity."

GRADING: STANDARDIZED PATIENT DATA-GATHERING CHECKLISTS

History Checklist

- ☑ **S**ymptom: Ask about 3 Ps (polyuria, polydipsia, polyphagia)
- ☑ **S**ymptom: Ask how often patient checks sugar and how readings have been
- ☑ **S**ymptom: Ask if patient has had any problems since the last checkup
- ☑ **I**ntensity: Find out how the chronic disease is affecting his life
- ☑ **O**nset: How long has he had diabetes?
- ☑ **A**ssociated symptoms (CVS): Chest pain, SOB, headache, claudication
- ☑ **A**ssociated symptoms (neuro): Vision changes, peripheral sensory changes (tingling, numbness), weakness, foot hygiene
- ☑ **A**ssociated symptoms (kidney): Changes in urinary frequency, appearance of urine
- ☑ **A**llergies: NKMA
- ☑ **M**edication: Has there been any recent change in medicine dose? Check compliance.
- ☑ **P**ast medical history: Hospitalizations, surgery
- ☑ **R**eview of symptoms: Sleep, urinary if not previously asked in HPI, weight change
- ☑ **S**X: Not sexually active, sexual dysfunction?
- ☑ **S**H: Alcohol, smoking, living arrangements

Physical Exam Checklist

- ☑ General appearance
- ☑ HEENT: Visual acuity
- ☑ HEENT: Pupils
- ☑ HEENT: Fundi
- ☑ CV: Carotid artery
- ☑ CV: Radial, dorsalis pedis, posterior tibial pulses
- ☑ CV: Auscultate the heart, PMI
- ☑ CV: JVD
- ☑ Chest: Auscultation of lungs
- ☑ Neuro: Motor strength all four extremities
- ☑ Neuro: Sensory exam of feet
- ☑ Neuro: Gait
- ☑ Joints: Inspection and palpation of feet

SAMPLE PATIENT NOTE

History: Include significant positives and negatives from history of present illness, past medical history, review of system(s), social history, and family history.

CC: *Patient is here for 6-month diabetes checkup*

HPI: *50-year-old diabetic male with no specific complaints. Did have episode with diaphoresis when hiking and felt tired for next week. Pt checks sugars twice a day. 70–120 readings. Weight stable at 170 lb. No polyuria, polydipsia, polyphagia. Denies chest pain, SOB, palpitations, or headache. No peripheral sensory changes. No episodes of change in vision or focal weakness. Allergies NKDA. Meds Humulin 70/30. No recent change in dose. Lovastatin.*

PMH: *DM × 20 yrs. S/P cholecystectomy. Last year hospitalized with cellulitis of leg. No change in diet, weight, sleep, or urinary patterns.*

SX: *Not currently sexually active*

SH: *Lives alone (brother does expect call every A.M.). No drugs or smoking. Drinks 2/wk.*

Physical Exam: Indicate only pertinent positive and negative findings related to patient's chief complaint.

VS: *WNL*

GA: *NAD*

HEENT: *PERRL. Fundi flat without hemorrhage. V/A 20/30 OU. Pharynx clear.*

CV: *JVD. PMI not displaced. S1 S2 WNL, no murmur or gallop. Pulses: carotid, radial = 2/4 B/L; dorsalis pedis & posterior tibial = 1/4 B/L*

Chest: *Clear to auscultation*

Abd: *Soft and nontender; + old scar RUQ*

Ext: *Site of old cellulitis well healed. No redness or tenderness to feet.*

Neuro: *Alert. Motor 5/5 all 4 ext., gait WNL. Decreased light touch, sharp, and vibration sensations below knee B/L.*

Differential Diagnosis: In order of likelihood (with 1 being the most likely), list up to five potential or possible diagnoses for this patient's presentation. (In many cases, fewer than five diagnoses are likely.)

1. *Diabetes mellitus*
2. *Ischemic heart disease*
3. *Peripheral neuropathy*
4. *Hyperlipidemia*

Diagnostic Workup: List immediate plans (up to five) for further diagnostic workup.

1. *CBC, lytes, BUN, Cr, glucose*
2. *HbA1c; U/A for microalbiuminuria*
3. *Fasting cholesterol, HDL, LDL, triglycerides*
4. *ECG, cardiac stress test*

CASE DISCUSSION

Notes about the History-Taking

The initial history may begin as follows:

Doctor: "How can I help you today?"

Mr. Sugar: "I'm here for my 6-month checkup, and I need more syringes."

Doctor: "Sure, I can get you more syringes. Are you having any other problems I can help with?"

Mr. Sugar: "No."

The doctor in this exchange does a good job of answering the patient's concerns about more syringes. She also determines that there is no other medical complaint. Had the patient said "I had chest pain last week," the entire case would have been different and you would focus on doing SIQORAAA on the chest pain.

This man, however, has no complaints, so ask about his diabetes in more detail: How often does he test his blood sugar? How high have his sugars been? Are there any other diabetic complications? The intensity could be measured by the DEATH (*see* Section 1) questions for the more severely disabled, or simply find out how the chronic disease is affecting his life. The onset and duration of this patient's diabetes are also very important.

Ischemic heart disease is very common in long standing diabetics. So when a patient like this notices any sort of change, even as nonspecific as weakness or nausea, it is worthwhile to obtain an ECG. The associated symptoms for this case can simply be all the complications that diabetics experience including the myocardial infarct questions.

Doctor: "Mr. Sugar have you had any shortness of breath?"

Mr. Sugar: "No."

Doctor: "How about any chest pain, especially when you were hiking?"

Mr. Sugar: "No."

Doctor: "Any palpitations in the chest?"

Mr. Sugar: "No."

Doctor: "Have you had any sudden or brief loss of vision?"

Mr. Sugar: "No."

Doctor: "How about weakness on just one side of the body?"

The past history is important to find out the medications used and to check compliance. Review of symptoms will sometimes reveal hidden health problems in cases where there is no specific chief complaint. If you have been a diabetic for 20 years, you have a very high risk for a vascular catastrophe. Sexual history would be important because erectile dysfunction is a common complication of the neuropathy and vascular disease associated with diabetes.

Notes about the Physical Exam

The physical for a diabetic who comes in for a checkup must include the eyes and the feet. Had this diabetic patient presented with shortness of breath, chest pain, or unstable vital signs, you could skip the funduscopy and concentrate the physical on the cardiovascular system. In this case, you have a stable patient who at this moment feels fine. Be sure to examine the eyes and feet. Placing makeup on the bottom of the SP's foot to simulate a diabetic foot ulcer would be an outstanding way to mimic real life. Only if you remove the patient's socks (after getting permission) would you find the problem and make the diagnosis.

In this case you found abnormality in the light touch of the lower extremities. Once you find one abnormality it is likely that there are other problems in the same location. Mr. Sugar also has decreased sharp sensation and decreased vibration sense from his diabetic neuropathy. Peripheral neuropathy is often unnoticed by patients, especially when it is in the early stages, so his simply denying any changes in sensation during the history doesn't mean that there aren't any sensory changes.

Comments about the Patient Note

If you collect a historical fact from the SP during the HPI (in this case, the history of 20 years of diabetes) you are not obligated to write it in the HPI section of the note. You may document your findings in any section of the note that is relevant. The weight is important. In this case it was documented as part of the history, but it would have been equally correct at the beginning of the Physical Exam section.

The diagnosis of peripheral vascular disease is supported from the physical finding of decreased pulses. The neuropathy is suggested because of the sensory findings. The diagnosis of hyperlipidemia is made by the history.

Renal function and U/A are always correct answers in diabetics as they are target organs. The lipid panel as ordered is standard for most adult patients getting a checkup.

Case 27: **Domestic Violence**

DOORWAY INFORMATION

Opening Scenario

Kim Turner is a 29 y/o female with 2 months of abdominal pain, fatigue, and just not feeling well. This is her third visit in 2 months.

Vital Signs

- Temp: 37.0°C (98.6°F)
- BP: 120/80 mm Hg
- HR: 80/min
- RR: 16/min

Examinee Tasks

1. Obtain a focused history.
2. Perform a relevant physical examination. Do not perform rectal, pelvic, genitourinary, female breast, or corneal reflex examinations.
3. Discuss your initial diagnostic impression and your workup plan with the patient.
4. After leaving the room, complete your patient note on the given form.

BEFORE ENTERING THE ROOM

1. Cues: There could be several reasons why a patient makes multiple return visits. This patient presents with an acute problem each visit. The multiple visits could be just following up at the doctor's request after test results are back or treatment is reevaluated. The underlying condition may be something unusual that has so far eluded diagnosis such as rheumatologic problem. Or there may be a social problem that has yet to be elucidated. The history will require you to ask some direct and possibly sensitive questions.

2. Clinical Reasoning: Fatigue is a common symptom and there are many conditions to consider. Any chronic illness can make a patient fatigued. Doing a thyroid exam, ordering a TSH and using hypothyroidism as a diagnosis will always be correct in this situation. Also consider anemia, diabetes, and depression as additional common problems.

You may not yet know the cause of this patient's abdominal pain but one of the first things you should recognize before entering the room is that her vital signs are stable. With 2 months of pain and currently normal vital

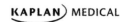

signs, it is not likely that this is going to be an acute abdomen or a surgical problem. However, it is important to keep an open mind about possible differentials when asking SIQORAAA on the abdominal pain. You should be deducing a differential diagnosis that helps to explain all (or almost all) of the patient's symptoms.

FROM THE STANDARDIZED PATIENT

History

HPI: Ms. Turner states that she has had abdominal pain off and on for the past 6 months. It started slowly, and can last anywhere from minutes to days. It can occur in any or multiple quadrants of her abdomen. It feels crampy. It is 10/10 when it happens. Other times, the pain is milder. It never radiates to the back or groin. She sometimes takes an Ativan tablet (benzodiazepine), which seems to help.

The pain is significantly aggravated when she is not getting along with her son's father, especially after they argue. No fever, chills, anorexia, vomiting, diarrhea, jaundice, or dysuria. Prior to the last 6 months, she has not had any problems with abdominal pain.

When asked about allergies, she jokes that she is allergic to "men."

Ms. Turner takes Ativan now and then when she feels really fatigued and not well. She gets them from multiple sources, including the Internet. She takes benzodiazepines now just about every day.

PMH: She was hospitalized in the past for a blowout fracture of the orbit a couple of years ago when she tripped off a curb. Last year she was hospitalized for a rare condition. She carries the hospital discharge papers with her. She pulls them out of her purse when asked.

> **Ms. Turner:** "Oh, I was hospitalized last year with a rare condition."
>
> **Doctor:** "What was it?"
>
> **Ms. Turner:** "I had some type of bleeding problem. Here—I have the papers with me."

She hands you a paper that says "Idiopathic retroperitoneal hemorrhage." No surgery other than to reconstruct her face. If you ask about trauma, she will tell you "No" at this point.

FH: No one in her family has the same constellation of symptoms that she does. There is no family history of hemophilia or bleeding disorder.

Ob/Gyn: Her last menstrual period was 2 weeks ago and was normal. She is G2P2. Her youngest child is 7 years old.

SHx: Is not sleeping well and wakes up frequently. Her weight and diet have not changed. She is sexually active with her son's father when he stays with them. She does use the Pill. She has never had a sexually transmitted disease. Her son's father lives about half the year with them and spends a lot of time somewhere else. She is chronically stressed about the relationship. She smokes 1 pack per day. Denies alcohol or recreational drugs.

Physical Exam

Patient appears to be in no acute distress, although she is not smiling. Her head is normocephalic. She does still have some chronic pain in the cheek where her facial bones were broken, but says that it's a lot better and healing well. Her pharynx is normal. Her neck is supple.

Chest: There are ecchymoses on her anterior chest wall. Her respiratory excursion is normal. There is tenderness to the left posterior ribs with additional ecchymosis. Percussion, tactile fremitus, and auscultation of the lungs are normal. If asked, she says it does hurt when she takes a deep breath. Her heart tones are normal.

Abdomen: Free of any rash or ecchymosis. Bowel sounds are normal. Her abdomen is a little tender all along the left side. No rebound. There is no CVA tenderness. Her extremities appear normal. She is alert. Her gait is normal. Motor strength is equal in all four extremities. She denies feeling sad, helpless, or hopeless.

THE CLOSING

Doctor: "Ms. Turner, I have finished your physical exam. I'd like to review our meeting with you. You told me you have this abdominal pain. On your exam I found you are tender in the tummy and have large bruises on your chest. I am concerned that when you were injured you may have hurt your chest or belly."

Ms. Turner: "Yes, that's really why I'm here."

Doctor: "Ms. Turner, many women are victims of domestic violence. If anyone is hurting you, I can help keep you safe." *(Patient looks down at the floor, gets tearful, and will not speak)*

Doctor: "I know it's difficult to talk about. Remember, I am here to help."

Ms. Turner: "He is really a good man. But sometimes he loses his temper."

Doctor: "No one has the right to hurt you." *(Patient nods in agreement)*

Doctor: "I'd like you to see our counselor to help. Also I want to be sure you have a safe place to go when you feel you are in danger."

Ms. Turner: "He has a key—it's his house."

Doctor: "I'll bring you a list of shelters that you can use. And thank you for telling me. Of course, the most important thing is to be safe in the future. I also want to take an x-ray of your chest and belly to look for any bleeding inside the body. Then we will meet again to discuss the results and to see how you are doing with the counselor."

Ms. Turner: "Yes, Doctor, thank you."

Doctor: "Do you have any questions for me?" *(Patient shakes her head)* "Okay, I'll call you tomorrow with the test results."

CHALLENGING QUESTIONS

Ms. Turner: "Please call me on my cell phone so he won't know I was here."

Answer: "Sure."

CASE DISCUSSION

Notes about the History-Taking

The patient will not tell you about domestic violence unless you express empathy and understanding and talk about confidentiality and safety.

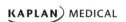

GRADING: STANDARDIZED PATIENT DATA-GATHERING CHECKLISTS

History Checklist

- ☑ Site/symptom
- ☑ Intensity
- ☑ Quality
- ☑ Onset
- ☑ Radiation
- ☑ Aggravating factors
- ☑ Alleviating factors
- ☑ Associated symptoms
- ☑ PMH: Hospitalizations
- ☑ PMH: Major illness
- ☑ PMH: Surgery
- ☑ PMH: Trauma
- ☑ Ob/Gyn: LMP; para gravida scoring
- ☑ SH: Who she lives with and what stressors are

Physical Exam Checklist

- ☑ General appearance
- ☑ HEENT: Inspection
- ☑ HEENT: Palpation
- ☑ HEENT: Thyroid
- ☑ Chest: Inspection
- ☑ Chest: Palpation
- ☑ Chest: Fremitus
- ☑ Chest: Percussion
- ☑ Chest: Auscultation
- ☑ CV: Auscultation of heart
- ☑ Abd: Inspection
- ☑ Abd: Palpation
- ☑ Abd: Check CVA and inspect back
- ☑ Neuro: Mental status/psychiatric screen for depression

1. Empathy: If the patient feels that you are not caring, the SP will not admit to the domestic violence.
2. Statement of confidentiality: If, somewhere in the interview (usually right before the Ob/Gyn Hx), you do not inform the patient that the interview is confidential, the patient will not admit to domestic violence.
3. Safety statement: You must speak to the patient's unmentioned concerned about her safety. You must tell the patient that you can help keep her safe.

Notes about the Physical Exam

Once you find the bruise on the anterior chest, you should realize it is necessary to check the entire body for additional simulated physical findings. Also, a bruise over the chest would indicate that you should do as complete a chest exam as time will allow.

It is necessary to ask additional history during the physical exam when you find the rather dramatic bruising. Ask about chest pain and shortness of breath. You will also want to ask how the fresh bruises got there.

Doctor: "I see a lot of bruises here on your side."

Ms. Turner: "Oh, I must have bumped myself."

Doctor: "It must have been a hard bump!"

Ms. Turner: "Or maybe I fell down the stairs."

Be sure to consider physical injuries on a domestic violence case.

SAMPLE PATIENT NOTE

History: Include significant positives and negatives from history of present illness, past medical history, review of system(s), social history, and family history.

CC:	Fatigue, weakness, abdominal pain for 2 months
HPI:	29 y/o female states has intermittent abdominal pain for 2 months. It can last hours to days and is migratory to all 4 Q. Described as crampy, mild to severe in nature. Better when she takes Ativan, worse with arguing with her son's father. No diarrhea, vomiting, anorexia, fever, dysuria, or jaundice.
	Denies SOB or chest pain. She denies feeling sad, feeling hopeless or guilty.
	Allergies: None
	Meds: Ativan, oral contraceptives
PMH:	No prior episodes. Hosp/surg = fracture orbit from fall 2 years ago. Hx of "idiopathic retroperitoneal hemorrhage" last year.
ROS:	Has not been sleeping well, no recent change in weight
Family Hx:	No hx of bleeding disorder
SX:	Active, one partner. No hx of STD. LMP 2 wks ago NL. G2P2.
SH:	Lives with son. Son's father in household about ½ time. Stressed over relationship + Smokes. – Drugs/alcohol.

Physical Exam: Indicate only pertinent positive and negative findings related to patient's chief complaint.

VS:	WNL
GA:	NAD. Pt not smiling.
HEENT:	PEERL, pharynx clear. Some tenderness remains on face from old fracture. Thyroid: Not enlarged, without tenderness.
Chest:	Bruise along L thoracic posterior ribs. Mildly tender, NL respiratory excursion. No flail chest. Normal, fremitus, percussion, and auscultation. Also bruise on anterior chest wall.
CV:	S1 S2 WNL. No rub, murmur, or gallop.
Abd:	No ecchymosis. BS+, mild LUQ, LLQ tenderness. No mass or rebound. No CVA pain.
Extremities:	Appear NL
Neuro:	Alert. Motor 5/5 all ext. Gait NL.

Differential Diagnosis: In order of likelihood (with 1 being the most likely), list up to five potential or possible diagnoses for this patient's presentation. (In many cases, fewer than five diagnoses are likely.)

1. Domestic violence
2. Hemopneumothorax
3. Splenic hematoma
4. Benzodiazepine dependence
5. Hypothyroidism

Diagnostic Workup: List immediate plans (up to five) for further diagnostic workup.

1. Pelvic and rectal exam
2. CBC, INR
3. CXR, U/A
4. CT Abd
5. TSH

Comments about the Patient Note

The SP will put on purple-blue makeup to simulate a bruise or ecchymosis. This physical finding may have been caused by trauma or bleeding disorder. All patients with any bruising need a CBC. A CBC will give you the patient's hemoglobin level as well as the platelet count. Checking the PT/PTT or INR as a screen for a bleeding disorder is also indicated. Looking at a peripheral blood smear is also correct.

If the patient will not admit to the diagnosis of domestic violence, you can still use it as a differential diagnosis. Write "Suspect domestic violence."

Certainly, the focus on a domestic violence case is not only to arrange for counseling but also to diagnose and work up any injuries.

Many patients refer to oral contraceptives as "the Pill." The patient's history of idiopathic retroperitoneal hemorrhage was from undiagosed trauma from domestic violence in the past.

Case 28: **Child with Vomiting and Diarrhea**

DOORWAY INFORMATION

Opening Scenario

Donna Martin is an 18-month-old female child whose mother wishes to talk to you about the child's vomiting and diarrhea.

Vital Signs

There are no vital signs taken in this case.

Examinee Tasks

1. Obtain a focused history.
2. You will not be required to perform a physical examination in this case.
3. Discuss your initial diagnostic impression and your workup plan with the patient.
4. After leaving the room, complete your patient note on the given form.

BEFORE ENTERING THE ROOM

1. Cues: There will be no child SPs present on test day. Pediatric cases will be represented via a surrogate (mother or caretaker who will speak with you in person or by phone). Since you will not be required to complete a physical exam during the encounter, you may spend the extra time completing the pediatric history.

2. Clinical Reasoning: Diarrhea may have several different causes: bacterial infection, parasitic infections, medications, or viral diarrhea. Rotavirus, the most common cause of diarrhea in pediatrics, has an incubation period of 2 days, and can cause vomiting and watery diarrhea for 3 to 8 days associated with fever and abdominal pain.

This case is intended to test your ability to obtain a history that helps elucidate the cause of the diarrhea. In addition, since you do not know the patient's vital signs, you will need to ask questions that may help you determine the severity of the child's condition and provide guidance to the mother/caregiver.

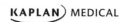

FROM THE MOTHER

History

HPI: Mrs. Martin calls you to tell you that her child is sick. It started about 48 hours ago with vomiting and fussiness. Donna has thrown up a total of 3 times a day for the past 2 days. The vomiting began with food. Now just water and mucus is coming up, as the baby will not eat or drink much. For the past day, Donna has had four episodes of diarrhea. The diarrhea is brown and watery. Donna seems to be hot, but Mrs. Martin does not have a thermometer and has not taken her temperature. At times, especially when she is having a bowel movement, the baby appears to be in pain. Donna won't smile or play, seems to be more tired than usual, and has not had a wet diaper from urine in 8 hours. Mrs. Martin isn't sure if any diapers contained both urine and stool due to the large amount of diarrhea. (Donna needed a quick bath after each episode of diarrhea, and her bottom is looking red already.)

This all began 3 days after returning from a play-date with a group of other toddlers. Tylenol seems to make Donna feel a little better, but the vomiting and diarrhea have not stopped. Drinking cow's milk seems to make the diarrhea worse, when the child is less active and playful. She prefers to sit quietly and watch TV. Constantly, she wants to be held and rocked gently. There is no rash or yellowing of the skin. No cough or runny nose, no shortness of breath.

PMH: Donna has never had this before. She has no known allergies to medication or food. Aside from pediatric vitamins, she takes no meds. She has had no hospitalizations, other than at birth for 24 hours. No surgery, major illnesses, or trauma. Donna finished a course of amoxicillin for otitis media just as the fever and vomiting began. Donna has a greatly decreased appetite, and has not been sleeping well.

FH: No one else in the family has a similar illness. Donna lives with her mother, father, and a golden retriever dog. Mrs. Martin is getting worried that Donna does not look so good, and worries that the child is dehydrated. There is no travel history.

Ped Hx: Mrs. Martin received prenatal care while pregnant with Donna and did not smoke or use drugs or alcohol. She carried Donna to full term but had a C-section after a 28-hour labor. Donna had no problems in the first days and weeks of life. She was breastfed for the first 8 months. Now Donna eats regular table food and cow's milk. Donna growth and development is normal. She started walking at 1 year, and was just starting to urinate in the potty during the daytime when she got sick. She gets regular checkups. Her immunizations are complete except that she has not had the new rotavirus vaccine.

Physical Exam

There is no physical exam in this case.

THE CLOSING

> **Doctor:** "Mrs. Martin, thank you for calling me today about Donna. Let me make sure I understand. On the last day of the amoxicillin that she was taking for an ear infection, she started with fever and vomiting. That was 2 days ago."
>
> **Mrs. Martin:** "Yes, Doctor."
>
> **Doctor:** "Then yesterday she started with diarrhea. It is likely that she has a new infection, probably a virus, making her sick. Her symptoms may also be from the antibiotics but this is less likely from what you have described to me."

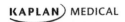

"I'd like you to stop milk for now and instead give her fluids such as Pedialyte, which will help. I will also need to see her as soon as possible for an exam. Can you bring her in to see me now?"

The key here is that you're always available and you want to see the patient. Naturally, if someone has called in only for a school physical, you would tell them just to make an appointment. If it sounds like a medical emergency, have her call 9-1-1 and tell her you will meet her at the hospital. In pediatrics, you generally want to see the child for any illness *today*. For the test, it is best to discuss with the caregiver the need to call an ambulance if the child sounds sick. You may also then say that you will meet her at the hospital. You may also be creative and say you will even make a house call!

There are two important counseling opportunities in this case. One is to counsel the mother to stop feeding Donna the cow's milk, as it is making the diarrhea worse. Instead, assure her that Donna is receiving adequate fluid and electrolyte replenishment. Second is to explain that infants can be dehydrated very rapidly and that Donna will need to be evaluated as soon as possible for any serious concerns with her condition.

GRADING: STANDARDIZED PATIENT DATA-GATHERING CHECKLISTS
History Checklist

- ☑ **S**ymptom: Diarrhea and vomiting
- ☑ **I**ntensity: Number of vomits, number of diarrheal stools, for how many days (frequency)
- ☑ **Q:** What color is the vomit and diarrhea?
- ☑ **O**nset: When did vomit and diarrhea begin?
- ☑ **O**nset (progression): Is it getting better or worse?
- ☑ **A:** What makes it better?
- ☑ **A:** What makes it worse?
- ☑ **A**ssociated symptoms: Any other signs of infection? Dysuria, cough, coryza
- ☑ **A**ssociated symptoms: Lethargy, arousability
- ☑ **P:** Prior illnesses of vomiting and diarrhea
- ☑ **A:** Allergies
- ☑ **M:** Medications
- ☑ **H:** Hospitalizations, major illness, trauma, surgery
- ☑ **R**OS: Diet currently
- ☑ **R**OS: Sleep pattern currently
- ☑ **F**H: Anyone else at home with the same symptoms?
- ☑ **S**H: Who lives in the family, and what is the stress level over the illness?

Prenatal History

- ☑ **P**renatal Hx
- ☑ **B**irth history
- ☑ **N**eonatal history
- ☑ **F**eeding history
- ☑ **G**rowth and development
- ☑ **R**outine care—immunizations and checkups

SAMPLE PATIENT NOTE

History: Include significant positives and negatives from history of present illness, past medical history, review of system(s), social history, and family history.

CC: 18-month-old with vomiting and diarrhea

HPI: 2 days of vomiting and being fussy and febrile. Vomited 6 times total, first just food, now clear. No blood. 1 day of diarrhea, 4 episodes, brown and watery. Seems to have cramps with BM. Fever better with Tylenol. Diarrhea worse when drinks milk. No cough, coryza, dysuria, or rash. Decreased play, more lethargic than usual. No difficulty with arousal.

           Allergies: NKMA

           Medications: Pediatric vitamins. Tylenol for fever. Recent course of amoxicillin for otitis media.

PMH: No prior episodes of vomiting and diarrhea. No hospitalization, surgery, trauma, or major illness. Just had recent ear infection and finished amoxicillin.

ROS: Child has decreased appetite and not sleeping well

FH: No one else in family has similar illness

SH: Donna lives with parents and dog. Mother worried about possible dehydration.

Ped Hx: Full-term child, mom received prenatal care, no drugs, no smoking or alcohol during pregnancy. C-section. No problems in neonatal period. Breast-fed until 8 mo, now on regular food and cow's milk. Mom states growth and development are normal. Immunizations are up-to-date except child has not received rotavirus vaccine.

Physical Exam: Indicate only pertinent positive and negative findings related to patient's chief complaint.

There is no physical exam in this case.

Differential Diagnosis: In order of likelihood (with 1 being the most likely), list up to five potential or possible diagnoses for this patient's presentation. (In many cases, fewer than five diagnoses are likely.)

1. Dehydration
2. Gastroenteritis
3. Rotavirus
4. Diarrhea from amoxicillin
5.

Diagnostic Workup: List immediate plans (up to five) for further diagnostic workup.

1. Physical exam
2. U/A
3. Lytes, glucose, BUN
4. Stool for rotavirus
5. Stool for C-diff

CHALLENGING QUESTIONS

Mrs. Martin: "Oh, I have no transportation and can't come today."

Answer: "Hmmm. It sounds like I need to see Donna today. I need to get a stool sample to check for infection and a blood test to check her for dehydration. Can you take a taxi or ask someone to drive you? If you cannot come in right away, please call the ambulance and have them bring you into the emergency room. I will meet you there."

CASE DISCUSSION

Notes about the History-Taking

Emphasis here is given on getting the number of times—and the color—of the vomiting and diarrhea. Since you cannot "see" your patient, it's helpful to get a description of the child's activity level. Is the baby floppy or listless? Is she interactive with her environment? A complete pediatric history will be expected on children younger than 2 years of age.

Notes about the Physical Exam

There was no physical exam in this case.

Comments about the Patient Note

In this case, the pediatric history is listed separately rather than integrated into the HPI and PMH. This is fine. If you run out of space on the History section of your note, it is okay to spill over into the blank Physical Exam section.

A diagnosis of viral diarrhea may also be made. You would also be correct in listing bacterial causes and parasitic causes of diarrhea in your differential.

Testing in this case includes checking for dehydration and checking the sugar. Children can easily become hypoglycemic if they are not eating. Certainly, checking the stool for the most common cause, rotavirus, is indicated. Stool for C-diff is to check for an overgrowth of *Clostridium difficile* from the amoxicillin.

Case 29: **Life Insurance Exam**

DOORWAY INFORMATION

Opening Scenario

John Brown is a 55 y/o male who comes to the office wanting a physical exam so he can buy life insurance.

Vital Signs

- Temp: 37.0°C (98.6°F)
- BP: 145/94 mm Hg, right upper limb sitting
- HR: 90/min, regular
- RR: 20/min

Examinee Tasks

1. Obtain a focused history.
2. Perform a relevant physical examination. Do not perform rectal, pelvic, genitourinary, female breast, or corneal reflex examinations.
3. Discuss your initial diagnostic impression and your workup plan with the patient.
4. After leaving the room, complete the standard patient form that is waiting for you at your desk.
5. Turn in the form that Mr. Brown gives you, but do not write on it.

BEFORE ENTERING THE ROOM

1. Cues: Write your mnemonics on your blue sheet. These will remind you of other questions to ask, and will ensure that you don't skip pertinent aspects of the history. Write down abnormal vital signs and keep them in mind during your encounter. Your diagnoses should explain these abnormal vitals. Read the doorway information. In this case you are told what to do with the form the SP gives you!

2. Clinical Reasoning: Life insurance policy means the insured person gives money annually to the insurance company each year. If the insured person does not die in that year the insurance company keeps the money. If the insured person dies during the year a family member designated by the policy holder gets a large sum of money. So life insurance companies will not give a policy if they think the patient is at risk of an early death.

The approach to this case is very similar to a periodic health exam in that you should ask yourself, What is likely to cause death in Mr. Brown in the next few years?

FROM THE STANDARDIZED PATIENT

History

HPI: Mr. Brown says he feels fine and needs a physical exam so he can buy life insurance. He denies having any shortness of breath, chest pain, weight loss, or blood in the stool. No chronic cough, no sores that won't heal, no fevers, hoarseness, or trouble swallowing.

PMH: No allergies. He is taking saw palmetto to help with a problem of frequent urination. He had his gallbladder removed 5 years ago. That was the last time he had his blood pressure or any blood tests taken. He denies diabetes, hypertension, or heart disease. He believes he has "white coat syndrome" and that this gave him an elevated reading for the last 20 years or so.

ROS: Patient sleeps more than usual, yet wakes up tired. Mr. Brown feels it is because his wife often wakes him because he snores. His diet consists of high-carbohydrate, high-fat meals, as he admits to eating a lot of fast food. He has gained about 50 lb in the last 5 years. He has been urinating a lot at night as well as during the daytime. He does drink a lot of bottled water because he is frequently thirsty. No burning with urination; no blood in the urine. No disturbance in flow of urine or hesitancy.

FHx: Dad and older brother died at age 58 of heart attack.

SX: Has not been sexually active recently. Has had problems maintaining an erection.

SHx: Lives with his wife. No unusual stress, he says. No recreational drug use. Has smoked 1 pack per day for the past 20 years. EtOH: has one or two drinks three times a week. Works as an air traffic controller.

Physical Exam

Mr. Brown states his weight is 100kg. He is 5 feet, 6 inches tall. He is in no distress. His vision is 20/30 in both eyes. His pupils are normal, and reactive to light. The fundoscopic exam reveals a normal red reflex. His Pharynx is normal. His neck exam reveals no carotid bruits or thyroidmegaly. He has no jugular venous distention. His chest appears barrel chested with an increased anterior-posterior diameter. His nail beds appear pink but he does have clubbing of the fingers. When you listen to the lungs he has a few rahles at the bases bilaterally that clear when he coughs. His heart sounds are normal. There are no rubs or murmurs heard. You cannot feel the point of maximum impulse, perhaps due to his obesity. His belly is soft, obese, nontender, and without masses. An old scar from the gall bladder surgery is located in the right subcostal abdomen. He has some edema of both lower extremities. Radial pulses are strong but the pulses in his feet are present but diminished. Mr. Brown is alert. He is able to walk normally. His strength is equal and strong in all 4 extremities. There is no redness or tenderness or open sores on the feet. He has decreased sensation below the knee to light touch in both legs.

THE CLOSING

As with all cases, it is important to explain your clinical impression to your patient and discuss the next steps in working up his condition. Your main task is to identify and treat all of the patient's risk factors for vascular disease and cancer.

> **Doctor:** "All right Mr. Brown. Let me just summarize what you have described to me. You have had weight gain over the last few years, a thirsty feeling, and the need to urinate frequently. Do I have this right?"
>
> **Mr. Brown:** "You make it sound bad. I'm just getting old!"

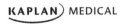

Doctor: "Well, I'd like to help you get a lot older. I'd like to see if you have high blood sugar, and also to run some basic tests for your heart, kidney, and cholesterol level."

Mr. Brown: "Is there anything else?"

Doctor: "We can talk about the results of these tests and determine if there are any medicines that would be beneficial. Can you come back this Friday at the same time and we can discuss the results?"

Mr. Brown: "Yeah, sure."

Doctor: "In the meantime, I'd like you to eat five servings of vegetables a day and minimize the amount of fatty foods and high sugar foods in your diet. Sometimes it's difficult to know how much fat is in takeout and fast foods, so it's best to avoid these in your diet. Also, for your ongoing health, I would recommend that you stop smoking. Here is the phone number for a Stop Smoking Class that many people find helpful in quitting. Quitting cigarettes is the single most important thing you can do for your health, as it prevents a large number of health conditions. I know that we've discussed a lot today, but I want to make sure that you understand all of these things. Do you have questions for me?"

CHALLENGING QUESTIONS

Mr. Brown: "Doc, could you just put down on the form that everything is normal? I really need this insurance."

GRADING: STANDARDIZED PATIENT DATA-GATHERING CHECKLISTS

History Checklist

- ☑ **S**ite/symptoms: Ask if he has any other problems you can help with
- ☑ **A**ssociated symptoms (CVS): Chest pain, excercise intolerance, shortness of breath, PND, claudication
- ☑ **A**ssociated symptoms (neuro): Headache, dizziness, weakness, sensory changes
- ☑ **P**ast medical history: Hospitalization
- ☑ **P**ast medical history: Major illness/ask about HTN specifically
- ☑ **P**ast medical history: Surgery
- ☑ **A**llergies
- ☑ **M**edicines
- ☑ **R**OS: Recent changes in weight
- ☑ **R**OS: Ask about diet
- ☑ **R**OS: Ask about urination (frequency, changes), bowel movements, blood in stool
- ☑ **S**exual history: Sexual function history
- ☑ **S**ocial Hx: Smoking history, recreational drug use, alcohol
- ☑ **S**ocial Hx: Stress level
- ☑ **S**ocial Hx: Exercise

Physical Exam Checklist

- ☑ General appearance
- ☑ HEENT: Pupils, visual acuity, funduscopy
- ☑ HEENT: Thyroid palpation
- ☑ HEENT: Check for JVD
- ☑ Chest: Inspect (front and back)
- ☑ Chest: Auscultate
- ☑ CV: Carotid pulse, auscultation and palpation
- ☑ CV: Radial, DP, PT pulse
- ☑ CV: Heart auscultation
- ☑ CV: Heart PMI
- ☑ Abd: Palpation
- ☑ Neuro: Motor strength four extremities
- ☑ Neuro: Gait
- ☑ Neuro: Sensation four extremities
- ☑ Neuro: Brachial DTR
- ☑ Joints: Inspect knees

SAMPLE PATIENT NOTE

History: Include significant positives and negatives from history of present illness, past medical history, review of system(s), social history, and family history.

CC: 55 y/o male presenting for an insurance physical

HPI: Mr. Brown denies any complaints but has noticed increased frequency of urination. He also is frequently thirsty and has 50-lb weight gain in 5 years. Pt nocturia. No dysuria or hematuria. No SOB, chest pain, cough, hoarseness, change in bowel habits, or blood in stool. No change in skin lesions. No headache, weakness, sensory changes or weakness.

Allergies: None

Meds: Saw palmetto

PMH: Hospitalized for cholecystectomy 5 yrs ago. No hx DM, no reported hx HTN (last BP check was 5 years ago, reported "white-coat" HTN for past 20 years). Never had sugar checked.

ROS: Diet—fast food, high fat. Sleep—snores, increased daytime sleepiness.

Fam Hx: Father and brother died age 58 MI

SX: + Erectile dysfunction

SH: Lives with wife. Smokes 1 ppd, EtOH 1–2 drinks 3x/wk. No drug use. States no unusual stresses.

Physical Exam: Indicate only pertinent positive and negative findings related to patient's chief complaint.

VS: NL except for BP = 145/94. Ht 5 ft 6 in, wt 220 lb.

GA: No distress

HEENT: PERRL, V/A 20/30 OU. Fundi: NL red reflex. No thryroidmegaly, − JVD.

Chest: Increased AP diameter, rales at bases that clear with cough, + clubbing

CV: Carotid upstrokes NL without bruit. Decreased pulses 1/4 DP, PT B/L, radials 2/4. S1, S2: WNL, PMI not palpable.

Abd: Soft, obese, nontender. No masses. Old R subcostal scar.

Neuro: Gait NL, motor 5/5 all 4 ext, decreased light touch below knees B/L. Light touch sensation intact both feet B/L.

Differential Diagnosis: In order of likelihood (with 1 being the most likely), list up to five potential or possible diagnoses for this patient's presentation. (In many cases, fewer than five diagnoses are likely.)

1. Diabetes, obesity
2. Elevated BP reading
3. Peripheral vascular disease
4. Peripheral neuropathy
5. Prostatic hypertrophy

Diagnostic Workup: List immediate plans (up to five) for further diagnostic workup.

1. Rectal and prostate exam
2. U/A, CBC, stool for FOBT
3. Lytes, BUN, Cr, glucose
4. Cholesterol, HDL, LDL, triglyceride
5. Prostate-specific antigen (PSA) test

Answer: "I'm afraid I can't do that. How about working together to make your health better?"

Mr. Brown has just requested that you lie. Apart from not committing insurance fraud, the key to this challenge is to stay calm, nondefensive, and nonjudgmental. If the patient is insistent about what he believes you should include in the form, simply give him back the blank form.

CASE DISCUSSION

Notes about the History-Taking

Do not get into the habit of skipping the bottom half of the Doorway Information. While it is usually the same in each case, it is different in some. Make sure to read the Examinee Tasks on every case.

Here, you receive directions on what to do if Mr. Brown hands you an insurance form he'd like you to send to his insurance company. You are asked not to write on any paper the SP hands you. You are instructed to write the standard Patient Note. To summarize: Read the Doorway Information and any paper the SP gives you, and do what it says.

The patient will open the encounter in a manner similar to the following:

> **Mr. Brown:** "Here is the insurance physical form I need you to fill out." *(He hands you a paper)*

> **Doctor:** *(Takes paper, reads it, and places it on his clipboard)* "Thank you. I'll fill it out and send it in after our visit."

> **Mr. Brown:** "Okay."

Mr. Brown's primary concern may be getting his insurance arranged, and he may not be as concerned about his overall health and well-being. You will need to concentrate on what to do to keep this patient alive and healthy, and relay to him any concerns about his risk factors.

At the beginning of this type of case there are no symptoms on which to do SIQORAA, so after your usual introduction, Mr. Brown will tell you about his insurance form. Be sure also to ask if there is anything else you can help with.

> **Doctor:** "Aside from the insurance form, do you have any other health concerns I can help with?"

> **Mr. Brown:** "No."

Since the answer is no, you can go directly to associated symptoms; had the answer been yes, you would do SIQORAA on whatever the complaint was.

What are the associated symptoms of someone with no medical complaints? This turns the case into a periodic health exam. Cardiovascular disease and cancer are the two things most likely to end this patient's life. The average adult may need treatment/counseling for hypertension, smoking, obesity, and diet, just to name a few. So the associated symptoms in this case will include asking some common symptoms of cardiovascular disease and cancer. If you receive any positive responses to the questions you ask, you may then go back and obtain more details with your SIQORAA mnemonic.

In this case, one clue is that Mr. Brown takes saw palmetto for his nocturia. This is the first medical complaint he has spoken about (by this point you have probably noticed his obesity, increased chest diameter, and possibly clubbing) so you should ask all your urinary questions. It is also appropriate to begin thinking about diabetes as a condition that he may have. After this, you'll need to complete the PAMHRFSS history. You may find that the patient has sleep apnea as well as erectile dysfunction. Erectile dysfunction may be a clue that he has vascular disease as well as neuropathy.

Comments about the Physical Exam

This is where height and weight are important. In general, ask height and weight for pre-employment physicals, pediatric cases, and other cases in which patients will want help with managing their diabetes, hypertension, or obesity.

The physical exam should be focused on the patient's urinary complaints as well as the target organs of diabetes mellitus and hypertension. For the urinary complaints, pay close attention to the genitourinary exam and palpation of abdomen (although do note that much of the genitourinary exam is forbidden on the Step 2 CS exam). For diabetes and hypertension, pay attention to the eyes, feet, and cardiovascular exam.

Comments about the Note

Even though you may not find out about Mr. Brown's problem with urination and weight gain until the ROS questions, it is fine to include this information in the HPI of the Patient Note. This will demonstrate that you are able to organize information from the patient history into a logical patient note, and shows the graders the important features that support your primary diagnosis, which, in this case, is diabetes.

Either way, though, you would get credit if you listed the urinary problem and the weight gain under the ROS section of the history. The most important thing is to document your findings on paper and not to worry so much about the absolute best heading under which to list it.

There are more possibilities for the differential diagnoses in this patient than you will have time or space to write. Certainly, sleep apnea, prostate cancer, prostatitis, and hypothyroidism are acceptable responses in the differential diagnosis. Write down the ones you think are most probable, and then make sure you have selected the basic tests that match these diagnoses. For example, had the doctor in this case listed hypothyroidism, then a TSH would be appropriate in the workup.

There are many more tests that this 55-year-old man will need soon: HbA1C, TSH, ECG, and a CXR. Eventually he may need a colonoscopy, stress test, sleep study, nerve conduction velocity of the lower extremities, and more. The advice is to get the general tests done first and add additional tests as time and space allow.

Case 30: **Obesity**

DOORWAY INFORMATION

Opening Scenario

Shirley Adams is a 15 y/o female whose mother has come to the clinic concerned about Shirley's weight gain.

Vital Signs

No vital signs are taken in this case, since the patient is not present.

Examinee Tasks

1. Obtain a focused history.
2. You will not be required to perform a physical examination in this case.
3. Discuss your initial diagnostic impression and your workup plan with the patient's mother.
4. After leaving the room, complete your patient note on the given form.

BEFORE ENTERING THE ROOM

1. Cues: The opening scenario gives you information that can begin your thinking about the case. However, in this case it is very brief, and you must keep an open mind as to what this entire case is about. Based on the introduction, this is a surrogate case that involves your speaking with the mother. As with other surrogate cases, you will need to order a physical exam on the patient note and you will need to take a pediatric/adolescent history. Also keep in mind that obesity is associated with depression and eating disorders, so you should ask about symptoms of depression.

2. Clinical Reasoning: There is an obesity epidemic in the United States. It is mainly attributed to large portions of high-calorie foods (high-fat and high-sugar meals) and a sedentary lifestyle. Secondary causes of obesity may also be considered, such as hypothyroidism, insulinoma, Cushing syndrome, and polycystic ovarian disease; however, these account for far fewer cases than general overeating and underexercising.

FROM THE MOTHER

History

HPI: Ms. Adams tells you that her daughter, Shirley, appears to have given up on her weight loss and feels defeated by the number of diets she has attempted. Shirley is 5 feet 2 inches and 220 lb. Her mother would like you to recommend a diet. Since the age of 8 months, Shirley has always been above the 95% for weight on the growth charts. By second grade she was the heaviest child in her class, and has remained so throughout her life. She has tried various popular commercial diets, but at best, they helped her to maintain the same weight for a few months. When she stopped a certain diet, her weight would typically increase.

According to Ms. Adams, Shirley carries most of her weight around her belly and even her upper back. Her arms and legs seem very skinny in comparison. Shirley is too large to play with other children outdoors, and it is affecting her self-esteem. Shirley seems sad and hopeless about her condition. She has never talked of harming herself but she frequently stands in front of the refrigerator and eats for hours into the night. Shirley recognizes that she often eats when bored, dissatisfied, or depressed. She has less energy than usual lately. She has a very poor body image. She never tries to make herself vomit.

She is allergic to PCN. She takes no medications.

PMH: Shirley has never been hospitalized. No surgery or trauma. Never diagnosed with diabetes.

SHx: Shirley has been sleeping more than usual lately. Her diet consists mostly of high-fat and processed foods. She eats many crackers, but few fruits and vegetables. Shirley lives at home with her mother and father. Shirley is a sophomore in high school with average grades. She does not drink alcohol, use drugs, or smoke cigarettes.

Family Hx: Everyone in Shirley's family is a little overweight, according to Ms. Adams, so it is possible she has a genetic predisposition.

Ob/Gyn: Shirley has never had a period. That is another thing that Ms. Adams is concerned about. Ms. Adams states that Shirley is not sexually active—in fact, she has never had a boyfriend and has very few friends at all. Shirley is also very self-conscious about her weight and the fact that she has some facial hair and bad acne.

Physical Exam

There is no physical exam in this case.

THE CLOSING

Doctor: "Thank you for coming to talk to me today, Ms. Adams. I would like to review what we talked about today." *(Ms. Adams nods)* "Shirley has been overweight her entire life. Now it is affecting her self esteem."

Ms. Adams: "Yes, that's the short version."

Doctor: "I'd like to examine Shirley as soon as possible. There are many conditions that can cause one to be overweight."

Ms. Adams: "Like what? I thought it was just from overeating."

Doctor: "That's usually the case. But sometimes there are hormonal problems. I'll need to take a blood test to check."

Ms. Adams: "She won't want to see you. Should I lie to her and trick her into coming to see you?"

Doctor: "No, we have found that telling the truth is always the best policy. Just tell her I want to help her with her weight. Tell her that she can talk to me confidentially."

Be sure to mention the patient (who is not in the exam room) by name. It is more personable and demonstrates empathy. The doctor in this exchange showed great concern for his patient.

CHALLENGING QUESTIONS

Ms. Adams: "I've read about new FDA-approved pills for weight loss. Can't you just give me a prescription?"

Answer: "I don't know if that medicine would be right for Shirley without a physical exam and a blood test. Let me know if she refuses to come to the appointment. I can call her at home, or perhaps set up some counseling for her."

As always, you cannot prescribe medication on this test without seeing the patient. You always need to see and examine the patient, and get test results back, to know if a medication is safe and indicated.

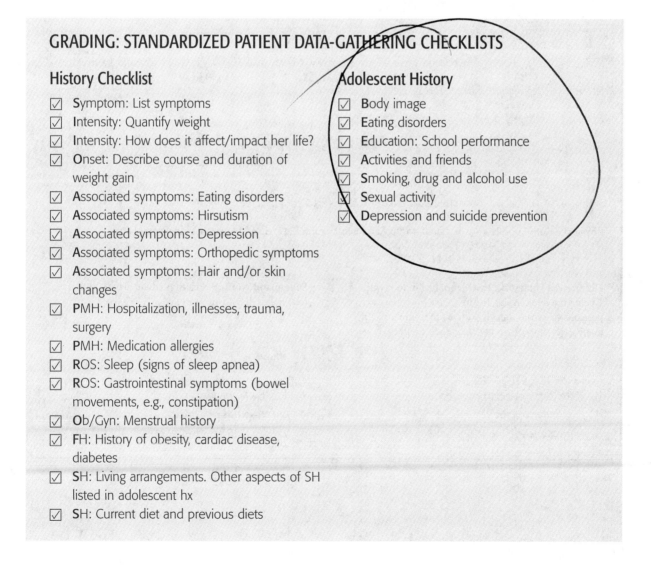

GRADING: STANDARDIZED PATIENT DATA-GATHERING CHECKLISTS

History Checklist

- ☑ **S**ymptom: List symptoms
- ☑ **I**ntensity: Quantify weight
- ☑ **I**ntensity: How does it affect/impact her life?
- ☑ **O**nset: Describe course and duration of weight gain
- ☑ **A**ssociated symptoms: Eating disorders
- ☑ **A**ssociated symptoms: Hirsutism
- ☑ **A**ssociated symptoms: Depression
- ☑ **A**ssociated symptoms: Orthopedic symptoms
- ☑ **A**ssociated symptoms: Hair and/or skin changes
- ☑ **PMH:** Hospitalization, illnesses, trauma, surgery
- ☑ **PMH:** Medication allergies
- ☑ **ROS:** Sleep (signs of sleep apnea)
- ☑ **ROS:** Gastrointestinal symptoms (bowel movements, e.g., constipation)
- ☑ **Ob/Gyn:** Menstrual history
- ☑ **FH:** History of obesity, cardiac disease, diabetes
- ☑ **SH:** Living arrangements. Other aspects of SH listed in adolescent hx
- ☑ **SH:** Current diet and previous diets

Adolescent History

- ☑ Body image
- ☑ Eating disorders
- ☑ Education: School performance
- ☑ Activities and friends
- ☑ Smoking, drug and alcohol use
- ☑ Sexual activity
- ☑ Depression and suicide prevention

SAMPLE PATIENT NOTE

History: Include significant positives and negatives from history of present illness, past medical history, review of system(s), social history, and family history.

CC: 15 y/o female with weight gain

HPI: Hx comes from mother. Pt has been above 95% for weight her entire life. Now 5'2", 100 kg. Has tried multiple commercial diets without success. Pt has poor body image. Ms. Adams describes that Shirley frequently eats large amounts of food late into the night. Triggers include boredom and feelings of hopelessness. Has decreased energy. Her diet consists of few fruits and vegetables and mostly high-fat processed foods and crackers. Most of her weight is in her trunk. Mother states pt's arms and legs look "skinny." No hx of self-harm ideation. Is an average student, a sophomore in high school. No recent change in grades. Does not have many friends. Mother reports pt has more acne and facial hair compared to her peer group.

Allergies: PCN

Meds: None

PMH: No hospitalizations, trauma, or surgery. No hx of DM, HTN, or orthopedic problems.

ROS: Sleeping more than usual lately

FH: Many overweight family members

Ob/Gyn: Has never had a period. Also has hirsutism and acne.

SX: Not sexually active

SH: Lives with mother and father. Does not smoke or use alcohol or drugs.

Physical Exam: Indicate only pertinent positive and negative findings related to patient's chief complaint.

There is no physical exam in this case.

Differential Diagnosis: In order of likelihood (with 1 being the most likely), list up to five potential or possible diagnoses for this patient's presentation. (In many cases, fewer than five diagnoses are likely.)

1. Obesity
2. Cushing's syndrome
3. Polycystic ovarian syndrome
4. Hypothyroidism
5. Nighttime eating disorder/depression

Diagnostic Workup: List immediate plans (up to five) for further diagnostic workup.

1. Physical exam
2. TSH, CBC lytes, BUN, Cr, Glu
3. FSH, LH, prolactin level
4. Ultrasound of ovaries
5. 24-hour urine-free cortisol

CASE DISCUSSION

Notes about the History-Taking

Ms. Adams (the patient's mother) is waiting for you when you enter the room. The term *obesity* is considered medical terminology. Use *obesity* in the note but not when talking to patients. Tell patients they are *overweight*. Also, stay away from calling patients *fat*.

The adolescent history includes asking about body image, eating disorders, education, friends, drugs, sex, smoking, and depression. Since no physical exam is possible—there is no patient present—use the time you would ordinarily spend on the physical exam filling in the details of the adolescent history you have not yet obtained. In this case, the adolescent history was merged and asked with the SIQORAAA PAMHRFOSS and written with the HPI and PMH. It would be equally correct to ask the adolescent history questions at the end of the standard history. It would be equally correct to write a separate heading on the note for "Adolescent Hx" and record your findings there.

Eating disorders that cause obesity include binge-eating disorder, nighttime eating disorder, and bulimia. They are commonly associated with depression but can occur without depression as well. With all of these disorders, the patient feels unable to control his/her eating. Specific eating disorders may be used as differential diagnoses in the obese patient. Binge-eating disorder manifests by eating large amounts of food over a 2-hour period. Patients with nighttime eating disorder, as the name implies, eat most of their daily calories in the period from after dinner to bedtime. Bulimia often causes patients to be overweight despite self-induced vomiting.

You may ask your patients about eating disorders by using the following questions:

- What are your eating patterns?
- Do you ever feel that you cannot stop eating when you want to?
- Do you eat mostly at night?
- Do you make yourself vomit after eating?

Notes about the Physical Exam

There is no physical exam in this case.

Comments about the Patient Note

In this case, there is no physical exam to perform. However, if this were an obese person coming for advice on weight loss, you would concentrate on the organ systems where obesity causes damage—namely, a good cardiovascular exam. Secondary organ systems could include the knees and the spine. Check the abdomen for gallstones (RUQ tenderness), and palpate the thyroid gland.

Be sure to include the current height and weight as well as a complete description of the patient's weight throughout her life. You will not be expected to calculate the Body Mass Index.

Polycystic ovarian disease typically has a workup to include follicle-stimulating hormone (FSH), luteinizing hormone (LH), and prolactin. The use of abbreviations is acceptable. An ultrasound would look at the ovaries.

Cushing syndrome is uncommon but is hinted at by the mother when she talks about Shirley's skinny extremities. A 24-hour urine collection for cortisol is a good first test. Remember, the graders for Step 2 CS are looking for initial tests to get the workup started.

Case 31: **Parkinson's Disease**

DOORWAY INFORMATION

Opening Scenario

Richard Wilson is a 70 y/o male with Parkinson's disease and fever.

Vital Signs

- Temp: 38.9°C (102.0°F)
- BP: 160/114 mm Hg, right upper limb sitting
- HR: 110/min, regular
- RR: 24/min

Examinee Tasks

1. Obtain a focused history.
2. Perform a relevant physical examination. Do not perform rectal, pelvic, genitourinary, female breast, or corneal reflex examinations.
3. Discuss your initial diagnostic impression and your workup plan with the patient.
4. After leaving the room, complete your patient note on the given form.

BEFORE ENTERING THE ROOM

1. Cues: Write your mnemonics on your blue sheet. These will remind you of other questions to ask, and will ensure that you don't skip pertinent aspects of the history.

2. Clinical Reasoning: Pay close attention to known chronic conditions. When the Doorway Information indicates that your patient has a particular chronic disease, you likely need to consider complications of that chronic disease in your differential diagnosis. Parkinson's patients are more prone to aspiration pneumonia, however complications from Parkinsonian medications can also cause fever.

For this case, consider the following common complications of Parkinson's disease before you walk into the room:

- Dysphagia (can lead to aspiration)
- Depression
- Sleep disorders

- Constipation
- Falls (subdural hematoma)
- Side effects from too much medication
- Increased Parkinson's symptoms from too little medication

FROM THE STANDARDIZED PATIENT

History

HPI: Mr. Wilson has 2 days of fever to 103°F. He has a cough productive of yellow sputum. Mild shortness of breath began last week, he believes, after he nearly choked on a piece of apple. Mr. Wilson has also had increasing problems walking over the past 2 weeks, and almost fell several times. In fact, today he really cannot walk at all and had to be carried into your office due to tremor and weakness. He complains of being very stiff. Tylenol controls the fever only for a few hours. He feels like he has been getting sicker every day this week and cannot tell why. He denies chest pain, headache or confusion.

Medications: Benztropine—dose increased one month ago. Levodopa—stopped taking 2 weeks ago because he ran out of medicine. No known drug allergies.

PMH: Mr. Wilson was diagnosed with Parkinson's 5 years ago. He was hospitalized for pneumonia 1 year ago, from which he made a full recovery. One month ago he was hospitalized because he was unable to urinate and had a full bladder. Mr. Wilson had many concussions in the past from boxing as a young man. No surgical history.

SH: Mr. Wilson has not been eating well because of increased drooling and, since the apple episode last week, the fear that he will choke on his food. He has not had any change in his sleep. He complains of difficulty swallowing. He frequently feels the need to urinate, but only a few drops come out each time. Often, he cannot get to the bathroom fast enough and so he wets his pants. Mr. Wilson lives at home with his wife. He does not smoke or use alcohol.

Physical Exam

When you enter the room, you observe that Mr. Wilson is diaphoretic, lying back. He appears to be very stiff and uncomfortable from tremors. His head is without bruising or tenderness. His pupils are round and reactive to light. Mucous membranes of the mouth and pharynx are very dry. He is alert and oriented to person, place, and time. His neck is rigid with passive movement.

Patient's lungs are clear to auscultation. He has normal respiratory excursion, tactile fremitus, and normal percussion. He is tachycardic. No abnormal heart tones are heard. Abdomen is soft. Bowel sounds are present. There is no suprapubic tenderness or masses. No CVA tenderness.

Mr. Wilson has severe bradykinesia and is too weak to walk. He is rigid in all four extremities with passive movement. His sensation is intact in all four extremities.

THE CLOSING

As with all cases, it is important to explain your clinical impression to your patient and discuss the next steps in working up his condition. You should provide some indication about the length of time he may be unable to walk, as this may affect his transportation and employment options. Be sure to answer any additional concerns he may have.

Doctor: "Mr. Wilson, I have finished my physical exam and would like to discuss what might be causing you to feel sick. First, I want to be sure I understand. You told me you have a high fever with yellow sputum. You ran out of levodopa about 2 weeks ago and now you feel very stiff and can't walk."

Mr. Wilson: "Yes."

Doctor: "I think you might have an infection in your chest. Stopping the levodopa might also be part of the problem. I'll need to take a picture of your chest and a sample of blood to look for infection. We can do those tests right now and I should have some answers for you in an hour. Then we will talk about treatment. Do you have any questions?"

In this case it is not appropriate to end the encounter by saying "We will meet again," as this patient obviously needs to be hospitalized. It is more appropriate to say that you will do the tests now and have the results back soon. Even though it is appropriate in other cases, it's best not to lecture this patient about the dangers of stopping his medication at this time: Right now he is simply too sick.

CHALLENGING QUESTIONS

Mr. Wilson: "Am I going to die?"

Answer: "What you have is serious, but I am going to get you the appropriate treatment and will do everything I can to help."

GRADING: STANDARDIZED PATIENT DATA-GATHERING CHECKLISTS

History Checklist

- ☑ Symptoms: Fever, cough, SOB
- ☑ Intensity: Ask "How is this affecting your life?"
- ☑ Quality of pain
- ☑ Onset of symptoms
- ☑ Alleviating factors
- ☑ Aggravating factors
- ☑ Associated symptoms: Motor changes (weakness, tremor, rigidity, ambulation)
- ☑ ROS: Changes in urination, bowel movement
- ☑ PMH: Hospitalizations
- ☑ PMH: Major illnesses
- ☑ PMH: Surgery
- ☑ Allergies
- ☑ Medicines: Hx of increased benztropine, and that pt stopped levodopa, tylenol
- ☑ Social HX: Who does he live with?

Physical Exam Checklist

- ☑ General appearance
- ☑ HEENT: Inspection to look for trauma from fall
- ☑ HEENT: Palpation to look for tenderness
- ☑ HEENT: Pharynx
- ☑ Chest: Inspection
- ☑ Chest: Respiratory excursion
- ☑ Chest: Tactile fremitus
- ☑ Chest: Percussion
- ☑ Chest: Auscultation
- ☑ CV: Auscultation
- ☑ Abd: Palpation
- ☑ Neuro: Mental status, orientation
- ☑ Neuro: Motor
- ☑ Neuro: Gait
- ☑ Neuro: Check neck for meningitis

SAMPLE PATIENT NOTE

History: Include significant positives and negatives from history of present illness, past medical history, review of system(s), social history, and family history.

CC: 70 y/o male. Fever

HPI: Pt with 2 days of fever up to 103°F. Has had a cough productive of yellow sputum after getting a bite of apple "down the wrong pipe" last week. Mildly SOB. No chest pain. Pt also has been getting increasingly stiff, with difficulty walking and almost fell several times. This is because of severe weakness, tremor, and rigidity. He is completely incapacitated and cannot move on his own. This has been for the last week as well. The fever goes down with Tylenol just for a few hours. Nothing in particular seems to make it worse.

Meds: Benztropine (dose was recently increased last month). Levodopa (has not taken in 2 weeks because ran out). NKDA.

PMH: Hospitalized for pneumonia last year and urinary retention last month. (Pt had Foley catheter removed 3 weeks ago.) Parkinson's for 5 years. Had multiple concussions due to boxing in his youth. No recent trauma. No surgery.

ROS: No change in his sleep pattern. Decreased food intake because of drooling and trouble swallowing. Complains of urinary hesitancy, urgency with frequency. No burning. Frequent incontinence.

SH: Lives with wife; denies tobacco, EtOH, or drug use

Physical Exam: Indicate only pertinent positive and negative findings related to patient's chief complaint.

VS: 160/114, 110, 24, 102°F

GA: Very rigid, diaphoretic

HEENT: Atraumatic, PERRL. Pharynx very dry. Neck supple.

Chest: Resp excursion NL, fremitus NL, percussion NL. Lungs clear to Auscultation.

CV: Tachycardia, S1 S2 NL

Abd: BS+, nontender all 4 quadrants and suprapubic. No CVA tenderness.

Neuro: Alert and oriented to person, place, and time. Motor hard to test, extremely rigid all 4 extremities to passive movement. + Bradykinesia. Pt too weak to walk. Sensation intact all 4 extremities.

Differential Diagnosis: In order of likelihood (with 1 being the most likely), list up to five potential or possible diagnoses for this patient's presentation. (In many cases, fewer than five diagnoses are likely.)

1. Pneumonia (secondary to aspiration)
2. Anticholinergic symptoms from medicine
3. Neuroleptic malignant syndrome
4. Prostatitis/Urinary tract infection
5. Urinary retention

Diagnostic Workup: List immediate plans (up to five) for further diagnostic workup.

1. CBC, blood culture, sputum culture
2. CXR
3. U/A, urine culture
4. Lytes, BUN, Cr
5. CPK

CASE DISCUSSION

Notes about the History-Taking

This is a complex history in that the patient has two equally important complaints: pneumonia and the worsening Parkinson's symptoms. Usually the two illnesses portrayed will be related—one being a complication of the other—as it is in this case.

With multiple complaints you may not be able to do SIQORAAA on each complaint separately. This is sometimes confusing in this patient encounter because you have to make decisions and collect only the most relevant history of each complaint instead of strictly following the mnemonic.

One approach for patients with multiple disparate chief complaints is as follows: Make sure you understand the SQO (site/symptom, quality/quantity, and onset) for each complaint. R (radiation) is usually needed only when the patient has pain. Then, after you have identified all the major complaints, do the Intensity ("How is this illness affecting your life?") and AAA (aggravating, alleviating factors, and associated symptoms) once for all the major symptoms together.

Notes about the Physical Exam

This case demonstrates what to do when an SP is portraying a very ill patient. The history is highly suggestive of pneumonia, yet the SP portraying the case reveals no physical findings of pulmonary consolidation! It is impossible to simulate dullness to percussion, increased fremitus, or rales and rhonchi. So what you will document is exactly what the real physical findings are, as well as physical findings that are obviously simulated. However, when you get to the diagnosis, put more weight on the history. It is the history that gives you the diagnosis in most cases.

Comments about the Patient Note

This patient has separate issues discussed in the HPI. First is a discussion of his pneumonia-like symptoms with the history of the apple aspiration. Sputum and shortness of breath are used for the associated symptoms of his pneumonia. His other complaint is his worsening Parkinson's symptoms. The onset and course of his slow movement, tremor, and weakness are discussed.

Parkinson's consists of the triad of (1) resting tremor, (2) rigidity, and (3) bradykinesia. Also look for dementia and depression in a Parkinson's case.

The workup of this patient is that of any older person with high fever. Blood, urine, and sputum culture as well as CXR will always be correct. The CPK is to look for muscle destruction, which you would see from increased muscle rigidity associated with neuroleptic malignant syndrome (NMS). NMS can occur after stopping levodopa suddenly, as this patient did.

The medication history is very important in this case. Benztropine can also be used to treat Parkinson's, and it has anticholinergic properties.

You may also consider ordering an ultrasound to look for urinary retention.

It would also be correct to add "Foley catheter with residual volume" to your Diagnostic Workup. Foley catheter may be considered a treatment that is forbidden on the USMLE exam; however, in this situation you are placing the Foley to make a diagnosis of urinary retention. Similarly, it would be acceptable to place an NG tube if its purpose was to determine if blood from the rectum is from an upper gastrointestinal source. Cardiac catheterization may also be ordered as it is the best test to determine patency of the coronary arteries. Just do not order angioplasty; angioplasty is a treatment and is never done for the purpose of diagnosis.

Case 32: **Breaking Bad News**

DOORWAY INFORMATION

Opening Scenario

Paul Harris is a 50 y/o male who had a colonoscopy last week. He is here with his wife, Mary, to get the results of the pathology report on the polyp that was removed. The test shows he has adenocarcinoma of the colon.

Your task is to tell this patient that he has adenocarcinoma of the colon. There will be no Patient Note on this encounter.

Vital Signs

No vital signs given in this case.

Examinee Tasks

1. Tell the patient he has colon cancer.
2. There is no history or physical exam in this case.
3. There is no note in this case.

BEFORE ENTERING THE ROOM

1. Cues: The Doorway Information always contains the tasks that are asked of you. For this case you are told that there will be no Patient Note. For this case you are told there is no history or physical exam. A case that involves breaking bad news to a patient may take up the entire 15 minutes. If you are asked to do a history and write a note, you can still use the "telling bad news" technique, but do the six steps involved more briefly. It is less likely you'll be asked to do a telling bad news case like this that also requires a physical exam.

2. Clinical Reasoning: The S-P-I-K-E-S protocol is a strategy to tell bad news. The six steps are S—Setup, P—Perception, I—Invitation, K—Knowledge, E—Emotions, and S—Strategy and Summary. (*Reproduced with permission from Dr. Walter F. Baile and Dr. Robert Buckman.*)

Using the techniques of the SPIKES protocol would be an excellent way to approach a "telling bad news" case in Step 2 CS. Of course since there is no treatment in Step 2 CS you would not go into detailed explanation of treatment optons as you would in real life. The rest of this case is mostly based on the original SPIKES protocol but is slightly adapted for the Step 2 exam.

- **Step 1: Setup:** Enter the room, look the patient in the eye, and do your standard introduction. If there are two SPs in the room and you aren't sure who the patient is, you can find out by asking. Try to address most of your conversation to, and make the most eye contact with, the patient and less eye contact with the family member.

> **Doctor:** "Hello, Mr. Harris?"
>
> **Mr. Harris:** "Yes, Doctor. I'm Paul Harris."
>
> **Doctor:** "My name is Dr. First-Name Last-Name. I will be helping you today."

Next, you need to introduce yourself to other people in the room, in this case, Mrs. Harris. Do not simply assume that the man and woman seated before you are husband and wife. You need to know everyone's name and how they are related. Handshakes would generally be in order with the patient and adult family members. Since the patient is wearing normal street clothes and not a patient gown, no drape is given.

> **Doctor:** "Mr. Harris, could you please introduce me?"
>
> **Mr. Harris:** "Oh, I'm sorry. This is my wife, Mary Harris."
>
> **Mrs. Harris:** "Hello, Doctor."
>
> **Doctor:** "Hello, Mrs. Harris."

In this type of case, you should sit down and conduct the interview.

The next part of the setup is to ensure privacy. Two sample lines are:

> **Doctor:** "I've scheduled a full 15 minutes and asked that my staff not interrupt us."

or

> **Doctor:** "I have turned off my pager and asked that we not be disturbed."

Using either of these phrases subtly tells the patient that this is not going to be a normal, routine doctor visit. The patient will have a sense that something important is about to happen. You can pretend to turn off an imaginary pager. If you are still in the room when the overhead announcement tells you the case is over at the end of 15 minutes, simply say "I'm sorry—I have to answer this overhead page. I'll be back as soon as I can."

The next part of the setup entails figuring out which family members the patient wants to have present while you have this conversation. The patient almost always brings a family member along for support, and that person should not be encouraged to leave. Coming in to receive biopsy results is a special situation and is different from a first visit, where you generally interview the patient alone, in private.

If you ask the wife to leave, it will mostly likely go like this:

> **Doctor:** "Mrs. Harris, would you please step out while I go over the test results with Mr. Harris?"
>
> **Mr. Harris and Mrs. Harris, in unison:** "Oh no, Doctor!"
>
> **Mrs. Harris:** "I want to stay."
>
> **Mr. Harris:** "Doctor, I want my wife to stay."
>
> **Doctor:** "Oh, ok, sure, you may stay."

A better approach is to look at the patient and say the following:

Doctor: "Would you like your family member to stay or step out while we discuss the results today?"

Mr. Harris: "Of course I want her to stay."

It is also correct to ask if the patient wants anyone else (not currently present) included in the conversation.

Doctor: "Is there anyone else we should call in to discuss the results?"

Mr. Harris: "No."

If the patient says yes, the conversation could go something like this:

Doctor: "Is there anyone else we should call in to discuss the results?"

Mr. Harris: "Yes, my daughter."

Doctor: "Is she here?"

Mr. Harris: "No."

Doctor: "Would it be all right if she came next visit? I'd still like to talk with you today. I will be happy to talk to your daughter on the phone also."

Mr. Harris: "Yes, that's fine."

- **Step 2: Patient perception:** The next step is to find out what the patient thinks about his health problem, and what he understands so far about the workup of his condition. At this point, you should correct any misunderstandings the patient may have. For example, a patient who had a colonoscopy may not remember that he had a polyp removed. He might have been told immediately after the procedure, but forgot because he was on so many medications. Since the examinee tasks asked you to obtain a focused history, it is appropriate to take a few moments to obtain and summarize the history to date.

Doctor: "Do you remember why we did this test?"

and/or

Doctor: "What have you been told about your symptoms?"

If you know the symptoms, you could ask the patient when he first had the symptom and what he thought it might be. Or you could ask at what point the patient thought something serious was going on.

If the patient has been seeing multiple physicians, it is fine to ask the patient what the other doctors have told him about his condition.

In this example the exchange might go something like this:

Doctor: "Mr. Harris, do you remember why we did the colonoscopy?"

Mr. Harris: "Yes, to find out why I was having blood in my stool."

Doctor: "That's right. What did you think the bleeding was from?"

Mr. Harris: "Well, I thought my hemorrhoids were acting up again."

Doctor: "Did you think it was something serious when you saw the blood?"

Mr. Harris: "Not really, but I got scared one night when I really saw a lot of blood."

Doctor: "Have you seen any other physicians for this problem?"

Mr. Harris: "Yes, the night I saw a lot of blood I went to the emergency room to get checked out."

Doctor: "And what did they tell you?"

Mr. Harris: "They told me I was 'stable' but that I needed to do the colonoscopy."

Doctor: "Do you remember the doctor talking to you immediately after the colonoscopy?"

Mr. Harris: "Not really, I was little groggy."

Doctor: "The doctor removed a tiny piece of skin from the inside of the bowel during your colonoscopy."

Mr. Harris: "Oh! I didn't know that."

Mrs. Harris: "I was there, dear, when the doctor told you."

Doctor: "It is normal not to remember everything you are told immediately after receiving sedatives. Removing a small piece of skin or tissue is called a biopsy."

- **Step 3: Invitation:** Even though the patient came in specifically to get the test results, it's best not to blurt out the result when it is bad news. It is much better to tell the patient you are ready to go over the results today. Then get the patient's permission to tell the news, and have some idea about the level of detail the patient is expecting. Different patients have different needs for the level of detail they wish to know.

  Doctor: "I have the test results back. Would you like to go over them now?"

  Mr. Harris: "Yes."

  Doctor: "Would you like basic information or all the details?"

  Mr. Harris: "The details, I guess."

  Doctor: "So if it turns out to be something serious, you would like to know."

  Mr. Harris: "It is serious, isn't it?"

By going through this process, the patient already has a good idea of what the problem is even before you tell him about the cancer. This technique of "telling the whole truth and nothing but the truth, but in small doses" gives the patient time to comprehend the life-changing news you are delivering.

- **Step 4: Give knowledge:** You need to explain to the patient precisely what the problem is. Give the news in small doses.

  Doctor: "Yes, Mr. Harris, I'm sorry to have to tell you that the pathology report shows that what you have is serious and will require treatment."

  Mr. Harris: "Really?"

  Doctor: "Yes, the biopsy showed a tumor."

  Mr. Harris: "A tumor! Like a growth, you mean?"

  Doctor: "Yes, exactly."

  Mr. Harris: "Huh . . ."

  Doctor: "When we looked at the tumor with a microscope, we saw that the tumor is cancerous. What we mean when we say something is cancerous is that the growth is uncontrolled."

  Mr. Harris: "Cancerous?"

  Doctor: "Yes, the test shows that you have colon cancer."

  Mr. Harris: "That report must be wrong!"

  Doctor: "I'm sorry to have to tell you that the report is correct. The pathology reports that you have cancer of the colon."

You will notice that the word *sorry* is acceptable. Also, the doctor in this exchange kept away from medical terms such as adenocarcinoma or metastasis. If there were metastasis to tell the patient about, you would tell the patient that the cancer has spread.

Telling the patient that he has cancer is not the end of the "Give knowledge" section. You must also tell the patient about future treatment plans. For Step 2 CS, you do not need to know the 5-year survival statistics or even if a particular cancer is a medical or surgical problem. Give the SP a few seconds to respond, then say the following:

> **Doctor:** "I know this is serious news. But I want to tell you that there are treatment options available for your condition."

> **Mr. Harris:** "It's curable?"

> **Doctor:** "The type of cancer you have does have treatment options. You will have a specialist that is an expert in dealing with this sort of cancer and you will get the best care available for your condition."

From the moment you tell the patient he has cancer, there has to be a lot of repetition of facts and the counseling you give the patient. That is because the patient will have a difficult time remembering and concentrating on what you are saying. An SP who asks the same questions over and over at this point is giving a realistic performance. It is not because he doesn't understand you.

Go on at this point and give additional knowledge about the treatment plan. Besides indicating that there is treatment available, tell the patient more about the cancer specialist in addition to you. It is important that the patient understands that you will remain the primary care physician and that you are not abandoning him to the specialists.

> **Doctor:** "You will be treated by a team of doctors. I will remain your primary physician, of course, and I am referring you to a cancer specialist named Dr. Brown. She has many years of experience in managing colon cancer. I'll bring you her number, and I have already made an appointment for you. I would then like to see you again back here in my office. Okay?"

- **Step 5: Manage emotions:** The patient will probably make some comment to indicate that he can't believe this is true or that he doesn't understand. If this happens, explain again about the positive pathology report (in nonmedical terms) and how you have medication and treatment options available, how the patient will be meeting a cancer specialist, and how you will remain his regular doctor.

If the patient is tearful or crying, this is a good time to use the appropriate touch on the shoulder or forearm and say something like the following:

> **Doctor:** "I can see you are upset. I was upset also when I got the results."

Certainly you can offer the patient a tissue or sip of water, or just sit quietly with him for a few seconds while the information soaks in. If the patient says, "Am I going to die?" or "What is my 5-year survival?," the answer is always the same.

> **Doctor:** "What you have is serious, but we have medications and treatment available."

THE CLOSING

- **Step 6: Summarize:** Summarizing the encounter consists of getting the patient to paraphrase everything that you talked about today.

> **Doctor:** "Mr. Harris. I know I gave you a lot of information to remember today. I want to make sure you understand me correctly."

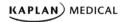

Mr. Harris: "Okay."

Doctor: "Can you repeat back to me what I have told you today?"

Mr. Harris: "You told me I have colon cancer, that it is treatable, and that you want me to see an additional doctor to help treat it, and that I should continue to consider you my regular doctor."

Doctor: "That's right."

If the patient has any misconceptions, explain again what you want until the patient can repeat it back to you. Then ask about any additional questions.

Doctor: "Mrs. Harris, I haven't heard from you. Do you have any questions for me now?"

Mrs. Harris: "No, Doctor, I'm just kind of stunned, I guess."

Doctor: "You can call me anytime with questions, and of course come to our next appointment. And I'm looking forward to meeting your daughter also."

Doctor: "Mr. Harris, any questions for me?"

Mr. Harris: "No, not now."

Doctor: "Here is my phone number. Please call me if you have any questions before our next visit. You have an appointment scheduled for Tuesday. I would like to see you back here next week after your appointment. Is that all right with you?"

Mr. Harris: "Yes."

CHALLENGING QUESTIONS

Mrs. Harris: "If it's cancer that my husband has, please don't tell him."

Answer: The key to this challenge is not to get defensive or dismissive.

Incorrect:
Doctor: "Mrs. Harris, my responsibility is to my patient, not you, and I'm telling him."

Correct:
Doctor: "Why do you feel that way?"

Mrs. Harris: "Well, I think it would depress him."

Doctor: "We have found that if we don't tell patients they have cancer, they eventually find out anyway. Then they're often angry and resentful toward their doctors and family."

Mrs. Harris: "But what about depression?"

Doctor: "It's best to get the news out in the open. If he gets depressed I can help treat that also. I'll ask Mr. Harris if he wants to know the test results. If he doesn't, I will speak only with you about it. If he does want to know, I need to tell him and we both can help support him."

Mrs. Harris: "I guess you're right."

CASE DISCUSSION

Notes about the History-Taking

There is no formal hx-taking in this case.

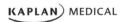

GRADING: STANDARDIZED PATIENT DATA-GATHERING CHECKLISTS

History Checklist

- ☑ **D**id the doctor introduce self to everyone in the room?
- ☑ **S**etup
- ☑ **P**atient perception
- ☑ **I**nvitation to give bad news
- ☑ **G**ive knowledge
- ☑ **M**anage emotions
- ☑ **S**ummarize; have SP paraphrase

Physical Checklist

Not applicable in this case.

Notes about the Physical Exam

There is no physical exam in this case.

Comments about the Patient Note

No patient note in this encounter.

Case 33: **Smoking**

DOORWAY INFORMATION

Opening Scenario

Brian Black is a 48 y/o male who wants to stop smoking.

Vital Signs

- Temp: 37.2°C (98.9°F)
- BP: 130/80 mm Hg
- HR: 84/min
- RR: 24/min

Examinee Tasks

1. Obtain a focused history.
2. Perform a relevant physical examination. Do not perform rectal, pelvic, genitourinary, female breast, or corneal reflex examinations.
3. Discuss your initial diagnostic impression and your workup plan with the patient.
4. After leaving the room, complete your patient note on the given form.

BEFORE ENTERING THE ROOM

1. Cues: Write your mnemonics on your blue sheet. These will remind you of other questions to ask and will ensure you don't skip pertinent aspects of the history. Be sure to make note of the elevated RR given in the doorway vital signs.

2. Clinical Reasoning: Looking at this Doorway Information you should realize that a complete smoking history is needed: when did the patient start to smoke, how many packs/day, number of years he has smoked. You should also find out what the patient has done to stop in the past and how successful he was. It is important to not be judgmental, and to be encouraging of the patient's desire to stop. Do not belittle his past failures in attempting to quit.

In this type of case you will also need to ask if the patient has any additional symptoms that he can describe. If he says no, you can use the SIQORAA mnemonic to find out all about the smoking history. When asking about associated symptoms, ask a few questions about the complications of smoking, e.g., shortness of breath, weight loss, cough, hemoptysis, and hoarseness, to name a few.

The vital signs are very important and should always be scrutinized for clues. Normal breathing rate in adults is 16 breaths/min. When you see respiratory rates in the 20s, ask a few questions to find out why the patient is breathing fast. Also, few patients in the real world have temperatures of exactly 98.6°F. Most clinicians define a fever as a temperature of greater than 100.4°F. Certainly, if the temperature is above this level, think of it as a fever case. If the temp is between 98.6°F and 100.4°F, ask a few questions about the patient having fever and chills at home. But generally, a temperature less than 100.4°F is not a fever.

Mr. Black's vital signs show that he is tachypneic but not febrile.

FROM THE STANDARDIZED PATIENT

History

Mr. Black states that his mother died last month from lung cancer and emphysema. He realizes it is time for him to stop smoking.

> **Doctor:** "How can I help you today?"
>
> **Mr. Black:** "I want to stop smoking."
>
> **Doctor:** "Great, I am glad you came to see me. I can help with that. Do you have any symptoms right now that I can help with as well?"
>
> **Mr. Black:** "No, I'm all right now. I just watched my mother die of emphysema and lung cancer over the last 6 months. I know I need to stop."

So in this case use the SIQORAA to get his entire smoking history.

Patient started smoking when he was 12 years old. By age 18 he was smoking one pack a day. By age 30 he smoked 2 packs/day until now. He has tried to quit several times in the past. He has tried going cold turkey, a nicotine patch, even bupropion a couple of years ago. At the most, he can stop smoking for a week or so before he restarts. He has noticed that he has a cough productive of greenish sputum for months at a time most winters. Mr. Black considers this a normal finding for smokers.

It is also affecting his life in that he stopped playing racquetball because he gets too winded and a little wheezy with intense physical exertion. He no longer runs for the commuter train when he is late because it would take the entire ride home to catch his breath. Once the conductor wanted to call an ambulance for him, but Mr. Black refused. He has had no fevers, and he has lost about 10 lb in the last 2 years. He is not on a diet. Occasionally, when he has a hard coughing spell, a tiny streak of blood comes up. He is not hoarse. He has no episodes of chest pain.

Mr. Black takes no medications and has no allergies.

He has never been hospitalized. He has had no trauma or major surgery. He did have pneumonia last winter, for which he received antibiotics. No history of DM, HTN, or heart or lung disease. He has never had any exposure to tuberculosis.

Mr. Black lives with his wife of 25 years. He works as a consultant. He states that his job is somewhat stressful, and says that's why he smokes. He does not drink alcohol or use recreational drugs.

Physical Exam

When you walk into the room you will see an SP demonstrating pursed-lip breathing and a prolonged expiratory phase. The SP will probably simulate this physical finding for only the first minute or two of the case. His color is pink. The pharynx is normal. There is no supraclavicular or cervical adenopathy. His chest appears normal. Palpation and respiratory excursion, tactile fremitus, percussion, and auscultation will all be normal. He has no jugular venous distension. His heart tones are regular. There is no cyanosis or peripheral edema. Mr. Black does have clubbing. He is awake and alert.

THE CLOSING

Doctor: "Mr. Black, I have finished your physical exam and would like to talk to you about how you can stop smoking."

Mr. Black: "Good."

Doctor: "It sounds to me like you are also having some symptoms from smoking: the cough and sputum, the time you had pneumonia, and the short-of-breath feeling that has stopped you from playing racquetball."

Mr. Black: "Well, that's all just normal smoking stuff."

Doctor: "It is likely related to smoking. On your exam I see that you are breathing a little fast at rest. We need to take a picture of your chest and have you take a breathing test. I want to see if the smoking has done any damage to the lungs."

Mr. Black: "Do you think I'm too late?"

Doctor: "No, no. Every day is a good first day to be smoke-free. I'd like you to start attending the smoking cessation classes here at the hospital immediately. When the tests are back, I'll call you. It's great that you are here today. It shows you are serious about stopping, and I'll help however I can."

CHALLENGING QUESTIONS

Mr. Black: "But I've failed so many times before!"

Answer: "It's better to think positively. Now you have another opportunity, with help from me and the stop-smoking classes."

CASE DISCUSSION

Notes about the History-Taking

In this case it is important to get the amount of cigarettes smoked. Find out when he started smoking as well as the course and duration of tobacco use. Ask if the patient ever got treatment and was able to stop. Asking about complications of tobacco use such as heart, lung disease and symptoms of cancer would be appropriate.

Notes about the Physical Exam

This case requires a complete chest exam as well as some of the cardiovascular exam. Focuing the most attention on the lungs is based on his history of sputum and dyspnea.

GRADING: STANDARDIZED PATIENT DATA-GATHERING CHECKLISTS

History Checklist

This case is complex in that there really are many additional problems that need to be included in the HPI as well. For example, Symptoms: shortness of breath, cough, sputum, smoking are included in the HPI.

☑ **S**ymptoms

☑ **I**ntensity: How it is affecting the pt's life? Can no longer exercise

☑ **O**nset: When did shortness of breath start? When did pt start smoking?

☑ **O**nset: Course of smoking, course of dyspnea

☑ **P**rogression of symptoms

☑ **P**revious attempts to quit smoking

☑ **A**ssociated symptoms: Ask about heart disease, COPD, and cancer

☑ **A**llergies

☑ **M**edications

☑ **P**MH

☑ **F**H: Mother died 6 mo from emphysema

☑ **S**H: Living arrangement, stress

☑ **S**H: Alcohol, recreational drug use

☑ **A**ssociated symptoms (resp): cough, sputum production, presence of blood, hoarseness

☑ **A**ssociated symptoms (CVS): Chest pain, dyspnea on exertion, PND

Physical Exam Checklist

☑ **G**A: Notice the pursed-lip breathing

☑ **H**EENT: Pharynx

☑ **H**EENT: Adenopathy

☑ **C**V: Heart auscultation, PMI

☑ **C**V: JVD

☑ **C**hest: Inspection

☑ **C**hest: Palpation/respiratory excursion

☑ **C**hest: Tactile fremitus

☑ **C**hest: Percussion

☑ **C**hest: Auscultation

☑ **E**xtremities: + Clubbing. No edema or cyanosis.

Comments about the Patient Note

As smoking was discussed in detail in the HPI, there is no need to mention it again in the social history. It is important to note that although your SPs will not have any "real" acute findings, you may have patients that do have symptoms of chronic illnesses. It would not be unusual to have an SP with changes in the chest wall (e.g., increased chest AP diameter) and possibly signs of clubbing. Don't be surprised to find real physical findings as well as simulated.

Emphysema and Chronic Obstructive Pulmonary Disease would also be accepted as correct diagnoses. One pack-year (pk-yr) is defined as smoking one package of cigarettes a day for one year.

SAMPLE PATIENT NOTE

History: Include significant positives and negatives from history of present illness, past medical history, review of system(s), social history, and family history.

CC: Dyspnea, wants stop smoking

HPI: Pt presents wanting to stop smoking. Has smoked since age 12. ~50 pk-year hx. Has tried nicotine patch and bupropion without success. Feels he smokes due to stress of job.

            + Cough productive of sputum for several months each winter, occasional streak of blood

            + SOB, DOE that prevents exercise

            + 10-lb weight loss,

            − Chest pain, hoarseness, fevers

            NKMA, no meds

PMH: No hospitalizations, trauma, or surgery. Had pneumonia last year Rx as outpt.

FH: Mother died of emphysema and lung Ca

SH: Lives with wife, works as consultant. No alcohol or recreational drugs.

Physical Exam: Indicate only pertinent positive and negative findings related to patient's chief complaint.

VS: NL except RR = 24

GA: Looks mildly SOB, pursed-lip breathing

HEENT: Pharynx is clear. No abnormal cervical or supraclavicular adenopathy.

Chest: Prolonged expiratory phase. Chest with increased AP diameter. NL respiratory excursion. Normal tactile fremitus, percussion, and auscultation.

CV: S1, S2 WNL; no murmur, rub, or gallop. No JVD. PMI not displaced.

Ext: No cyanosis or edema. + Clubbing.

Differential Diagnosis: In order of likelihood (with 1 being the most likely), list up to five potential or possible diagnoses for this patient's presentation. (In many cases, fewer than five diagnoses are likely.)

1. Emphysema
2. Chronic bronchitis
3. Lung Ca
4. Tuberculosis
5. Pneumonia

Diagnostic Workup: List immediate plans (up to five) for further diagnostic workup.

1. CXR
2. CBC
3. Pulmonary function test
4. PPD
5. CT chest

Case 34: **Schizophrenia**

DOORWAY INFORMATION

Opening Scenario

Ken Lee is a 22 y/o male graduate student. He is brought to you because he is "not acting right."

Vital Signs

- Temp: 37.2°C (99.0°F)
- BP: 140/80 mm Hg
- HR: 90/min
- RR: 16/min

Examinee Tasks

1. Obtain a focused history.
2. Perform a relevant physical examination. Do not perform rectal, pelvic, genitourinary, female breast, or corneal reflex examinations.
3. Discuss your initial diagnostic impression and your workup plan with the patient.
4. After leaving the room, complete your patient note on the given form.

BEFORE ENTERING THE ROOM

1. Cues: Altered mental status indicates that you will need to complete a neuro exam and a psychiatric exam as well. When you enter the room this patient will be wearing street clothes so no physical exam will be possible. Do not give the drape to standardized patient wearing street clothes. You still should do a complete Mini Mental Status exam.

Mental status changes can be caused by psychiatric illness as well as causes that are considered more organic, such as recreational drug use and encephalitis.

2. Clinical Reasoning: The psychiatric exam consists of the following:

- General appearance
- Orientation to person, place, and time
- Speech
- Recent and remote memory

- Attention and concentration
- Mood and affect
- Thought process
- Hallucinations, delusions, or paranoia
- Suicidal/homicidal ideations
- Insight

General appearance is no different from any other case. Simply describe how the patient looks, any poor hygiene, disorganized appearance, and anything out of the ordinary.

A large part of the psychiatric exam is simply the Mini Mental Status exam. In addition to Mini Mental Status, you will need to comment on the patient's speech, mood, and affect, and the presence or absence of hallucinations and/or delusions. Finally, no psychiatric chart is complete without commenting on suicidal ideations.

Speech can be described as normal, pressured, or rapid. Feel free to comment on the volume, rate, tone, and accent, and any stuttering or idiosyncratic features.

Mood is what the patient reports:

Doctor: "How do you feel?"

Whatever the patient says in response to this is considered his mood.

Affect is the emotional state that you (as the physician) observe: euthymic, neutral, euphoric, dysphoric, flat, and blunted are all psychological terms. Simply describe, in your own terms, what you see.

Thought process is the organization of the patient's thought process: logical, loose associations, flight of ideas, tangential, and circumstantial are all common descriptors.

Hallucinations

Doctor: "Sometimes people see or hear things that are not really there. Does this ever happen to you?"

Delusions

Doctor: "Do people ever tell you that you have very unusual ideas about yourself or the world?"

Insight is what the patient thinks he needs in terms of treatment.

Doctor: "What do you think about your symptoms (illness)?"

FROM THE STANDARDIZED PATIENT

History

HPI: Mr. Lee is brought to you by the police. Of course, the police have left before you arrive and are unavailable for interview. Mr. Lee is fully dressed so you know a physical exam involving heart, lungs, and abdomen will not be needed on this case. When you enter the room he is standing, staring at the wall. His clothes are torn and dirty. It looks like he hasn't showered in a week. He appears to be staring intently at a small spot on the wall.

When you call his name he startles and turns to stare at you. To your surprise, he answers questions quite bluntly and efficiently. He tells you he is not sure why he was brought to the doctor. He states that he "on a mission" to stop the university from making any additional mistakes and thereby "save the solar system." He tells you he is a graduate student in astrophysics at the university. Or rather, he *was* a student until he was expelled for his thesis idea that no one else could understand. He states that he made such a breakthrough while in communication with Alpha Centaurians. He has felt this way for several months. Prior to this he was not so sure about the alien communication, but now he has proof. He tells you that at one time he fit into the establishment and got a full-ride scholarship to the university right out of high school. But over the years, as he concentrated on his work to the exclusion of all social contact, he made this discovery. Nothing has made the voices better or worse. He has felt sad, hopeless, or guilty at times. He is somewhat angry about being forced out his apartment and living on the street.

He has no allergies and is not taking any medications.

PMH: Mr. Lee says he has never felt like this before. He states he has no allergies. He takes no medications because there "may be a government plot preventing [him] from saving the solar system."

He was hospitalized once for 3 days last month when he was found talking to himself in the park. The hospital released him with a bottle of pills that he discarded to prevent government eavesdropping. No trauma. No surgery. No history of high blood sugar or high blood pressure.

ROS: He has not been sleeping more than an hour or two a night. He has lost 20 to 30 lb.

PH: There is no family history of psychiatric disease. His father died last year at age 72.

SH: He is not sexually active. He has no family. He does not smoke or use alcohol. He has recently stopped drinking alcohol—last week—because he found it blocked communications. He has found that the use of PCP and LSD in a 1:1 ratio aids in hearing the Alpha Centaurians' instructions. His last drug use was yesterday. Hopefully, he can get the instructions clearly soon.

Mr. Lee is oriented to person, place, and time. He seems intelligent. He frequently uses novel new words and has to explain their meaning. His recent and delayed memory are intact. He will not spell the word *world* backwards to test attention and concentration. He feels that is beneath someone of his stature. He states that he feels elated and honored to be the contact person for the aliens. He looks agitated. He does not feel he needs the attention of a physician because nothing is wrong. His work must not be interrupted. He has no plans to harm himself or anyone else.

Physical Exam

In this case you have only general appearance, vital signs.

THE CLOSING

> **Doctor:** "Mr. Lee, thank you for speaking with me. Thank you for telling me about the voices and the communications you have been receiving. I think part of what you have been hearing may be just from the LSD and PCP you have taken. It is possible that the stopping alcohol suddenly could be part of it also. How much alcohol were you drinking a day when you stopped?"

> **Mr. Lee:** "About a fifth *(i.e., one-fifth of a gallon)* of vodka a day."

> **Doctor:** "I want to get a blood test to check your sugar and look for any chemical imbalance that is causing your symptoms."

CHALLENGING QUESTIONS

> **Mr. Lee:** "I don't want any tests. I don't want you to inject me with any monitoring devices."

Answer: "I'm here to help and would never do anything to harm you. I also want you to stop using drugs immediately. I'll have the counselor come and speak to you now. Do you have any questions?"

GRADING: STANDARDIZED PATIENT DATA-GATHERING CHECKLISTS

History Checklist

- ☑ Symptoms
- ☑ Intensity
- ☑ Onset
- ☑ Aggravating factors
- ☑ Alleviating factors
- ☑ Associated symptoms
- ☑ Allergies
- ☑ Medications
- ☑ Hospitalizations, major illness, trauma, surgery
- ☑ ROS: Sleep
- ☑ ROS: Diet
- ☑ Family history
- ☑ Social Hx: Alcohol
- ☑ Social Hx: Drug use
- ☑ Social Hx: Living arrangements—homeless

Psychiatric Checklist

- ☑ Orientation
- ☑ Memory
- ☑ Attention and concentration
- ☑ Language
- ☑ Obeys commands
- ☑ Mood
- ☑ Affect
- ☑ Speech
- ☑ Thought process
- ☑ Hallucinations
- ☑ Suicidal ideations
- ☑ Insight

CASE DISCUSSION

Notes about the History-Taking

This patient is blatantly psychotic and is very verbal about what he experiencing. Many patients with schizophrenia have much less speech. The Board, however, will not give you a patient with catatonia (there would be no way to test your interpersonal skills and English proficiency).

Many patients are reticent to speak about the voices, and it may take a few minutes for you to realize that the patient is having auditory hallucinations, tangential thinking, loose associations, or bizarre thoughts.

A good way to ask about psychosis if it is:

> **Doctor:** "Sometimes when people are under a lot of stress, they hear or see things that other people do not. Has this ever happened to you?"

Comments about the Patient Note

Always read the Doorway Information carefully, as it will say what the tasks are and if a note and physical are wanted. This patient is wearing street clothes and you will need to include a physical exam in the workup. This is because a patient who is to be examined must first change into a gown. In real life it is proper for the doctor to step out of the room while the patient is changing. On this test, once you leave the room, you cannot go back in.

Do not worry where you write the psychiatric exam—either the History section or the Physical Exam section of the note is correct. *Where* you write it is not important. *What* you write—and your legibility—is important.

SAMPLE PATIENT NOTE

History: Include significant positives and negatives from history of present illness, past medical history, review of system(s), social history, and family history.

CC: *On a mission to save the solar system*

HPI: *22 y/o male brought in by police. Pt is hearing voices. Has plan to save solar system. Recently lost his housing. Is a former university student who states he is in communication with aliens. Ceased regular EtOH intake last week.*

This has been continuous for at least 3 months but has been slowly worsening for years. Nothing has made it better, including a brief hospitalization last month. Voices are "clearer" with rec drug use. Pt states at times feels sad and hopeless, at other times is angry over loss of housing and possible government eavesdropping.

PMH: *No previous psychotic episodes*

NKMA, noncompliant with any medication

Hospitalized last month for similar symptoms. Denies trauma, DM, HTN, or surgery.

ROS: *Not sleeping, 1–2 hours/day, 20-lb weight loss*

FH: *No hx of psychiatric illness. Father died last year at age 73.*

SH: *Homeless, no alcohol for past week. Uses PCP and LSD. Last used yesterday.*

Physical Exam: Indicate only pertinent positive and negative findings related to patient's chief complaint.

GA: *Pt is dirty and staring at wall*

VS: *WNL*

Psychiatric
history: *Pt is alert and oriented to person, place, and time*

Speech is rapid and pressured

Recent and remote memory intact

Not cooperative to check attention and concentration

Mood: Expansive, elated

Affect: Agitated, jittery

Thought process: Delusional

+ Psychosis, hearing voices of the "aliens"

Denies suicidal intent

Differential Diagnosis: In order of likelihood (with 1 being the most likely), list up to five potential or possible diagnoses for this patient's presentation. (In many cases, fewer than five diagnoses are likely.)

1. *Schizophrenia*
2. *Bipolar with psychosis*
3. *Psychosis 2nd to LSD, PCP*
4. *Alcohol withdrawal*
5. *Hyperthyroidism*

Diagnostic Workup: List immediate plans (up to five) for further diagnostic workup.

1. *Physical exam*
2. *CBC, lytes, BUN, Cr, Ca, glucose*
3. *TSH*
4. *Drug screen*
5. *E to H*

Case 35: **Pediatric Temper Tantrum**

DOORWAY INFORMATION

Opening Scenario

Betty White is the grandmother of Amy White (age 24 months). She wants to speak to you about the child's emotional problems.

Vital Signs

There are no vital signs in this case.

Examinee Tasks

1. Obtain a focused history.
2. You will not be required to perform a physical examination in this case.
3. Discuss your initial diagnostic impression and your workup plan with the patient.
4. After leaving the room, complete your patient note on the given form.

BEFORE ENTERING THE ROOM

1. Cues: Since this is a pediatric case you already know there will be no patient to examine and you will have the entire 15 minutes for the history. A pediatric history will be important. This case could be done as a phone case, or the caretaker of the child may come and speak to you in person, as in this case. Assume that you have permission for discussion and treatment of all patients on this test.

2. Clinical Reasoning: Most temper tantrums are part of normal growth and development. They occur in pre-verbal or minimally verbal children who cannot express themselves. These spells occur mostly in the presence of the primary caretaker. They happen more often when the child is tired, hungry, bored, in physical discomfort, or just having a day that is different from the normal routine.

Temper tantrums start suddenly and are characterized by the child crying or screaming, turning red in the face, looking very upset or mad, and flailing all four extremities. The child is conscious, and this is not a seizure. These tantrums last only a minute or two (though it seems a lot longer if you are the parent).

FROM THE GUARDIAN

History

Mrs. Betty White made an appointment to meet with you regarding Amy, her grandchild. She tells you that she lives with Amy and Amy's mother (Lisa White). Betty is the primary caregiver and Lisa works two jobs to provide income for the three of them. Betty states that she is happy to help out raising the child, but at times Amy is hard to control.

Approximately twice a week Amy seems to have a sudden crying spell, where she is crying as loudly as she can while kicking, screaming, and moving her arms about wildly. It is very embarrassing because it often happens when Mrs. White has taken Amy with her to a 2-hour church service or when they are out shopping. She tries to comfort the child, and the tantrums generally stop after a minute or so. Immediately before and afterward, the child's behavior is normal, and she never faints or harms herself in any way. The child does not "turn blue." These spells or episodes started happening a couple of months ago. Nothing seems to make them less frequent, and nothing can be done to stop an episode once it starts.

Amy takes no medicine other than pediatric vitamins, and has an allergy to strawberries.

Amy has never been hospitalized other than at birth. Lisa had an uneventful labor and a normal delivery. The whole time in the hospital was 30 hours, but they are still paying the bill off for a 2-day hospital stay. Amy has never had surgery and only rarely gets sick. Last month she had an ear infection, and she has had a couple of colds in her lifetime. Amy sleeps through the night, 11 hours. She was reliably taking two naps a day, but now some days will take only one nap. Betty has noticed that Amy is more likely to have a crying spell if she misses her nap altogether. Amy is recently toilet-trained but she still wears a diaper at night "just in case." She does not appear to be in any pain when she urinates. She is growing and gaining weight.

Mrs. White recalls that her daughter, Lisa, also had crying spells, but states, "I was a lot younger then and could handle it better." Betty never feels like she is going to lose control of herself and hit or shake the baby. When the "episodes" happen, Mrs. White tries to console the child with a hug, but the baby just kicks harder. The three of them are generally happy with their life, but both Lisa and Betty wish that Lisa had more time to spend with Amy.

No one in the household smokes. Betty is primary caregiver. Lisa, the child's mother, works two jobs to make ends meet. The father is no longer in contact with the family.

Amy was a full-term baby and had no problems after birth. Lisa did get prenatal care and did not smoke or use alcohol. Amy was 7 lb 3 oz at birth and has had no problems with breathing, no turning yellow, and no fevers. She was bottle-fed with Enfamil and Similac until age 1 year. She started with vegetables and cereals at 5 months of age. Now Amy eats normal table food and drinks cow's milk without any problems.

Amy's immunizations are up to date. She has had regular checkups. She started walking and speaking words at age 11 months. She now says 200 words or so, and is starting to use sentences.

Physical Exam

There is no physical exam in this case.

THE CLOSING

Doctor: "Mrs. White, I'd like to review what you have told me. You are the primary caretaker for your grandchild, Amy." *(Mrs. White nods in agreement)* "Amy has been having episodes where she is screaming and crying and is inconsolable that last for a couple of minutes. In between episodes, everything is fine with her."

Mrs. White: "Yes, that's correct."

Doctor: "What you are describing sounds like temper tantrums. I do want to see Amy for a physical exam to be sure."

Mrs. White: "What can we do about them?"

Doctor: "They usually happen when a child is tired, hungry, or not doing something that is in her regular routine. All you can do is sit quietly with her until it passes. Punishment doesn't work to prevent tantrums. Usually children grow out of them as they get older. Would it help you to know that temper tantrums are a normal part of growing up?"

Mrs. White: "Yes."

Doctor: "Do you have any questions?"

The key to the closing here is to counsel the caretaker that tantrums are normal. You also say that to be sure, you want to see the child for a physical exam. It is key to elicit the caretaker's response to the tantrums. If someone tells you he/she is punishing a child, you need to correct his/her parenting skills.

Guardian: "Whenever my 2-year-old has a temper tantrum, I send him to bed without dinner."

Doctor: "We have found that punishment does not work for temper tantrums. It would be much better if you could just put your child in 'time-out' for a minute. Once the tantrum and the time-out are over, forget about it and pretend it never happened."

Time-out is a popular parenting technique that seems to work to the advantage of the child and the equally frustrated parent. Pick a spot in the house or specific chair to be the time-out chair. (It can be a chair, a couch, a bed, or a spot on the floor.)

The parent should remain calm, take the thrashing toddler to the time-out chair or spot, and gently place him there. And then just wait for the tantrum to pass. Add on another 30 seconds or minute or so for the child to regain his composure. Once time-out is over, the parents should not hold any grudges and should just get on with life!

CHALLENGING QUESTIONS

Mrs. White: "Should I take Amy to a child psychologist?"

Answer: "No, but I'd like to examine Amy. Can you bring her to the office tomorrow?"

The grandmother has not told you anything to suggest that the child's behavior is abnormal. Temper tantrums are a normal developmental stage that is part of the human condition.

CASE DISCUSSION

Notes about the History-Taking

If you enter a room and are not sure if the person is the patient or not, ask the SP for his/her name.

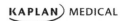

GRADING: STANDARDIZED PATIENT DATA-GATHERING CHECKLISTS

History Checklist

☑ **S**ymptoms: Get description of "emotional problems"

☑ **I**ntensity: Find out how Mrs. White responds to these episodes

☑ **O**nset: When did tantrums start?

☑ **D**uration: How long do the tantrums last?

☑ **P**rogression: What is the frequency? Is the number of tantrums changing with time?

☑ **H**ave you noticed anything that precipitates a tantrum? (What makes it worse?)

☑ **H**ave you noticed anything that makes them occur less often? (What makes it better?)

☑ **A**ssociated symptoms: You want to ask about any fainting spells, turning blue, or if the child ever gets hurt during a tantrum

☑ **P**MH: Past hospitalizations, trauma, major illness, and surgery

☑ **R**OS: Sleep history, any problems urinating, dietary history

☑ **F**H: This is not a genetic condition, but might be a good time to see if the grandmother can remember her own daughter's childhood. It's likely that daughter Lisa also had temper tantrums at this age.

☑ **S**Hx: Who lives in the household? Is there any new or excessive stress at home? What is Mrs. White's reaction to the temper tantrums? Screen for any worries about child abuse.

Pediatric History Checklist

☑ **P**renatal Hx:

☑ **P**ed Hx: Did mom get prenatal care? Did she refrain from smoking and alcohol?

☑ **B**irth Hx: Birth full-term? Normal delivery or C-section?

☑ **N**eonatal Hx:

☑ **F**eeding Hx:

☑ **G**rowth and development

☑ **R**outine care: Immunizations and checkups

Doctor: "Hello, My name is Dr. First-Name Last-Name. What is your name?"

Mrs. White: "I am Mrs. Betty White. I am Amy's grandma."

Sometimes patients' stories are complicated, with multiple family members being important. It is important for CIS and SEP to ask questions, and paraphrase until you understand that Betty White is the grandmother, Lisa White is the mother, and Amy is the grandchild and patient.

Primary care physicians caring for children should ask about secondhand smoke, smoke detectors, firearms in the home, car seats, and being sure poisons are locked out of reach. These are all good preventative medicine questions. If you have a case of a child being brought in for a school physical or general checkup, go ahead and

SAMPLE PATIENT NOTE

History: Include significant positives and negatives from history of present illness, past medical history, review of system(s), social history, and family history.

HPI: Onset a couple of months ago, 1–2 episodes a week of crying, screaming, and generally thrashing about. Lasts 1–2 minutes. Nothing makes it better, seems to be more frequent when child is tired. No fainting, turning blue, or breath-holding spells. Child does not injure herself during tantrums.

Allergies: Strawberries

Meds: Pediatric vitamins. Immunizations are up-to-date.

PMH: Mother had prenatal care, no alcohol or cigarettes during pregnancy. Full term, NSVD. No problems in neonatal period. No hospitalizations, trauma, or surgery.

ROS: Sleeps 12 hr/nite, down to 1 nap a day on most days. Toilet-trained, does not appear uncomfortable urinating.

SH: Grandmother is primary caretaker, mother works 2 jobs, and patient in household. Denies unusual stresses. Caretaker is not worried she will harm the infant.

Ped Hx: Regular prenatal care. Full term normal vaginal delivery. No neonatal complications. Initially bottle-fed on Enfamil and Similac, now on table food and cow's milk. Started walking at 11 mo. Toilet-trained at 2 yrs. Speaks about 200 words. Regular checkup. Immunizations up-to-date.

Physical Exam: Indicate only pertinent positive and negative findings related to patient's chief complaint.

There is no physical exam in this case.

Differential Diagnosis: In order of likelihood (with 1 being the most likely), list up to five potential or possible diagnoses for this patient's presentation. (In many cases, fewer than five diagnoses are likely.)

1. Temper tantrums
2. Normal development
3.
4.
5.

Diagnostic Workup: List immediate plans (up to five) for further diagnostic workup.

1. Physical exam
2. No tests indicated
3.
4.
5.

ask these questions. If the case has a chief complaint of a site or symptom, concentrate on learning about the chief complaint first.

Notes about the Physical Exam

There was no physical exam in this case.

Comments about the Patient Note

If the guardian seems unduly stressed or feels that he/she may harm the child, offer a meeting with a counselor. You can also offer a support group.

> **Parent/Guardian:** "Sometimes I feel so frustrated when my child has a tantrum. I like the time-outs because it gives me a chance to cool down too."

> **Doctor:** "Are you ever worried that you might hurt or shake the child?"

> **Parent/Guardian:** "To tell you the truth, I did scare myself a couple of times but no, I never have."

> **Doctor:** "Thank you for telling me. Your feelings are not unusual. I'd like to give you the number of a parenting support group. It helps to talk to others in the same situation."

The danger signs of temper tantrums are if they are starting or getting worse after 4 years of age. Sometimes this can be an indication of depression, autism, or attention deficit disorder. Consider these diagnoses only with tantrums that are getting worse after age 4.

> **Doctor:** "Does your child pass out?"

Ask about any fainting. If the child faints, consider seizure or arrhythmia as a possibility and get the appropriate tests of EEG (electroencephalogram) and neuroimaging. For arrhythmia, of course, you need an ECG, perhaps an echocardiogram, and a Holter monitor.

> **Doctor:** "Does your child ever get hurt during an episode?"

Ask about self-harm. In an uncomplicated temper tantrum, the child does not hurt himself.

> **Doctor:** "Does your child hold her breath?"

Lastly, ask about breath-holding spells. You can also ask if the child's color changes. (Blue is bad.)

For these types of behavioral cases, it is essential to find out if there is any new stress in the family. Also, get the parents' reaction to the temper tantrum and counsel them on dealing appropriately with the behavior.

The doctor in this exchange wrote much of the pediatric history under the headings of HPI and PMH. It would be just as correct to write all the history under the Ped Hx heading, or to omit the Ped Hx heading entirely. As long as the relevant and critically important information is on the note, the graders will not be concerned with exactly where you convey it.

A physical exam is always indicated. Some children have more tantrums when they have physical discomfort that they cannot communicate to the adults. Kids are more cranky if they have untreated otitis or a UTI. Writing "No tests indicated" tells your examiner that you recognize that this condition needs no testing to confirm the diagnosis.

In this note, the correct answer was only one diagnosis because you were expected to recognize that tantrums are a normal part of growth and development.

| SECTION THREE |

Appendixes

Appendix A: **Abbreviations**

Use abbreviations sparingly. For clarity, it is always better to spell out the acronym or abbreviation.

yo or y/o	year old
m	male
f	female
b	black
w	white
L	left
R	right
hx	history
h/o	history of
c/o	complaining/complaints of
NL	normal limits
WNL	within normal limits
Ø	without or no
+	positive
–	negative
abd	abdomen
AIDS	acquired immune deficiency syndrome
AP	anteroposterior
BUN	blood urea nitrogen
CABG	coronary artery bypass grafting
CBC	complete blood count
CCU	cardiac care unit
cig	cigarettes
CHF	congestive heart failure
COPD	chronic obstructive pulmonary disease
CPR	cardiopulmonary resuscitation
CT	computed tomography
CVA	cerebrovascular accident
CVP	central venous pressure
CXR	chest x-ray
DM	diabetes mellitus
DTR	deep tendon reflexes
ECG	electrocardiogram
ED	emergency department

EMT	emergency medical technician
ENT	ears, nose, and throat
EOM	extraocular muscles
EtOH	alcohol
Ext	extremities
FH	family history
GI	gastrointestinal
GU	genitourinary
HEENT	head, eyes, ears, nose, and throat
HIV	human immunodeficiency virus
HPI	history of present illness
HTN	hypertension
IM	intramuscularly
IV	intravenously
JVD	jugular venous distension
KUB	kidney, ureter, and bladder
LMP	last menstrual period
LP	lumbar puncture
MI	myocardial infarction
MRI	magnetic resonance imaging
MVA	motor vehicle accident
Neuro	neurologic
NIDDM	non–insulin dependent diabetes mellitus
NKA	no known allergies
NKDA	no known drug allergy
NSR	normal sinus rhythm
PA	posteroanterior
PERRLA	pupils are equal, round, and reactive to light and accommodation
po	orally
PT	prothrombin time
PTT	partial prothrombin time
RBC	red blood cells
SH	social history
TIA	transient ischemic attack
U/A	urinalysis
URI	upper respiratory tract infection
WBC	white blood cells

Appendix B: Communications and Interpersonal Skills (CIS) Component of the Exam

As described in Section I of this book, after each patient encounter the standardized patient will evaluate your interpersonal and communications skills. This is best thought of as a checklist since there are particular mannerisms which help convey these appropriate skills. The following table is designed to give you an idea of what you're likely to be evaluated on with respect to communications and interpersonal skills. Section I of this book describes these items in greater detail.

No	Yes	Interpersonal/Communication Skills Feature
		1. Examinee **knocked** before entering
		2. Appeared professional in **dress/grooming/hygiene**
		3. **Introduced self** by name
		4. Made comfortable **eye contact**
		5. Focused **attention and concentration** on patient
		6. Conveyed a **respectful and nonjudgmental** attitude
		7. Used appropriate **draping** technique
		8. Used **transitional** phrases and references
		9. Expressed **empathy** (reflected patient's feelings) and made appropriate **reassurances**
		10. Gave patient time to think and answer **without interrupting**
		11. Asked **open-ended** questions
		12. Used **nonleading** questions
		13. Asked **one question at a time** (clear and concise)
		14. Used **lay language** (volunteered explanation)
		15. Effectively **listened** and **paraphrased** information throughout the encounter
		16. Was **connected** and **purposeful** during the physical examination
		17. **Summarized** significant information in closing, and clearly explained **diagnostic plans**
		18. Placed patient **at ease** and communicated information **without alarming** the patient
		19. **Asked** if patient had questions, and **answered appropriately**

Kaplan Medical's Five Essentials

- Introduction—sets the tone for the encounter
- Empathy—reflects the patient's feelings
- Reassurance—aids the patient's feelings
- Paraphrasing—clarifies patient's information and allows note taking while paying attention to the patient
- Closing—crucial for exam success

Appendix C: **Doorway Information Flashcards**

NOTE FROM THE AUTHOR

The following flashcards are to be used as an exercise and preparation tool for approaching a standardized patient based on doorway information. They are not to be used as an authoritative text of differential diagnoses and management.

The importance of a complete history and physical examination in determining an order of likely diagnoses cannot be undervalued. Because these cards do not give complete history or examination findings, you will not find the differential diagnoses listed strictly in order of likelihood. Use the history and physical examination findings as a guide and consult a textbook of medicine when managing patient care issues.

Please be aware, however, that for your USMLE Step 2 CS exam, you must list your differential diagnoses and workup in order of likelihood and relevance.

i.e. a 72yo male with chest pain

Differential Diagnosis	Diagnostic Workup
1. Unstable angina	1. ECG
2. Acute MI	2. CK-MB, troponin
3. GERD/PUD	3. EGD & biopsy
4. DES	4. Esophageal manometry
5. Costochondritis	5. Chest XR

Good luck!!

—Eric Deppert, M.D. and Henry Ostman, M.D.

27yo ♀ with non-traumatic DVT

28yo Irish ♀ with unexplained
abdomen pain for "years"
& negative workup

42yo caucasian G3P3 with c/o
frequent urination & "accidents"

73yo ♂ c/o "blacking
out" while eating

27yo ♀ married for >3yr
is having difficulty getting
pregnant for last 18 months

63yo ♂ c/o favorite meal is not
appealing anymore and has
loss of taste [Dysgeusia]

Differentials

Irritable bowel syndrome
IBD
Celiac sprue
Depression
Domestic violence
PID
Porphyria
Endometriosis

Work-Up

Rectal for occult blood
Pelvic exam for culture/
   sensitivity
CBC
Antiendomesial Ab
Antigliadin Ab
24hr urine for
   Porphobilinogen
EGD/colonoscopy & biopsy
MRI Pelvis

Differentials

Risk Factors for DVT:
Cigarettes
Extended travel
Hx of DVT
OCP's
Immobilization
Trauma
Obesity
Malignancy
Pregnancy
Familial hypercoagulable state

Work-Up

d-dimer
Venous Doppler of extremities
Urine analysis
β-hCG
ESR, cRP
Factor V Leiden
Prothrombin G20210A
   mutation
Protein C & S levels [function
   & activity]
aPTT for lupus anticoagulant
Homocysteine
Lipoprotein a

Differentials

Deglutitional syncope
Post-prandial syncope
Aspiration
TIA / CVA
Arrhythmia
Seizures
Valvular heart disease
Acute MI/ unstable angina

Work-Up

ECG
CK-MB / Troponin
CXR
CT head
MRA brain stem
EEG
2-D Echocardiogram
EP study
Carotid U/S

Differentials

UTI
hyperglycemia
Atrophic vaginitis
Urge incontinence
Stress incontinence
Mixed incontinence
Overflow incontinence
pregnancy

Work-Up

Pelvic exam
Urine analysis & culture/
   sensitivity
Fasting glucose
Chem-7
Voiding cystourethrogram
β-hCG

Differentials

Smoking
Hot liquids
Dental disease
Sjögrens syndrome
Bell's palsy
Ramsay Hunt syndrome
CPA tumors
Medications
Hypogonadism
Hypothyroidism
Uremia
Hepatitis
Frontal lobe tumor
   (i.e.meningioma)
Depression

Work-Up

ANA
Anti-Ro/anti-La antibodies
MRI brain/brainstem
LH, FSH, Testosterone
TSH
Chem-7
LFT
Audiogram

Differentials

A. Male factors
Erectile dysfunction—medical
   vs. psychiatric
Oligospermia
Abnormal volume/viscosity
Varicocoele
Cryptorchidism
Ductal obstruction
Testicular failure [mumps]
Hypospadia

B. Female Factors
Congenital anomaly
PID
Amenorrhea
Anovulation
Endometriosis
Leiomyoma
Asherman's sydrome

Work-Up

A. Male genital/testicular exam
Semen analysis
Testosterone level
LH/FSH level
Prolactin
TSH

B. Pelvic/bi-manual exam
Serum progesterone
Hysterosalpingography
   Endometrial biopsy
LH/FSH level
Prolactin
TSH

28yo ♂ with complaint that his girlfriend says his breath "stinks"

23yo ♀ IVDA with back pain & arthralgias

32yo ♂ auto mechanic with 2 days of low back pain

38yo ♂ executive with 10 days of fever & negative outpatient workup

37yo ♂ with h/o alcoholism comes in with 3 episodes of vomiting blood

18yo ♀ Olympic gymnast with 1yr of diarrhea

Differentials

Infective endocarditis with
  septic emboli
Hepatitis A/B/C viremia
HIV arthropathy
Pyelonephritis
Psoas abscess
Perinephric abscess
Trauma- back
Seronegative
  Spondyloarthropathy
Lupus
Nephrolithiasis

Work-Up

Rectal exam for tone
2D-echocardiogram
CBC,
HIV test
Hepatitis serologies
Blood cultures x 3 sets
Urinalysis & culture
CT abdomen/pelvis
X-Ray L/S spine
ESR, RF

Differentials

Periodontal abscess
Sinusitis/ tumor of
  GERD
Zenker's diverticulum
Dysmotility
Lung abscess
Sialodenitis
Tonsillitis/tumor of
Renal/hepatic failure
DKA

Work-Up

Dental exam
X-Ray sinuses
Barium swallow
CXR or CT chest
Esophageal manometry
Upper endoscopy
Chem-7, LFT
Serum ketones & β-
  Hydroxybutyrate

Differentials

Occult abscess
EBV
CMV
Syphilis
HIV
Malaria / Ehrlichiosis
Babesiosis
Infective endocarditis
Still's disease
Collagen vascular disease
Alcoholic hepatitis
Drug fever—prescription vs.
  illicit
Solid Tumor
Hematologic malignancy

Work-Up

Tagged WBC scan
EBV/CMV titer
RPR
HIV
Peripheral blood smear, CBC
Blood cultures x 3 sets
2-D echocardiogram
ANA, RF
cRP, ESR
LFT's & GGT
Carbohydrate deficient
  transferrin
CT Chest/Abdomen/Pelvis

Differentials

Lumbosacral strain
Herniated disc
Petit's hernia – lumbar triangle
Ankylosing spondylitis
Referred pain 2°
  nephrolithiasis
Discitis/osteomyelitis
Vertebral fracture
Pott's disease

Work-Up

Rectal exam for tone
X-Ray Lumbar spine
ESR
Urine analysis
CBC
PPD/CXR

Differentials

Secretory
  Zollinger-Ellison syndrome
  Cholera
Osmotic
  Laxative abuse
  Malabsorption – ↓ surface
  area
  Maldigestion
Motility
  Irritable bowel syndrome
  – 2° to stress
  Meds- erythromycin,
  metoclopramide
Exudative
  IBD
  Infectious disease

Work-Up

Digital Rectal Exam & FOBT
Stool studies
CBC
PT/INR
Carotene level
Vitamin D level
d-Xylose test
Endoscopy & colon Biopsy

‡Remember there are "*SOME*"
  causes of diarrhea

Differentials

Gastritis
Peptic ulcer disease
Esophageal varices
Gastric varices
Mallory-Weiss tear
Boorhaeve's sydrome
Splenic vein thrombosis
AVM
Hemoptysis
Epistaxis
Laryngeal CA
Head & Neck CA

Work-Up

CBC
PT / aPTT
Upper endoscopy
Bleeding scan
CXR / X-Ray abdomen [for
  free air under diaphragm]
CT abdomen
Laryngoscopy

A 24yo medical resident returns from relief mission in the Philippines with diarrhea and weakness

24yo ♂ with 1 year diarrhea, weight loss, and skin rash

52yo ♀ with c/o food "gets stuck in my chest"

40yo ♂ comes in for hypercalcemia noted on routine labs during his annual check-up

33yo ♀ with headaches & palpitations, BP 190/110 mm Hg

30yo ♀ with joint pain, weakness, and fatigue for 1 year

Differentials

IBD
Celiac sprue
Whipple's disease
HIV
Lactose intolerance
Irritable bowel syndrome
    Infectious diarrhea
Laxative abuse
'SOME' causes of diarrhea

Work-Up

Digital Rectal Exam & FOBT
CBC, ferritin, TIBC,
    transferrin
PT/INR
Calcium, B_{12} level
Vitamin D level
Stool WBC / fecal fat
Stool C & S / ova & parasites
Antiendomesial Ab
Antigliadin Ab
Anti-*Saccharomyces cerevisiae*
    Ab
p-ANCA
HIV test
Small bowel Biopsy

Differentials

Infectious Diarrheas:
Bacterial—*E. coli, Salmonella,*
    Shigella, Campylobacter,
    Yersinia
Parasitic—*Giardia*, nematodes,
    trematodes, flukes
Viral—rotavirus, Norwalk,
    Hepatitis A

Tropical sprue
Whipple's disease
IBD

Work-Up

Digital Rectal Exam & FOBT
Stool studies – WBC, Ova &
    Parasites
CBC
LFT
Chem-7
Anti-*Saccharomyces cerevisiae*
    Antibodies
P-ANCA
Flexible sigmoidoscopy
EGD / small bowel Biopsy

Differentials

ATN – recovery phase
Sarcoidosis
Hyperthyroidism
Immobilization
Thiazides diuretics
Familial hypocalciuric
    hypercalcemia
Acidosis
Hemo**C**oncentration
Endocrinopathies
Hypervitaminosis **D**
Lithium
Intoxication -Milk alkali
Malignancy/myleoma
Hyper**P**arathyroidism

Work-Up

Ionized Calcium, PTH
Chem-7
CBC
24hr Urine calcium
25-OH vitamin D; 1, 25 OH-
    vitamin D levels
TSH, free T4
CXR
KUB X-ray

Differentials

Esophageal stricture / web
Schatzki's ring
Esophageal CA
Diffuse esophageal spasm
achalasia
Cervical spine osteophyte
Extrinsic compression—
    i.e., lymph node or mass

Work-Up

Digital Rectal Exam & FOBT
CBC

Barium swallow:
If positive, then EGD, CT
    Chest & Abdo, CXR
If negative , then esophageal
    motility study

Differentials

Fibromyalgia
RA
SLE
Lyme disease
parvovirus B19
Adrenal insufficiency
Hypothyroidism
HIV
IBD
Obstructive Sleep Apnea
Depression
Domestic violence
EBV, CMV
Hepatitis B/C

Work-Up

Digital Rectal Exam & FOBT
CBC
Chem-7
TSH, Free T_4
RF
ANA
LFT
ESR, c-RP
HIV
ACTH stimulation test
Hepatitis B/C serology
X-Ray hands
Sleep study

Differentials

Affective/panic disorder
Substance abuse
Hyperthyroidism
Pheochromocytoma
Renal artery stenosis
Hyperaldosteronism
Pregnancy
Domestic violence

Work-Up

Chem-7
Urine drug screen
TSH, free T_4
Plasma metanephrines &
Plasma normetanephrines
Aldosterone/renin ratio
MRI adrenals
β-hCG

Complaint/Patient Scenario

45yo obese ♂ with c/o
polyuria and confusion

Complaint/Patient Scenario

51yo ♂ alcoholic with
acute confusion

Complaint/Patient Scenario

28yo ♀ with c/o swollen glands
in her neck for 1 month

Complaint/Patient Scenario

58yo ♀ dry mouth for 1 year

Complaint/Patient Scenario

21yo college football player with c/o:
"I feel like I'm drunk when I walk"

Complaint/Patient Scenario

22yo ♀ complains of
recurrent mouth sores

Differentials

Hepatic encephalopathy
DT's/ alcohol withdrawal
Drug intoxication
Subdural hematoma
Seizure
Wernicke's encephalopathy
Spontaneous Bacterial
  Peritonitis
Meningitis
Constipation
Hypokalemia
Hepatorenal syndrome
Acute schizophrenia

Work-Up

Fecal occult blood—r/o
  GI bleed as cause for
  encephalopathy
Urine drug screen
Chem-7
LFT
CBC
Ammonia level
Ascitic fluid protein, albumin,
  cell count
CT brain
EEG

Differentials

Nonketotic hyperglycemia
Urosepsis
Diabetes insipidus
Pneumonia
Meningitis
Acute renal failure
Hypernatremia/hyponatremia
Hypercalcemia
CVA
Seizure
Arrhythmia/Atrial fibrillation
Substance abuse

Work-Up

Chem-7
CBC
Urine analysis, Urine C&S
Urine drug screen
CXR
LP & CSF studies
CT brain
EEG
ECG

Differentials

Drug toxicity
Alcoholism
Sjögrens syndrome
Granulomatous infiltration
NIDDM/IDDM
Diabetes insipidus
Autonomic neuropathy

Work-Up

Fasting glucose, Chem-7
ANA
Anti-Ro Ab
Anti-La Ab
Urine analysis & specific
  gravity
CXR
Schirmer test
Rose-Bengal stain

Differentials

Epstein-Barr virus
CMV
Syphilis
HIV
Toxoplasmosis
TB
Hepatitis A/B/C
Hodgkin's / NHL
ALL
SLE / collagen vascular disease
Sarcoidosis

Work-Up

CBC
EBV/CMV
RPR, FTA-Ab
HIV
LFT
Toxoplasma titer
PPD
CXR
ANA,ds-DNA
ESR , c-RP
Cervical node biopsy

Differentials

Aphthous stomatitis
Iron/folate/B_{12} deficiency
Herpes Simplex virus
SLE
IBD
Reactive arthritis
Pemphigus
Behçet's syndrome
Trauma

Work-Up

Stool for occult blood
Pelvic exam for ulcers
Ferritin, TIBC, transferrin
B_{12}, folate levels
ANA, ds-DNA
ESR, c-RP
Tzanck prep
Oral ulcer biopsy
Colonoscopy/biopsy

Differentials

Concussion
Subdural hematoma
Vertebral artery dissection
Subarachnoid hemorrhage
Epidural hematoma
Labyrinthitis
CNS tumor—posterior fossa
Substance abuse

Work-Up

CT brain
MRI brain
MRA neck & brainstem
Urine drug screen

Complaint/Patient Scenario

42yo ♂ drug abuser with purple bumps on legs x 2 weeks

Complaint/Patient Scenario

38yo ♀ cc: itching all over

Complaint/Patient Scenario

27yo ♀ with 1 week Hx of swollen right leg and U/S & for DVT

Complaint/Patient Scenario

82yo Black ♂ c/o L leg swelling and pain with SOB for 1 week U/S & for DVT, CT scan & for PE

Complaint/Patient Scenario

24yo ♀ with 1 year diarrhea, weight loss, and skin rash

Complaint/Patient Scenario

16yo ♂ passed out after running the 400-yard dash at a track meet

Differentials

Xerosis
Atopic dermatitis
Contact dermatitis
Drug reaction
Iron deficiency anemia
Lymphoma
Cholestasis
Primary biliary cirrhosis
pregnancy
Psoriasis
HIV
Scabies
Carcinoid
Urticaria/ dermatographia
ARF (uremic frost)
Hyperthyroidism
Polycythemia rubra vera
Hot tub foliculitis
Depression
Delusion of parasitosis

Work-Up

CBC & peripheral smear
Ferritin, TIBC, transferrin,
LFT
β-hCG
HIV
Chem-7
TSH
Erythropoietin level
Anti-mitochondrial Ab
Skin biopsy

Differentials

Cryoglobulinemia
Chronic active hepatitis
HIV
Scurvy
Connective tissue disease
Hypersensitivity vasculitis
Henoch-Schonlein purpura
IBD
Amyloidosis
Waldenstrom's
    macroglobulinemia
Primary biliary cirrhosis

Work-Up

Stool for occult blood
CBC
Chem-7
Cryglobulins
RF ANA
C3/C4/CH50
SPEP
Hepatitis B/C serology
HIV test
Anti-*Saccharomyces cerevisiae*
    Ab
p-ANCA
Anti-mitochondrial Ab

Differentials

Occult malignancy
Myeloproliferative disorder
Waldenstrom's
    macroglobulinemia
Multiple Myeloma
TTP
Vasculitis
PNH
Anticardiolipin Ab
Antiphospholipid Ab
Protein C/S deficiency
ATIII deficiency
Meds- Heparin

Work-Up

Rectal exam & FOBT
CBC & peripheral smear
SPEP
Sucrose lysis
Anticardiolipin Ab
Factor V Leiden
aPTT
Protein C & S
ATIII

Differentials

Factor V Leiden
Prothrombin mutation
Protein C/S deficiency
ATIII deficiency
Methylenetetrahydrofolate
    reductase mutation
Anticardiolipin Ab
Antiphospholipid Ab
Trauma
OCP's
Pregnancy
Vasculitis
↑ Homocysteine
↑ Lipoprotein a
Occult malignancy
Medications- heparin
TTP/HUS

Work-Up

Factor V Leiden
Prothrombin G20210A
Protein C & S
ATIII
Anticardiolipin Ab
aPTT
β-hCG
ANA, ds-DNA,ESR, c-RP
Homocysteine
lipoprotein a level
CBC & peripheral smear
Heparin Antibodies
Chem-7

Differentials

IHSS/hypertrophic obstructive
    cardiomyopathy
Arrhythmia [WPW syndrome]
Prolonged QT syndrome
Abnormal coronary
    vasculature
Electrolyte disturbance
Hypoglycemia
Vasovagal syncope
Seizure

Work-Up

2D echocardiogram
ECG
Exercise stress test
Chem-7
EEG

Differentials

IBD
Celiac/tropical sprue
Whipple's disease
Irritable Bowel Syndrome
lactose intolerance
Infectious diarrhea
Laxative abuse

Work-Up

Rectal exam & Heme test of
    the stool
CBC/ Ferritin, TIBC,
    transferrin/ B_{12}/folate
PT/INR
Ionized Calcium, Vitamin D
    level
Antiendomesial Ab
Antigliadin Ab
Stool for C/S, O & P
Stool for WBC's, fat
Small bowel Biopsy

34yo Italian ♂ with c/o
"I'm turning yellow"

20yo ♂ with several hours
of nose bleeding

70yo W ♂ with c/o tingling
in hands and feet

30yo ♀ with joint pain, weakness,
and fatigue for 1 year

22yo ♀ with chest pain
and palpitations

68yo ♀ acute onset nausea
and head 'spinning'

Differentials

Trauma
HTN
sinusitis
von Willebrand's disease
Idiopathic thrombocytopenic
 purpura
HIV
Acute leukemia
Aplastic anemia
lymphoma
Marrow infiltration/
 malignancy
DIC
SLE
Thrombocytopenia [drug
 induced]
Domestic violence
Drug abuse – cocaine
Wegener's granulomatosis

Work-Up

CBC
Peripheral blood smear
PT/aPTT/fibrin split products
HIV
ANA
Urine drug screen
Platelet aggregation studies
U/S abdomen [splenomegaly]
BM biopsy

Differentials

Gilbert's disease
G6PD
Pyruvate Kinase deficiency
Acute viral hepatitis
Cholangitis
Carotenemia
Drug induced hepatitis
Hemochromatosis
Non-alcholic fatty liver disease
Zieve's syndrome- (alcoholic
 hepatitis & hemolysis)
Wilson's disease
autoimmune hepatitis
Hemolysis- drug exposure,
 infection, toxin
Autoimmune hemolytic
 anemia

Work-Up

CBC & Peripheral smear
Cerruloplasmin
Haptoglobin,
LDH
LFT, Chem-7
SPEP
Anti-LKM Ab
U/S RUQ

Differentials

Fibromyalgia
Depression
RA
SLE
Hepatitis B/C
Lyme disease
HIV
Parvovirus B19
EBV
Adrenal insufficiency
Hypothyroidism

Work-Up

CBC
RF
ANA, ESR, CRP
Hepatitis B & C serologies
Chem-7, LFT's
Lyme titer
EBV titers
Parvovirus B-19 serologies
ACTH stimulation test
TSH, free T4
X-Ray hands

Differentials

DM type 1 and 2
Alcoholism
Vitamin B_{12}, folate deficiency
Amyloidosis
Multiple myeloma
Waldenstrom's
 macroglobulinemia
Chronic inflammatory
 demyelinating
 polyneuropathy Collagen
 vascular disease
ESRD
HIV
INH toxicity
Vitamin B6 deficiency

Work-Up

CBC & peripheral smear
Chem-7
Vitamin B_{12}, B_6 & folate levels
SPEP, UPEP
Urine analysis
RPR
ESR, c-RP
ANA, RF
HIV
Hepatitis B & C serologies
Nerve conduction study
LP with CSF studies

Differentials

Vestibular neuritis
Labyrinthitis
Benign Positional Vertigo
Meniere's disease
Wallenberg's Syndrome
Posterior fossa tumor
Temporal lobe epilepsy
Acoustic neuroma
Vestibulotoxic drugs
Perilymphatic fistula
Cogan's sydrome
Syphilis
Multiple sclerosis
Basilar migraine

Work-Up

MRI & MRA brain/brainstem
EEG
Audiometry
Electronystagmogram
RPR, FTA-Abs
ANA, ESR, c-RP
Anti-cochlear Ab
HIV test

Differentials

Mitral Valve Prolapse
Generalized anxiety disorder
Hyperthyroidism
Substance abuse
Domestic violence
Pregnancy
WPW/SVT
Pulmonary hypertension
Pheochromocytoma
Costochondritis
Spontaneous pneumothorax

Work-Up

2D echocardiogram
TSH, free T4
Urine drug screen
β-hCG
ECG
Holter monitor
Plasma & urine
 metanephrines,
 normetanephrines
CXR

42yo ♂ severe pain in
right eye for 4 hours

Mother c/o "my 4yo son is not
talking like he should for his age"

60yo ♂ c/o tremor in right
hand and frequent falls

22yo ♀ c/o twitching in her left
arm and then she passed out

40yo ♂ c/o "tingling feet and leg
weakness" after a trip to Cancún

27yo ♀ presents with pre-
employment physical
with c/o fatigue

Differentials

Deaf
Fetal alcohol syndrome
Autism
Lead poisoning
Congenital hypothyroidism
Fragile X
Down's syndrome
Klinefelter syndrome
Renpenning syndrome

Work-Up

Audiometry
Chromosomal analysis
Lead level
Free erythrocyte
   protoporphyrin level
TSH

Differentials

Acute angle closure glaucoma
Cluster headache
Anterior uveitis
Corneal abrasion
Conjunctivitis

Work-Up

Schiotz tonometry
CBC/ESR/ANA
Smear of discharge if present
Slit lamp biomicroscopy
Fluorescein stain

Differentials

Seizure
Pseudoseizures
Metabolic cause of seizure
Drug toxicity
Brain tumor
AVM
CVA
Meningoencephalitis

Work-Up

HIV
Prolactin level
CT brain
Urine drug screen
EEG
LP & CSF analysis & opening
   pressure
CBC
Chem-7
HIV test

Differentials

Parkinson's disease
Striatonigral degeneration
   [combined system disease]
Progressive Supranuclear palsy
Wilson's disease
Epilepsy
Substance abuse
Normal Pressure
   hydrocephalus
Essential tremor

Work-Up

MRI brain
CBC
Chem-7, LFT's
Ceruloplasmin level
Urine drug screen
EEG

Differentials

Hypothyroid
Iron deficiency anemia
Folate deficiency
B_{12} deficiency
Depression
Pregnancy
Substance abuse
SLE
Domestic violence
Sleep apnea
Autoimmune hemolytic
   anemia

Work-Up

TSH, free T4
CBC
Peripheral smear
B_{12}, folate levels
Ferritin, TIBC, transferrin
β-hCG
Urine drug screen
ANA, ds-DNA
12 channel sleep study
LDH, Haptoglobin

Differentials

Poliomyelitis
Guillian-Barre Syndrome
Transverse myelitis
Botulism
Tick paralysis
Tetrodotoxin [puffer fish]

Work-Up

LP/CSF study
EMG
Nerve conduction studies CBC
Chem-7, LFT

48yo ♂ with c/o erectile
dysfunction for 4 months

A 62yo ♂ recently Dx with lung
CA presents to your office with c/o
"who are you and why am I here?"

19yo ♀ college student with
nausea & vomiting for 24 hours

42yo ♂ smoker with chest
pain and cough for 1 week

50yo ♂ with HTN and
high cholesterol and chest
pain for 2 hours

A 16yo ♀ with "worst
headache of her life"

Differentials

Brain metastasis
Paraneoplastic syndrome
Medication side effect
SIADH ($\downarrow$ Na+)
Hypercortisolism (Cushing's)
Hypercalcemia
Hypoxia
Meningitis
Paraneoplastic limbic encephalitis

Work-Up

CT brain
Chem-7
Urine sodium/urine osmolality
Urine free cortisol
Calcium level
O_2 sat
LP with CSF studies

Differentials

Hypothyroidism
PVD, CAD
DM
Depression
$\uparrow$ prolactin
Medications (B-Blockers, thiazides)
Alcohol & Liver disease
Hemochromatosis
Renal failure
Spinal cord tumor
Trauma (bicycle seat)

Work-Up

Genitourinary/Prostatic exam
TSH, free T4
Fasting cholesterol, Triglycerides, LDL, HDL
Free/total testosterone
LH/FSH
Chem-7, CBC
HbA_{1c}
Urine drug screen, alcohol level
LFT
Iron, ferritin, TIBC
Prolactin
Doppler U/S penis
Postage stamp test
Nocturnal penile tumescence test

Differentials

Bronchitis
Pneumonia- bacterial/viral
GERD/PUD
Pleuropericarditis
Unstable angina
Acute MI
Pneumothorax
SVT/WPW
Neoplasia
Anterior chest wall syndrome

Work-Up

CBC
Sputum Gram stain & culture
CXR
ECG
2D echocardiogram
CK-MB, Tn-I
24hr esophageal pH monitoring
Barium swallow
CT chest
Upper endoscopy

Differentials

Gastroenteritis
Alcohol intoxication
Drug overdose- unspecified acetaminophen salicylate
Pregnancy
Pyelonephritis/UTI
Nephrolithiasis

Work-Up

CBC
Chem-7, LFT's
ABG
Blood alcohol level
Urine drug screen
β-hCG
Urine analysis, culture & sensitivity
CT abdomen & Pelvis for nephrolithiasis

Differentials

Intracranial bleed
Migraine headache
Tension headache
Sinusitis
Meningitis
Ocular strain/refractive error
Intracranial tumor
Substance abuse
Caffeine/alcohol withdrawal
Pseudotumor cerebri
Chronic paroxysmal hemicrania

Work-Up

CBC
CT head/sinus
LP & CSF studies & opening pressure
Urine drug screen
Alcohol level
Snellen's chart

Differentials

Unstable angina
Acute MI
Aortic dissection
Pericarditis
GERD/PUD
Penetrating peptic ulcer
Diffuse esophageal spasm
Pulmonary embolism
Spontaneous pneumothorax
Acute cholecystitis
Anterior chest wall syndrome
Herpes zoster

Work-Up

ECG
CK-MB, Tn-I
CXR
2D echocardiogram
CBC, LFT
CT chest or transesophageal echocardiogram for aortic dissection
H. pylori testing
Barium swallow
24hr esophageal pH monitoring
V/Q scan
Tzanck prep
Rectal exam for occult blood
Upper endoscopy

Complaint/Patient Scenario

A 22yo ♂ substance abuser
with headache for 2 days

Complaint/Patient Scenario

A 72yo ♀ with fatigue & headache

Complaint/Patient Scenario

A 26yo ♀ with arthralgias
and RLQ pain

Complaint/Patient Scenario

A44yo ♂ alcoholic, smoker with
3 days of mid-epigastric pain

Complaint/Patient Scenario

52yo ♀ with 1 week of LLQ pain
and history of heart failure

Complaint/Patient Scenario

77yo ♂ with 1 day of bright
red blood per rectum

Differentials

Sinusitis
Tension headache
Giant cell arteritis
Intracranial bleed
Subdural hematoma
Meningitis
Glaucoma
Neoplasm
Myelodysplastic syndrome
Myeloproliferative disorder
Waldenstrom's
  macroglobulinemia
Cervical disc disease
Trigeminal neuralgia
Refractive error
Temporomandibular joint
  dysfunction

Work-Up

ESR, temporal artery biopsy
CT brain/sinus
CBC
LP & CSF studies
Goniometry
SPEP
X-Ray cervical spine
MRI – temporomandibular
  joint

Differentials

Substance or alcohol
  withdrawal
Tension headache
Migraine headache
Cluster headache
Intracranial bleed / Subdural
  hematoma
Meningitis- bacterial/viral/
  fungal
Encephalitis
Sinusitis- maxillary/frontal
Neoplasm
Nicotine/caffeine withdrawal

Work-Up

Urine drug screen
Alcohol level
CBC
CT brain/sinuses
LP & CSF studies
HIV testing

Differentials

Pancreatitis
Peptic ulcer disease
Gastritis
Hepatitis
Cholecystitis
Acute MI
Unstable angina
Lower lobe pneumonia
Aortic aneurysm
Nephrolithiasis

Work-Up

LFT, amylase, lipase
KUB X-ray
Hepatitis A, B, C serologies
CBC
U/S abdomen
ECG
CXR
CK-MB, troponin
2D echocardiogram

Differentials

IBD/terminal ileitis 2°
  infections, TB, Yersinia
Acute appendicitis
Ectopic pregnancy
Cystitis/pyelonephritis
PID/Tuboovarian abscess
Ovarian torsion
Nephrolithiasis
Incarcerated hernia
Domestic violence
Mesenteric lymphadenopathy

Work-Up

Pelvic exam & Cervical swab
Rectal exam for occult blood
CBC
Urine analysis & culture
PPD test
Anti-Saccharomyces cerevisiae
  Antibodies
Abdominal X-ray
Pelvic U/S
Stool for ova, parasites, WBC
β-hCG

Differentials

Hemorrhoids
Fissure
Infectious diarrhea
Diverticular bleed
Lower GI bleed
Upper GI bleed
Neoplasia
Proctitis
IBD
Ischemic bowel
AVM

Work-Up

Rectal exam for occult blood
Flexible sigmoidoscopy/upper
  endoscopy
CBC
CT abdomen/ pelvis
Bleeding scan
Arteriography

Differentials

Diverticulitis
Mesenteric artery ischemia
Mesenteric vein thrombosis
Adhesions
IBD
Pelvic inflammatory disease
Viral/ bacterial diarrhea
Appendicitis
Colon CA
Nephrolithiasis
Inguinal hernia

Work-Up

Rectal exam for occult blood
Pelvic exam
KUB X-ray
CT abdomen/pelvis
LDH
CBC
Urine analysis for blood
Stool studies
Chem-7

Complaint/Patient Scenario

81yo ♀ with 3 days of
back pain following a fall
from standing height

Complaint/Patient Scenario

42yo G2P2 has 1 wk worth
of grayish white nipple
discharge from both breasts

Complaint/Patient Scenario

8yo ♀ previously toilet trained
has 1 week of intermittent
bed soiling with stool

Complaint/Patient Scenario

18yo black ♂ c/o 1 month Hx penile
ulcer after a trip to Somalia

Complaint/Patient Scenario

28yo ♂ c/o headache and
fever after camping trip to
Cape Cod 1 week ago

Complaint/Patient Scenario

16yo ♀ 1 week Hx sore throat
fever, swollen glands, rash

Differentials

Lactation/pregnancy
Hyperprolactinemia
Pituitary adenoma
Breast neoplasm/ malignancy
Early menopause
Hypothyroidism
Heroine/marijuana use

Work-Up

Clinical Breast Exam
β-hCG
LH/FSH
Prolactin level
TFT
MRI brain/pituitary
U/S breast / mammogram
Urine drug screen

Differentials

Osteoporotic fracture of
    vertebrae
or ribs
Herniated disc
Spondylolisthesis
Metastatic CA
Epidural hematoma
Dissecting aortic aneurysm
Solid organ rupture of spleen,
    liver, kidney
Elder abuse

Work-Up

Rectal exam for tone
X-Ray Lumbosacral spine
CXR with rib series
CT abdomen
CBC
Urine analysis
Chem-7

Differentials

Chancroid
Lymphogranuloma venereum
Herpes simplex virus
Granuloma inguinale
Syphilis
Cancer

Work-Up

Genital exam
RPR/FTA Ab
Hepatitis B/C or HIV Urethral
    swab & culture of ulcer for:
    Gram stain
    Wright stain
    Dark field microscopy
(Potential exposure)

Differentials

Hirschsprung's disease
Anal defects- ↑ or ↓ tone with
    overflow
Meningomyelocoele
Iatrogenic sphincterotomy
Spinal cord injury
Anal atresia/fissure
Intestinal obstruction
Cerebral palsy
Pelvic mass
Hypothyroidism
Imperforate anus
Child abuse/sexual abuse

Work-Up

Rectal exam
TSH, free T_3/ T_4
CT abdomen/ pelvis
Back/spine exam
CT myelogram
MRI spinal cord

Differentials

Epstein-Barr Virus
Streptococcal pharyngitis
Cytomegalovirus
HIV
Toxoplasmosis
Hepatitis A/B/C
Syphilis
Lymphoma
Rheumatic fever

Work-Up

CBC, Monospot test
LFT
Throat culture & sensitivity
EBV, CMV titers
HIV
RPR
Lymph Node biopsy

Differentials

Lyme disease
West Nile virus
Ehrlichiosis
Babesiosis
Arbovirus
Syphilitic meningitis
Bacterial meningitis
Rocky Mountain Spotted fever
Acute HIV infxn
Intracranial bleed
Intracranial mass

Work-Up

Lyme ELISA
CBC
RPR/FTA Ab
CT/MRI brain
LP & CSF studies
HIV test

50yo ♀ with well-controlled
HTN for many years presents
for routine exam

42yo ♂ with Hx of type 2 DM
[insulin dependent] comes
in for routine exam

Telephone call for prescription refill

Beware of things you might forget

29yo ♀ c/o left nipple discharge

25yo ♀ c/o difficulty sleeping

Differentials

Identify disease complications

Identify comorbid illness:

   HTN

   CAD

   PVD

   Cardiovascular disease

   Hyperlipidemia

   Erectile Dysfunction

Lifestyle modification

Medication side effects

Cardiovascular exercise

Work-Up

GU exam

HbA1C, lipids

Urine analysis for
microalbumin

Chem-7

Dilated Ophthalmic exam

Visual acuity testing

ECG

EMG

Nerve Conduction Studies

Exercise stress test

Differentials

Assess lifestyle & identify
cardiovascular risk factors

Explore secondary causes of
HTN

Identify target organ damage:

   heart, brain

   kidneys

   PVD, retinopathy

Medication side effects

Over the counter medications

Smoking cessation

Cardiovascular exercise 3X/
week

Limit alcohol < 1-2 drinks/day

Work-Up

CBC

Chem-7

UA

Lipids

TSH

ECG

Fundoscopy

Visual acuity testing

U/S abdominal aorta

Differentials

Depression

Domestic Violence

Pregnancy

Work-Up

Don't forget Rectal/Pelvic
exam

Differentials

Think about disease
complications and adverse
drug effects

Medication allergies

Educate patients

Ask about over the counter
medications

Work-Up

Schedule appointment for
examination and routine
health maintenance and
screening

Differentials

Generalized anxiety

Bipolar disorder/ mania

Schizophrenia

Hyperthyroidism

Alcohol withdrawal

Domestic violence

Sleep apnea

Restless leg syndrome

Amphetamine use

pregnancy

Work-Up

TSH/free T4

Urine drug screen

Carbohydrate deficient
transferrin

Ferritin level

12 channel sleep study

β-hCG

Differentials

Pregnancy

Prolactinoma

Hypothyroidism

Breast CA

Duct ectasia vs. papilloma

Medications

Work-Up

Breast exam

β-hCG

Prolactin

TSH/ free T4

Mammogram

30 yo ♀ c/o vaginal discharge

72yo ♂ c/o weakness and facial droop

60yo ♀ low back pain and fever for 2 days

8yo ♂ previously toilet trained has been wetting his bed for the last 10 days

72yo ♀ complains of excessive night time urination and decreased sleep and urinary urgency with occasional wetting in public. She has HTN, mild CHF, and uses Lasix once a day.

43yo G3P3 with a BMI of 33 c/o involuntary urine loss when bending over to do laundry

Differentials

TIA
CVA
Hyperglycemia/hypoglycemia
Carotid dissection
Bell's palsy
Seizure

Work-Up

CT brain
Chem-7
ECG
Carotid U/S
2D Echocardiogram
EEG

Differentials

Trichomoniasis
Vulvovaginal candidiasis
Bacterial vaginosis
Acute cervicitis
Retained foreign body
Pregnancy

Work-Up

Bimanual/speculum exam
Swab & smear for culture &
   sensitivity
KOH & wet prep
Pap smear
β-hCG
CBC

Differentials

Secondary enuresis:
   delayed CNS development
   Vesicoureteral reflux
   small bladder
UTI
Spinal cord injury
ADH deficiency
Psychiatric
Epilepsy
DM type 1
Child abuse

Work-Up

ADH level
Fasting glucose
Urine analysis & culture/
   sensitivity
MRI spinal cord
EEG
Intravenous pyelogram
Cystoscopy

Differentials

Pyelonephritis
Urosepsis
Infective endocarditis
Retroperitoneal abscess
   Nephrolithiasis
Discitis
Osteomyelitis
Ovarian torsion/cyst
Aortic aneurysm

Work-Up

GU/Pelvic/rectal exam
Urine analysis, urine C & S
CBC, chem-7
Blood cultures x 3 sets
KUB X-ray
CT abdomen/pelvis
X-Ray thoracolumbar spine
MRI lumbar spine

Differentials

Stress incontinence
Sphincter incompetency
Early menopause w/ atrophic
   vaginitis
Multiparous uterus
Medications [α-blockers]UTI
DM
Iatrogenic urethral
   injury [radiation,
   instrumentation]

Work-Up

Rectopelvic exam
LH/FSH
Urine analysis
Chem-7
Voiding cystometrogram

Differentials

Urge incontinence
Detrussor hyperreflexia
Diuretic use
CVA
Alzheimer's disease
Parkinson's disease
Multiple sclerosis
DM
UTI
Normal pressure
   hydrocephalus

Work-Up

Urine analysis
Fasting glucose
Cystoscopy with bladder
   manometry
Neuropsychiatric exam for
   dementia
MRI brain

52yo ♂ c/o left knee and
foot pain for 1 day

28yo ♀ with "years of constipation"

82yo ♂ nursing home patient
with 2 week Hx of diarrhea

18yo ♂ c/o "my urine is foaming"

54yo ♂ farmer c/o diarrhea
& polyuria for 1 week

40 yo ♀ c/o upper belly
fullness and heart burn

Differentials

Low residue diet
Motility disorders
Anal fissure/hemorrhoids
IBD
Irritable Bowel Syndrome
Colorectal CA
Hypercalcemia
Hypokalemia
Hypothyroidism
Hirschsprung's
Spinal cord tumor
Trauma
Amyloidosis
Scleroderma
Medications
Depression

Work-Up

Rectal exam & fecal occult blood
Chem-7
TSH, free T_4
Anal Manometry
Colonic motility studies
Colonoscopy with biopsy
Defecation fecography

Differentials

Acute gout
Psuedogout
Septic arthritis
Rheumatoic arthritis
Osteoarthritis
Trauma

Work-Up

Arthrocentesis & fluid analysis
X-ray knee & foot
CBC
Uric acid, chem-7
ESR

Differentials

Minimal change:
  NSAIDS
  Hodgkin's
Membranous GN:
  Solid tumor
  Hepatitis B
  Malaria
  Syphilis
  Gold, Penicillamine
MPGN:
  Hepatitis C
  NHL
  SLE
  cryoglobulinemia
FSGS:
  HIV
  Heroin
  Obesity
  Vesicoureteral reflux

Work-Up

U/A
Chem-7
LFT
CBC
Hepatitis B/C serology
RPR/FTA-Abs
HIV
ANA
C3 C4 CH50
SPEP/UPEP
Renal U/S ± biopsy
24hr urine protein & creatinine
Urine drug screen
CXR (systemic disease)

Differentials

Infections, *C. difficile*
Obstruction (impaction with overflow)
IBD
Ischemia
Food poisoning Lactose intolerance
Medications
Carcinoid
Colon Cancer

Work-Up

CBC
Stool osmolar gap
Stool WBC, culture, Ova & Parasites, *C. difficile* toxin
Chem-7
X-ray abdomen
Colonoscopy
24hr urine for 5-HIAA

Differentials

GERD
PUD
Stomach CA
Cholelithiasis
Cholecystitis
Dysmotility, Malabsorption
Chronic pancreatitis
RV failure & visceral congestion
Unstable angina
pregnancy

Work-Up

Digital rectal exam for occult blood
LFT
CBC
Chem-7
U/S Abdomen or CT Abdomen
EGD with biopsies for *H. pylori*
Motility studies
ECG
2D echocardiogram
EEG
B-hCG

Differentials

Diabetes Mellitus
"*SOME*" causes of diarrhea
Diabetes insipidus
Organophosphate poisoning
Cholinergic crisis

Work-Up

Fasting glucose
Stool osmolar gap
Stool WBC, culture, ova & parasites
Urine analysis
CBC
RBC cholinesterase level

Complaint/Patient Scenario

27yo ♀ presents with obesity
and excessive body hair
over the past 3 years

Complaint/Patient Scenario

50yo ♂ with double vision
while working late nights

Complaint/Patient Scenario

30yo ♀ c/o recurrent cough for
4 months. Pulmonary exam
reveals crackles at both bases

Complaint/Patient Scenario

27yo obese ♀ with newly
Dx HTN for 3 months now
c/o frontal headaches

Complaint/Patient Scenario

24yo ♀ with cough x 3 months

Complaint/Patient Scenario

60yo ♂ c/o my heart is
"jumping out of my chest"

Differentials

Myasthenia Gravis
    [incremental weakness]
Refractive error
Botulism
Periodic paralysis
Hypothyroidism

Work-Up

Tensilon test
Acetylcholine receptor Ab
Chem-7
TSH
EMG
Snellen chart

Differentials

Obesity
    Hypothyroidism
    Cushing's Syndrome
    Polycystic ovaries
    Insulinoma
    Lifestyle
Hirsutism
    Familial
    Idiopathic
    PCOS
    Ovarian CA
    Adrenal hyperplasia
    Adrenal CA
    Cushings's
    Porphyria Cutanea Tarda
Medications – Phenytoin
    (Dilatin)

Work-Up

Pelvic exam
TSH, free T4
24hr urine free cortisol & 17
    ketosteroids
Serum insulin levels, Chem-7
LH/FSH
DHEA
U/S ovaries
CT adrenals
Free & total testosterone
Plasma & urine porphyrin
    levels

Differentials

Renal artery stenosis
Fibromuscular hyperplasia
Pheochromocytoma
Hyperaldosteronism
Congenital adrenal
    hyperplasia Cushing's
    disease
Essential HTN
Coarctation of aorta
Hyperthyroidism
Alcohol/ ubstance abuse
Sleep apnea
Pregnancy

Work-Up

Chem-7
Renal U/S & arterial dopplers
U/A
Plasma metanephrines and
    normetanephrines
24hr urine free cortisol
17-hydroxyprogesterone
TSH
2D echocardiogram
Polysomnography
β-hCG

Differentials

S- Sarcoid
H- Hypersensitivity
    pneumonitis
I- Idiopathic Pulmonary
    fibrosis
T- TB
F- Fungal
A- Ankylosing spondylitis
C- Collagen vascular disease
E- Eosinophilic granuloma
D- Drugs

Work-Up

CXR PA & Lateral view
ACE level
PPD
AFB sputum Culture
ANA
CBC
ESR
c-RP
Quantitative IgE
Aspergillus precipitans
Fiberoptic bronchoscopy ±
    biopsy

Differentials

Atrial Fibrillation
Multifocal atrial tachycardia
SVT
Cardiomyopathy
Pulmonary embolism
Hyperthyroidism
PVC/PAC
Hypoglycemia
Panic attack
Anxiety
Drug toxicity
Drug ingestion

Work-Up

ECG
2D echocardiogram
Chem-7
Magnesium
TSH, free T4
ABG
CK-MB, Tn-I
Urine drug screen
24hr Holter

Differentials

Post nasal drip
Allergic rhinitis
Asthma
GERD
Bronchitis
Meds [ACE-i]
TB
Atypical pneumonia

Work-Up

PFT's with methacholine
    challenge
CXR PA/lateral
PPD
CBC
Esophageal pH monitor

60yo ♂ "my chest & stomach hurt while I'm eating"

74yo ♀ with h/o CAD & MI x 4 comes in with acute onset SOB

49yo ♂ c/o swollen legs

20yo ♀ c/o "my vision is blurry" and confusion after a long day of fun at the beach

40yo ♀ presents to your office with weight gain and fatigue

62yo ♂ presents for annual check up c/o "weak and tired" for 6 months, "I'm beginning to feel my age"

Differentials	Work-Up
Acute MI	ECG
Unstable angina	CK-MB, Tn-I
Acute pulmonary edema	2D echocardiogram
Arrhythmia	ABG
Valvular rupture	d-dimer
Papillary muscle rupture	V/Q scan
Aortic dissection	
PE	
Generalized anxiety disorder	

Differentials	Work-Up
Peptic ulcer disease	Fecal occult blood
Esophageal spasm	ECG
GERD	CK-MB, Tn-I
Unstable angina	CXR
Acute MI	Upper endoscopy
Dissecting Aortic aneurysm	CT chest & abdomen
Pericarditis	
Gastritis	

Differentials	Work-Up
Multiple sclerosis	CBC
Heat exhaustion	Chem-7
Heat stroke	U/A
Meningitis	UDS-7
Drug intoxication	LP & CSF studies
Severe dehydration	MRI brain
Rhabdomyolysis	
Sepsis- bacterial, viral	
Hypernatremia/hyponatremia	
Hyperglycemia/hypoglycemia	

Differentials	Work-Up
Nephrosis	U/A
Cirrhosis	albumin
Low albumin	CBC
Idiopathic cardiomyopathy	LFT
Valvular heart disease	CXR
Alcoholic cardiomyopathy	ECG
Ischemic cardiomyopathy	2D echocardiogram
IHSS	Chem-7
Sleep apnea	TSH
Cor pulmonale	Polysomnography
IVC clot/DVT	U/S legs for DVT
Myxedema	CT abdomen/pelvis
Pelvic mass	
Medications – amlodipine	

Differentials	Work-Up
Hypothyroidism	Rectal exam for occult blood
Iron deficiency anemia	CBC & peripheral smear
Macrocytic anemia	Ferritin, TIBC, transferrin
Depression	Chem-7
Sleep apnea	TSH
Metastatic CA	PSA
Structural brain disease	Cosyntropin stimulation test
Adrenal insufficiency	CT brain
Diabetes mellitus	Polysomnography
Hematologic malignancy	

Differentials	Work-Up
Pregnancy	Pelvic exam
Depression [DDx includes]:	β-hCG
brain tumor	CBC
SLE	TSH
Syphilis/Lyme/HIV	ANA
sleep apnea	RPR
hypothyroidism	ESR
Cushing's Syndrome	HIV
Adrenal insufficiency	Chem-7
B_{12} deficiency	LFT
domestic violence	B_{12} level
seasonal affective disorder	Cosyntropin stimulation test
Nephrosis	Dexamethasone suppression test
CHF	Polysomnography
Ovarian CA – Meig's Syndrome	
Malignancy – solid tumor vs. hematologic	

27yo ♀ sudden onset SOB

24yo ♀ professional sex worker presents with "burning when I urinate"

60yo ♂ executive with c/o 3 month Hx memory loss and accounting errors

66yo ♀ c/o several day Hx of ↑ swelling and erythema of L leg from knee down to ankle

24yo sexually active ♂ presents with painful L testicle

74yo ♀ presents with new onset dyspnea with pleuritic chest pain

Differentials

Gonococcal urethritis
Non-gonococcal urethritis
Trichomoniasis
Cystitis
Pelvic inflammatory disease
Nephrolithiasis
Reiter's syndrome

Work-Up

Pelvic exam
Culture of urethra for GC
DNA probe for GC/Chlamydia
RPR/FTA Ab
HIV
Urine analysis
Urine culture
KUB X-ray

Differentials

Asthma
generalized anxiety disorder
Arrhythmia
Pneumothorax
Pneumonia
Bronchitis
Pulmonary HTN
Pulmonary embolism
Myocarditis
Cardiomyopathy

Work-Up

CXR
ECG
CBC
ABG
Spirometry & lung volumes
V/Q scan
2D echocardiogram

Differentials

Cellulitis
DVT
Lymphangitis
Ruptured Baker's cyst

Work-Up

CBC
ESR
Venous Doppler leg
X-ray knee

Differentials

Multi-infarct dementia
Alzheimer's disease
Pick's Disease
Lewy body dementia
Normal pressure
    hydrocephalus Creutzfeld-
    Jacob disease
Brain tumor
Sub-dural hematoma
Alcoholism
Vitamin B_{12} deficiency
Hypothyroidism
Pellagra
HIV/syphilis/Lyme
SLE
depression

Work-Up

CT/MRI brain
LP & CSF studies
Vitamin B_{12} level
RPR/FTA Ab
TSH
ANA
ESR
cRP
Carbohydrate deficient
    Transferrin
Lyme titer
HIV test
UDS-7

Differentials

Pulmonary embolism
Unstable angina, myocardial
    infarction
Pneumonia with
    parapnuemonic effusion
acute pulmonary edema
arrhythmia
Viral pleurisy
Tuberculous pleurisy
Lung cancer

Work-Up

d-dimer
ECG
CK-MB, Tn-I
Sputum culture & sensitivity
Chest X-ray/Decubitus films
2D echocardiogram
ABG
V/Q scan
CT chest

Differentials

Epididymitis/ orchitis
Testicular torsion
Torsion of appendix testes
Inguinal hernia
Hydrocoele
Varicocoele
Spermatocoele
Testicular cancer
Trauma

Work-Up

Genital/Scrotal exam
Urethral swab
Urine analysis & culture
CBC
ESR
cRP
Scrotal U/S
AFP
β-hCG